Progress in Pain Research and Management
Volume 13

Chronic and Recurrent Pain in Children and Adolescents

Mission Statement of IASP Press®

The International Association for the Study of Pain (IASP) is a non-profit, interdisciplinary organization devoted to understanding the mechanisms of pain and improving the care of patients with pain through research, education, and communication. The organization includes scientists and health care professionals dedicated to these goals. The IASP sponsors scientific meetings and publishes newsletters, technical bulletins, the journal *Pain*, and books.

The goal of IASP Press is to provide the IASP membership with timely, high-quality, attractive, low-cost publications relevant to the problem of pain. These publications are also intended to appeal to a wider audience of scientists and clinicians interested in the problem of pain.

We will achieve high-quality publications through careful selection of subjects and authors, well-focused editorial work at several levels of production, and a smooth flow of materials. In addition, we believe that we can restrain costs and prices by employing the administrative resources of the IASP central office and by obtaining grant support for selected publications.

Because we will keep the price of our books low and their value high, they will reach a wider audience than do similar books published by for-profit companies. Furthermore, our access to leaders in the field of pain research and treatment guarantees an outstanding selection of material and excellent editorial oversight.

Previous volumes in the series
Progress in Pain Research and Management

Progress in Pain Research and Management
Volume 13

Chronic and Recurrent Pain in Children and Adolescents

Editors

Patrick J. McGrath, PhD

*Departments of Psychology, Paediatrics, and Psychiatry,
Dalhousie University, Paediatric Pain Service,
IWK Grace Health Centre, Halifax, Nova Scotia, Canada*

G. Allen Finley, MD, FRCPC

*Departments of Anaesthesia and Psychology,
Dalhousie University, Paediatric Pain Service,
IWK Grace Health Centre, Halifax, Nova Scotia, Canada*

IASP PRESS® • SEATTLE

Library of Congress Cataloging-in-Publication Data

Chronic and recurrent pain in children and adolescents / editors,
   Patrick J. McGrath, G. Allen Finley.
      p.   cm. — (Progress in pain research and management ; v. 13)
   Includes bibliographical references and index.
   ISBN 0-931092-27-2 (alk. paper)
   1. Pain in children. 2. Pain in adolescence. 3. Chronic pain.
I. McGrath, Patrick J. II. Finley, G. Allen, 1954–   .
III. Series
   [DNLM: 1. Pain—therapy—Adolescence. 2. Pain—therapy—Child.
   3. Chronic Disease—therapy. 4. Recurrence.   WL 704 C5562 1999]
   RJ365.C48 1999
   616' .0472' 083—dc21
   DNLM/DLC
   for Library of Congress   99-23564
                                                                              CIP

Published by:

IASP Press
International Association for the Study of Pain
909 NE 43rd St., Suite 306
Seattle, WA 98105 USA
Fax: 206-547-1703

Printed in the United States of America

Contents

Contributing Authors

K.J.S. Anand, MD, PhD *Departments of Pediatrics and Anesthesiology, University of Arkansas for Medical Sciences, and Arkansas Children's Hospital, Little Rock, Arkansas, USA*

Lynn Breau, BSc *Department of Psychology, Dalhousie University, Halifax, Nova Scotia, Canada*

Mary Ann Campbell, MA *Department of Psychology, Dalhousie University, Halifax, Nova Scotia, Canada*

Anthony H. Dickenson, PhD *Department of Pharmacology, University College, London, United Kingdom*

G. Allen Finley, MD, FRCPC *Departments of Anaesthesia and Psychology, Dalhousie University, and the Paediatric Pain Service, IWK Grace Health Centre, Halifax, Nova Scotia, Canada*

Bo Larsson, MD *Department of Public Health and Caring Sciences, Uppsala University, Uppsala, Sweden*

Patrick J. McGrath, PhD *Departments of Psychology, Pediatrics and Psychiatry, Dalhousie University, and the Pediatric Pain Service, IWK Grace Health Centre, Halifax, Nova Scotia, Canada*

Gunnar Olsson, MD *Department of Anesthesia, St. Göran's Hospital, Stockholm, Sweden; currently Pain Treatment Services, Astrid Lindgren Children's Hospital, Karolinska Hospital, Stockholm, Sweden*

Wahida Rahman, PhD *Department of Pharmacology, University College, London, United Kingdom*

Navil Sethna, MD *Department of Anesthesia, Harvard University, and Pain Treatment Service, Boston Children's Hospital, Boston, Massachusetts, USA*

Neil Schechter, MD *Developmental and Behavioral Pediatrics, University of Connecticut School of Medicine, and Department of Pediatrics, St. Francis Hospital and Medical Center, Hartford, Connecticut, USA*

Heather Schellinck, PhD *Department of Psychology, Dalhousie University, Halifax, Nova Scotia, Canada*

Anna Taddio, MSc, PhD *Departments of Pharmacy and Paediatrics, Division of Clinical Pharmacology and Toxicology, Hospital for Sick Children, and Faculty of Pharmacy, University of Toronto, Toronto, Ontario, Canada*

Anita Unruh, PhD *School of Occupational Therapy, Dalhousie University, Halifax, Nova Scotia, Canada*

Lynn S. Walker, PhD *Division of Adolescent Medicine, Department of Pediatrics, Vanderbilt University School of Medicine, Nashville, Tennessee, USA*

Acknowledgments

We are privileged to be part of an international community of pediatric pain researchers and clinicians. The work presented in this volume is under the authorship of specific individuals but is, in a large way, the result of the collective effort of that community. We thank all of you for making this such an exciting research area.

This volume is based on the second biennial International Forum on Pediatric Pain, held September 24–27, 1998, at White Point Beach, Nova Scotia, Canada. The meeting was generously sponsored by McNeil Consumer Products, Canada. We thank McNeil for their commitment to advancing knowledge in pediatric pain.

The IWK Grace Health Centre and Dalhousie University have been most encouraging of our efforts in pediatric pain. Patrick's participation in this volume has been supported by a Distinguished Scientist Award of the Medical Research Council of Canada. Allen has been similarly supported by a Clinical Research Scholar Award from the Faculty of Medicine at Dalhousie University.

We are delighted with the commitment of the IASP Press to publish high-quality, low-cost books. We are honored to have this volume join *Measurement of Pain in Infants and Children*, Volume 10 in this series.

We would like to also thank our spouses, Anita and Linda, and our children, Mika, Linnet, Nigel, and Meghan for their patience, understanding, and support.

Our patients and yours provide the impetus and the reason for this book. We are all in debt to them for their courage and determination. We hope that this volume on the science of chronic and recurrent pain helps current and future patients everywhere.

PATRICK J. MCGRATH, PHD
G. ALLEN FINLEY, MD, FRCPC

Chronic and Recurrent Pain in Children and Adolescents, Progress in Pain Research and Management, Vol. 13, edited by Patrick J. McGrath and G. Allen Finley, IASP Press, Seattle, © 1999.

1

Chronic and Recurrent Pain in Children and Adolescents

Patrick J. McGrath[a,c] and G. Allen Finley[b,c]

Departments of [a]Psychology, Paediatrics, and Psychiatry, and [b]Anaesthesia and Psychology, and [c]Paediatric Pain Service, IWK Grace Health Centre, Dalhousie University, Halifax, Nova Scotia, Canada

Chronic and recurrent pain in children and adolescents is a significant problem with high prevalence that inflicts a significant burden on sufferers and their families. Research on chronic and recurrent pain in children and adolescents has expanded dramatically over the past decade as a result of attempts to find help for families. Although some of the research has been based on work with adult pain, children and adolescents suffer from different pain disorders than do adults and new directions have been needed. Even when the disorders appear to be the same, such as in migraine, adult treatment may not be effective with children.

New approaches to pediatric pain have crossed disciplinary boundaries. Pain, especially in conjunction with developmental issues, is clearly too complex to be understood by one discipline or by using one set of analytical tools. Physicians, psychologists, nurses and other health professionals, and scientists have led the advances in chronic and recurrent pain research and management. Whereas multidisciplinary teams to treat chronic pain in children and adolescents were virtually unheard of a decade ago, they are now an important component of tertiary health care and have become the standard of care.

Textbooks in pediatric medicine have changed dramatically. A decade ago, pain was not mentioned in the standard texts. Today every text has chapters devoted to pain management, and pediatric pain is considered a science. The problem of chronic and recurrent pain is beginning to yield to concentrated research programs by scientists and clinician-scientists at institutions around the world.

However, serious problems remain. A significant proportion of children and adolescents suffer from repeated bouts of recurrent pain or have constant chronic pain. For example, even young children experience migraine, and a small but important number of adolescents have daily tension-type headache. Many children experience "growing" pains in their legs. Less commonly, some adolescents have debilitating neuropathic pains that in some cases prevent walking and other activities. Most children with arthritis have pain. About half of children with sickle cell disease suffer excruciatingly painful crises that are often unpredictable. Because of its severity and tendency to strike at any time, the pain dominates every aspect of their lives.

The vast majority of children and adolescents with significant chronic and recurrent pain continue to "do their jobs" by attending school, perhaps because of natural psychological and biological resiliency, because staying at home does little good, or because school attendance is mandatory. However, these children pay a considerable price in restriction of their activities. Learning, playing, and the formation and development of social relationships suffer. The quality of life in a child or adolescent with significant pain is markedly diminished.

Most children and adolescents with significant chronic or recurrent pain do not consult a pain specialist, and the reactions of primary health care providers frequently are not helpful. Children typically are not asked about their pain, even if they are suffering from a disease that has a documented high level of pain. It is not unusual for otherwise competent, kindly, and helpful medical personnel to ignore expressions of distress by their young patients. Those with pain that cannot be traced to a specific cause are routinely dismissed as having pain that is psychogenic or "all in the head." If the pain persists and continues to elude the search for the lesion, especially if pain is widespread, unusual, or changing, the child will be labeled as "pain prone," as if the pain is the child's own fault. These declarations are often made in the absence of any evidence of psychological cause.

Parents are put in a difficult position. The health care system does not acknowledge their expert knowledge of their child. They may be suspected of causing or prolonging their child's pain by their solicitude. They may see the pain ignored or dismissed as trivial. Their role in helping their child is rarely clearly appreciated or delineated.

This dismissive attitude about chronic and recurrent pain in children and adolescents extends beyond the individual patient. Although few providers would say that children and adolescents cannot feel pain or that their pain perception is markedly reduced, the myth persists that chronic and recurrent pain is unusual and likely to occur only in the context of significant physical or psychological disease. Paradoxically, the reverse argument is also heard—that pain is "part of growing up," "everyone has it," and therefore it is not serious and should not be treated.

Children and adolescents frequently adopt the belief that nothing can be done but "suffer in silence." When medication is prescribed, children and adolescents and their parents often do not take it in a timely manner, but delay until pain is severe because of a general reluctance to take drugs and a fear of tolerance and addiction.

In situations when psychological treatment could be helpful, it is seldom available. Many psychologists do not understand the complexities of significant pain, and few clinicians have a psychosocial orientation. Often, psychological services are limited by the payment system of the family's health care coverage.

The tendency of health care providers to dismiss pain assumes a more malignant character when it is combined with underlying racism, class bias, and sexism. Children and adolescents with sickle cell disease pain are mostly of African descent and frequently poor. They are denied adequate medical care, cast into an adversarial position, and often suspected of drug abuse when they need opioids for their pain, especially in the case of adolescent males. Young women are seen as "neurotic" if they require medication for menstrual pain.

The burden of chronic and recurrent pain may be increased over time because of biological sensitization. Central sensitization may increase sensitivity to pain and reduce pain thresholds. There are also potential psychological sequelae. The patterns of psychological coping and strategies of medication use that develop in childhood are likely to continue into adulthood.

Most aspects of recurrent and chronic pain have been inadequately researched. Many of the conditions we discuss here are difficult to study because both the pathology and the pain outcomes are difficult to measure. Pain that occurs intermittently may show improvement from treatment only after months or years of follow-up. The social and behavioral impact of chronic disease in adolescents confounds assessment of the pain, which may be only one of many problems that cause suffering. Because chronic and recurrent pain in children and adolescents does not have immediate economic impact, there is little public policy incentive to fund research. Also, given the relatively small market and the difficulties of research with children, the pharmaceutical industry has shown little interest, despite evidence that we cannot simply extrapolate from adult studies.

As in most areas of research, there is a significant lag between research discoveries and incorporation of findings into clinical practice. Diagnoses are frequently missed and proven treatments are often withheld. However, progress now seems inevitable, with a more complete body of knowledge, a more aware public, and a cohort of researchers and clinicians committed to finding solutions. Funding agencies are beginning to recognize the validity of pediatric pain research. Within the next few years, we should see positive results from a flood of new insights and new treatments in the areas that have been most resistant. This volume, we hope, will contribute to this wave of change.

Correspondence to: Dr. G. Allen Finley, MD, FRCPC, Department of Paediatric Anaesthesia, IWK Grace Health Centre, Dalhousie University, 5850 University Avenue, Halifax, Nova Scotia, Canada B3J 3G9. Tel: 902-428-8251; Fax: 902-428-2911; email: allen.finley@dal.ca.

Chronic and Recurrent Pain in Children and Adolescents, Progress in Pain Research and Management, Vol. 13, edited by Patrick J. McGrath and G. Allen Finley, IASP Press, Seattle, © 1999.

2

Mechanisms of Chronic Pain and the Developing Nervous System

Anthony H. Dickenson and Wahida Rahman

Department of Pharmacology, University College, London, United Kingdom

MECHANISMS OF PAIN TRANSMISSION

PAIN TRANSMISSION IN THE ADULT

Pain involves many neuronal systems, often organized into complex networks; they use a multitude of chemical mediators and transmitters, both at the site of injury in the periphery and within the central nervous system (CNS). The final sensation and the accompanying psychological aspects of the sensory message of pain will depend on interactions among these transmitters. However, to understand these interactions we need to understand the roles of the receptors for these transmitters. A universal principle is that activation of receptors is necessary for the actions of transmitters and mediators. Some receptors are excitatory, others inhibitory. Some interactions between transmitters and receptors produce dramatic or rapid changes in neural activity, whereas others cause mild or slow changes. A consequence of the mix of excitatory and inhibitory receptors is a balance between excitation and inhibition. Thus, activation of excitatory receptors will cause the release of transmitter and neuronal firing. By contrast, activation of inhibitory receptors will decrease firing, reduce transmitter release, and render neurons less excitable. Excitatory receptors are critical to the generation of pain and its transmission, whereas analgesia can be produced either by activation of inhibitory systems or by blocking excitatory systems (Yaksh and Malmberg 1994; Dickenson and Besson 1997).

The early ideas of specific, unchanging systems in pain have faded away, and now the transmission of pain is no longer viewed as a simple process but as messages arising from the interplay of several transmitter systems, both excitatory and inhibitory, at many levels of the CNS, especially the spinal cord. One consequence is that the relation between the stimulus and the response to pain is not always clear. Thus, any increases in activity in excitatory systems would tend to enhance pain (hyperalgesia). The same result could also be produced by reducing inhibitions so that excitations predominate. This plasticity results from the ability of pharmacological systems to quickly alter transmission in nociceptive systems and to modulate pain.

The concept that injury can induce both peripheral and central hypersensitivity has had important consequences for pain control strategies. Plasticity in excitatory and inhibitory transmitter systems is becoming reasonably well understood, and we can begin to see how changes induced in peripheral and central signaling systems can lead to chronic pain (McQuay and Dickenson 1990; Dubner and Ruda 1992; McMahon et al. 1993; Dickenson 1994a, Price et al. 1994; Woolf 1994). In the neonatal nervous system, transmitter systems are not the same as in the mature adult; transmission of nociceptive information from the spinal cord to higher brain centers could be markedly different in early postnatal life (Fitzgerald 1993, 1995, 1997). Plasticity and change are part of normal development.

DEVELOPMENTAL ASPECTS OF PAIN TRANSMISSION

Until quite recently, little priority has been given to elucidating the processing of nociceptive information in the immature animal or infant. This delay in research was due to the widely held misconception that infants do not feel pain (see Booker 1987; Schechter 1989). The reasoning was that the newborn child possesses an immature nervous system unable to respond to or interpret a painful stimulus in a manner similar to that of adults. Higher brain centers are required to perceive pain, and neonates were thought to have little cortical function. Also, as the newborn child has had little sensory stimulation and possesses little or no memory of such events, it was thought that a newborn would not remember an early painful experience. The presumed vulnerability of the infant respiratory system to depression by opioid analgesics and the long-term consequences of administering powerful analgesics, such as morphine, to a developing nervous system influenced the reluctance to prescribe them. Thus, many premature babies and young infants have been subjected to painful and traumatic events such as invasive procedures with little or no analgesia or anesthesia (Beyer et al. 1983; Schechter 1989).

It is now becoming accepted that babies and young infants do have the ability to respond to painful stimuli (see Craig et al. 1993; Grunau et al. 1994a,b; Fitzgerald 1995; Johnston et al. 1993, 1995), which they may not be able to verbalize but can display through specific facial expressions and body movements (Craig et al. 1993; Grunau et al. 1994a; Stevens et al. 1994). Boys who are circumcised will cry in a frequency relating to the painful elements during the procedure, and their behavior in the next 24 hours indicates their discomfort and pain, as seen in disruption of feeding patterns, adaptation, and bonding (Marshall et al. 1980). Studies on painful stimulation later, such as immunization at 3 months, have reported that circumcised infants display a much greater reaction long after the initial painful event (Taddio et al. 1995).

These studies indicate that infants remember painful procedures. Other research has shown that infants who experienced invasive procedures continued to display adverse behavior at the age of 18 months (Grunau et al. 1994a), which is indicative of a psychological consequence. Heel lancing is a routine procedure in neonatal wards. Fitzgerald et al. (1989, 1995) observed that the infant produces a vigorous behavioral response to repeated heel lances, including fast and protracted withdrawal of the limb and whole-body movements. The lower the postconceptional age, the greater the vigor of response with little or no habituation to the stimuli. These behavioral responses to repeated lancing were alleviated with topical EMLA cream (see Chapter 4 for a full discussion). Body movements are a form of pain behavior that can be reversed by the administration of analgesics. It appears that cortical awareness is functional in the newborn child, as evidenced by behavioral indices such as crying, defined facial expressions in response to painful stimuli, and ability to visualize and having spatial awareness of an object or person. Such responses indicate that areas of higher brain function are active in the neonatal period (see Booker 1987). These clinical data and numerous other studies reporting behavioral and physiological responses to painful stimuli leave little doubt that the neonatal infant is capable of responding to painful stimulation, but in an exaggerated and somewhat unspecific manner as compared to adults (see Fitzgerald 1995).

The nervous system of neonates is inherently more plastic than the adult nervous system because normal development is dependent on intrinsic structural and functional reorganizations. The development of the neonatal nervous system is not linear but includes several transitory functional stages before reaching the adult profile. This chapter reviews the general anatomical, physiological, and pharmacological changes that occur over the first three postnatal weeks in the rat CNS, with emphasis on the ontological developments within the spinal cord. It also addresses the roles of comparable systems in the adult, a topic with a considerable body of data. Relatively little is known about CNS development in the neonate and progression to the adult state, either in rats or humans.

A key point is that the receptor and transmitter actions that occur in the adult nervous system during information signaling play an additional role in the immature nervous system in that they are critical to the wiring of the developing networks. Thus, changes that occur in the relatively hard-wired adult that contribute to pain may evoke more widespread and dramatic changes in early life. However, it could equally be argued that the inherent plasticity of the young nervous system may lead to compensations that minimize permanent change.

PERIPHERAL TRANSMISSION OF PAIN

At peripheral levels, whether skin, muscle, or viscera, most nociceptive signaling of thermal and mechanical pain arises from the activation of polymodal nociceptors that are innervated by C-fibers. By contrast, the large myelinated Aβ-fibers convey innocuous information such as touch, pressure, and proprioception. The acute application of these modalities of stimuli results in a good relationship between the magnitude and location of the stimulus and the response. However, in the presence of inflammation or local tissue damage, which can result from a disease process such as arthritis or rheumatism, surgical procedures, or trauma, the fine unmyelinated C-fibers respond to local chemical stimulation and also become sensitized to chemical, thermal, and mechanical stimuli that lower their threshold for activation. During inflammation, blood vessels become leaky as a result of the actions of some of these chemical mediators so that other mediators gain access to the damaged site from the vasculature (Levine et al. 1993; Dray et al. 1994; Dray 1997). In the neonate, C-fibers are slow to make their final synaptic contacts in their terminal zones in the spinal cord (Fitzgerald 1985, 1987), and practically nothing is known about inflammatory mediators in early life. However, what is known is that Aβ-fiber stimulation can evoke exaggerated behavioral responses in early life. The flexor response, normally restricted to activation by high-threshold inputs in the adult, can be elicited by light touch in neonatal animals (Fitzgerald et al. 1987). A recent study demonstrated that C-*fos* protein is expressed in response to light touch stimuli (Aβ-fibers) and in response to noxious stimulation in the rat pup, whereas only the latter type of stimulus is effective in the adult (Jennings and Fitzgerald 1996). For a relatively long period postnatally, Aβ-fibers occupy and make synaptic contacts in the superficial laminae of the dorsal horn alongside the C-fiber terminals (Fitzgerald et al. 1995). It is possible that subthreshold depolarizations by the C-fibers may prime the spinal cord to subsequent Aβ-fiber inputs, which may contribute to the apparently enhanced input from the Aβ-fibers seen at early developmental stages.

Tissue damage generates the synthesis of arachidonic acid metabolites from adjacent membranes, the cleavage of the precursor of bradykinin to release the active peptide from the circulation, and the release of peptides such as substance P (SP) and calcitonin gene-related peptide (CGRP) from the C-fibers via the axon reflex. This inflammatory soup, which also contains 5-hydroxytryptamine or serotonin, potassium ions, and hydrogen ions, activates and sensitizes the peripheral endings and causes vasodilatation and plasma extravasation to elicit swelling, pain, and tenderness, the main signs of inflammation. The effects of these chemical mediators at the site of tissue damage contribute to peripheral hyperalgesia; pain is enhanced by their actions on the terminals of nociceptive peripheral sensory fibers. The mode of action of the aspirin-like drugs and the NSAIDs is to block the synthesis of the arachidonic acid metabolites. The recent synthesis of antagonists for the bradykinin receptors has provided good evidence for a role of both the B1 and B2 receptor subtypes in these peripheral events, with the latter receptor important in the early stages of persistent pain and the former induced with longer term stimuli (Dray 1997). The effects of other mediators, including the cytokines, nerve growth factors, catecholamines, and prostanoids (the latter also from the sympathetic nervous system), in addition to the more classical mediators mentioned above, means that the complexity of transmission at the peripheral level leading to hyperalgesia is greater than ever suspected (Dray et al. 1994; Dray 1997). Thus, the novel tetrodotoxin-insensitive sodium channel found in C-fibers is upregulated by inflammatory mediators (Gold et al. 1996). Clearly, persistent actions of these mediators at the peripheral level can underlie chronic pains. However, nerve growth factor (NGF) and related factors play exactly the role in early life that the name suggests (Goedert et al. 1981). Thus, an overexpression of NGF, such as occurs in the adult after tissue damage (McMahon and Bennett 1997), underlies some of the behavioral changes that occur and can change the phenotype of afferent nerves (Hokfelt et al. 1994) and conceivably alter the wiring of a young nervous system. Independently of these possibilities, a simple injury to the skin in the neonatal rat can lead to an enduring hyperinnervation of that area of skin (Reynolds and Fitzgerald 1995).

NERVE INJURY PAIN

The neurobiological basis for both understanding the causes and improving the treatment of nerve injury pain remains somewhat unclear (Fields and Rowbotham 1994). Studies that use several animal models of nerve injury, produced by manipulation of peripheral nerves in the rat, can help further understanding. Despite the many studies on the behavioral consequences of neuropathic interventions (Zeltser and Seltzer 1994), few electrophysiological data exist on the potential modification of central neuronal responses in these animal models. Several studies have shed light on the changes in peripheral nerves, but what occurs at the next relays? We could hypothesize that spinal neurons, located in the key relay between the peripheral nerve and the brain, will exhibit modified response profiles, which may aid understanding of some of the causes of neuropathic pain. Finding an answer will require a systematic investigation of the pharmacology of the spinal cord with both clinical drugs and experimental tools administered by various routes to probe receptors and channels (Bennett 1994).

Until recently, studies of the mechanisms of clinical pain syndromes have relied on data from animal studies involving the application of acute stimuli. The symptoms of pain arising from nerve injury, neuropathic pain such as allodynia (touch-evoked pain), spontaneous pain, hyperalgesia (enhanced pain to a given noxious stimulus), sensory deficits, and in some cases a sympathetic component are not replicated by acute models. Early animal studies of neuropathic pain used complete nerve section. More recent animal models are based on a restricted partial denervation of the hind limb following sciatic nerve injury (Bennett 1994). Two of the models constrict the sciatic nerve distal to the spinal cord, either by a tight ligation of a portion of the sciatic nerve (the partial ligation model; Seltzer et al. 1990) or by a loose ligation of the entire nerve (the chronic constriction injury [CCI] model; Bennett and Xie 1988). The most recent model uses tight ligation of two of the three spinal nerves that form the sciatic nerve (the spinal nerve ligation [SNL] model; Kim and Chung 1992). The behavioral consequences of these models mimic many of the symptoms of the human neuropathic state, although the extent and location of the injury differ, as does the degree of degeneration of different fiber types. Given the variability in the extent of peripheral nerve damage in patients, it is significant that many investigators report similar behavioral results, which suggests that common consequences can result from different peripheral changes. Almost no information exists on the behavioral consequences of nerve injury in young animals, but one study reports a rapid recovery after nerve damage when the ligation is performed early in life (Kim and Chung 1998). Evidence indicates that the aberrations in somatosensory processing that follow partial nerve injury are the culmination of several changes in the peripheral nervous system. Studies after nerve section (Wall and Devor 1983; Devor et al. 1992) suggest that the generation of ectopic discharges within the neuroma and the dorsal root ganglia (DRG) contributes to these changes. After partial denervation (CCI model), high-frequency spontaneous activity originating in the DRG targets the spinal neurons via injured A-fibers (Kajander and

Bennett 1992). In this same model, a novel "modified rapidly adapting" mechanoreceptor innervates the partially deafferented foot, suggesting changes in transduction processes (Na et al. 1993). A structural reorganization of large-fiber (Aβ) termination at the level of the spinal cord has also been reported (Woolf and Doubell 1994; Lekan et al. 1996), possibly allowing low-threshold inputs to gain access to spinal nociceptive transmission circuits. In early life, synaptic contacts occur between low-threshold afferents and neurons in what will be exclusively nociceptive zones of the spinal cord (Coggeshall et al. 1996).

Few electrophysiological studies have examined spinal neurons in nerve injury models, and none has used a range of test stimuli. In the CCI model, a high percentage of spinal neurons exhibit abnormal levels of spontaneous activity (Palacek et al. 1992; Laird and Bennett 1993; Takaishi et al. 1996), although many neurons have shown absent somatic receptive fields, which is unexpected in models of partial denervation. The number of neurons sensitive to low-intensity mechanical stimuli and the magnitude of mechanical evoked responses of the neurons were also reduced. Reduced thresholds of spinal neurons (and reduced magnitudes of responses) and spontaneous activity of spinal neurons after selective spinal nerve ligation have been reported (Chapman et al. 1998). It is still not clear how these changed peripheral and central neuronal responses contribute to the resultant pain states, but ongoing and evoked aberrant peripheral nerve activity must impinge upon altered peripheral and central signaling systems (Fields and Rowbotham 1994). Thus, anticonvulsants and antidepressants are used to control neuropathic pain (McQuay et al. 1995, 1996). These drugs are not used in other pain states; novel actions of some of these agents can been seen in the animal models (Chapman et al. 1998). The existence of peripheral mechanisms of hyperalgesia and nerve injury has a bearing on the induction of central hypersensitivity in the spinal cord because the block or reduction in generation of nociceptive messages at the first stage in the periphery would be expected to prevent some central alterations.

SPINAL TRANSMISSION OF PAIN

The number of transmitters and receptors found in the dorsal sensory horn of the spinal cord is considerable, and most of the candidate neurotransmitters and their receptors identified in the CNS are present in the spinal cord (Todd and Spike 1993; Dray et al. 1994; Dickenson and Besson 1997). The transmitters can be divided into those that are released in response to activity in the afferent peripheral fibers (local intrinsic spinal neurons) and chemicals liberated from the endings of descending fibers from the brain. However, no one transmitter has either an exclusive location or role, either in the spinal cord or the brain. Thus, it is unlikely that a "magic bullet" for pain will emerge. Most neurons are concentrated in the substantia gelatinosa, one of the densest neuronal areas in the CNS and a site crucial for the reception and modulation of nociceptive messages. Here incoming activity is altered by the local and descending pathways, and the final determination of the output message from the spinal cord can be dramatically different from the incoming signal—either hugely amplified and transformed or markedly attenuated, depending on the relative balance between excitation and inhibition (Dickenson et al. 1997). The actions of these transmitters at their spinal receptor can markedly alter the responses of the output cells and the relationship between stimulus and response.

The excitatory amino acids and several peptides fulfill many of the criteria required for neurotransmitters released from afferents, and there is considerable evidence for the involvement of both the excitatory amino acid, glutamate, and several peptides in nociceptive transmission in the dorsal horn of the spinal cord (Battaglia and Rustioni 1988; Dray et al. 1994; Hokfelt et al. 1994). In most peripheral C-fibers, glutamate coexists with a peptide, so dual receptor mechanisms are elicited after peripheral stimulation. Although afferent fibers contain many chemicals that are released after noxious stimulation, functional roles have been established only for the transmitters with antagonists for their receptors. The best strategy to study the roles of receptors is to determine whether an antagonist to a particular receptor can change the physiological response to pain (e.g., neuronal activity, behavior, or best of all, clinical pain ratings). Such changes provide good evidence that a receptor is involved in that particular response. This approach has permitted detailed study of the adult systems over time, and application of a similar approach will enhance our understanding of the development of pain and lead to improvements in analgesia.

PEPTIDE MECHANISMS

Substance P (SP), a member of a family of related peptides called either tachykinins or neurokinins, has long been implicated as one of the neurotransmitters involved in nociceptive transmission from C-fiber afferents. It is present in, and released from, C-fibers and also local spinal intrinsic neurons together with a release from descending fibers originating in the brain. Three receptors exist for these peptides: neurokinin-1 (NK-1), neurokinin-2 (NK-2), and neurokinin-3 (NK-3). SP is active at the NK-1 receptor (Otsuka and Yoshioka 1993). Interestingly, the release of both substance P and the related peptide, neurokinin A, is increased after peripheral inflammation (Duggan et al. 1988). SP can be detected in a much larger zone of the spinal cord after peripheral inflammation than in the normal state, whereas neurokinin A release into the cord can be substantial. Most of the dorsal horn can be reached by neurokinin A in normal animals. Antagonists at the tachykinin receptors are not yet fully characterized, but indications suggest that the NK-1 and -2 receptors may have roles, not in brief acute pains, but when the stimulus is more persistent, and thus may be important in central hypersensitivity. The evidence that these receptors contribute to afferent-produced increases in excitability of the spinal cord is strongest when the model involves inflammation, where it is known that the peripheral damage can upregulate the synthesis and consequently the spinal release of SP. This enhanced release of SP and the other neurokinins, at least in inflammatory states, may provide the mechanisms whereby the N-methyl-D-aspartate (NMDA) receptor for glutamate becomes more easily activated (Dickenson 1994a). As will be discussed later, antagonists of the neurokinins produce mild reductions in responses to noxious stimuli, indicating that they are not the exclusive transmitter systems.

Calcitonin gene-related peptide (CGRP) is released by noxious stimuli and excites dorsal horn neurons, but the lack of antagonists for the receptor(s) means that its role in pain processing is unknown. However, CGRP and SP share the same breakdown enzyme so SP can diffuse to large areas of the dorsal horn in the presence of CGRP because the latter occupies the degradative enzyme, allowing SP to escape break down and diffuse to more distant sites within the spinal cord. This, together with the increased synthesis of primary afferent peptides after inflammation, will increase the excitability of the spinal cord (Dray et al. 1994). Other peptides, such as somatostatin, neuropeptide Y, and galanin may be important, but development of selective antagonists is necessary to further understand the roles of these peptides.

Developmental aspects of peptide systems

Almost nothing is known about the pharmacology of developing spinal pain pathways, although it appears that the expression, distribution, and activity of excitatory neurotransmitters and their receptors within the spinal cord dorsal horn undergo remarkable postnatal changes. The development of the rat, expressed as postnatal (P) days, and the human share key basic similarities. However, as the species have different rates of development and the rat is born at a different developmental stage, it is difficult to produce a comparative list of developmental stages. However, the stages of postnatal life in the rat up to postnatal day (P) 21 correspond to the later stages of fetal life and early events in the newborn (Fitzgerald 1993).

The neuropeptides, SP, somatostatin, and CGRP all appear early in the DRG, although levels are initially low and increase throughout fetal life, with a marked increase perinatally to approach adult levels in rats by P14. Neuropeptides also appear early within dorsal horn cells of the spinal cord in rat pups and human fetuses (Charlton and Helke 1986; Marti et al. 1987), with the number of peptide-containing cells declining with postnatal age. Furthermore, analysis of SP receptors suggests similar changes in receptor binding (Charlton and Helke 1986).

Given the role of SP as a C-fiber neurotransmitter, it is of particular interest that SP receptors are diffusely distributed over the spinal cord gray matter up to P15 and become progressively more defined to specific nuclei as the rat matures. SP binding decreases with age so that at P260 the cord has one-sixth the binding sites present at P11 (Charlton and Helke 1986). Nothing is known about the functional effect of this receptor distribution on developing spinal pain pathways, but it could be envisaged that following peripheral activity there would be more widespread effects of SP in early life, with a larger neuronal population activated by the peptide. It is almost as if the role of the peptide in early life in the normal situation resembles its actions in the adult after inflammation.

EXCITATORY AMINO ACID MECHANISMS

It is now clear that the excitatory amino acids, glutamate and aspartate, are of utmost importance to the transmission of acute and chronic pains. Most neurons in the brain and spinal cord use glutamate as their major excitatory transmitter, and so side effects will most likely limit it as a potential target for analgesics. However, several receptors exist for glutamate, and the transmitter can produce different effects depending on which receptor is activated. The actions of glutamate are mediated via a particularly complex and unique receptor, the NMDA receptor, and by at least three other receptors. They are named after synthetic chemicals that are selective for the individual receptor. Glutamate, the natural transmitter, acts on all the receptors. The other three are the α-amino-3-hydroxy-5-methyl-4-isoxazolepropionic acid (AMPA) receptor, the metabotropic receptor, and the kainate receptor. Antagonists selective for all these non-NMDA receptors are aiding the discovery of their functional roles in pain processes (Dickenson 1994a, 1997; Price et al. 1994). Although the AMPA receptor clearly plays a role in both innocuous and noxious transmission through the spinal cord, the roles of the other two non-NMDA receptors are still unclear.

Many peripheral sensory fibers contain glutamate and aspartate, and

90% of fibers containing SP also contain glutamate (Battaglia and Rustioni 1988). This coexistence of more than one transmitter in a nerve fiber makes it highly likely that a noxious stimulus would induce a release of both peptides and excitatory amino acids into the spinal cord. We therefore suspected that these transmitters cooperate to activate spinal neurons in nociceptive pathways, a presumption that seems to be correct.

Much interest has centered on the involvement of the excitatory amino acids and their actions via the NMDA receptor complex in neuronal events in the spinal cord (Dickenson 1994a, 1995; Price et al. 1994). There is good evidence for an involvement of this receptor in other forms of increased excitability and long-term changes in the brain such as long-term potentiation (LTP) (Collingridge and Singer 1990). The marked and persistent elevations of activity induced in the hippocampus and other areas of the brain after NMDA receptor activation have implicated LTP in memory processes in the forebrain. However, it would be naive to expect that the same phenomenon occurs in sensory pathways, given their different biological function. The other transmitter systems acting on and around neurons containing the NMDA receptor will have a major influence on promoting and inhibiting activation of this receptor. These interactions are especially relevant to spinal sensory processing because sensory events can be transient, whereas memory is far more enduring. Thus, wind-up and sensitization of spinal neurons by peripheral stimuli decline after the cessation of afferent activity, whereas LTP in the brain persists after the end of the inducing stimulus.

The interest in the NMDA receptor has been prompted by its participation in synaptic transmission only when a certain number of events occur, a characteristic that has earned it the descriptor of "coincidence detector." These criteria for activation of the spinal receptor appear to occur only when peripheral input is of sufficient intensity and duration; this receptor and associated neuronal events thus may play a key role in persistent and chronic pains. Why? The ion channel for the NMDA receptor, when opened, allows vast amounts of sodium and calcium into the neuron, so much that the resultant increase in excitability of the neuron far exceeds that produced by activation of all other known receptors. Perhaps not surprisingly, the NMDA receptor is held in check so that it does not participate in "normal" transmission. The reasons are that activation of the NMDA receptor requires not just the release of glutamate and its binding to the receptor but also a sufficient level of glycine, elsewhere an inhibitory transmitter, to bind to an adjacent site where it acts as a required co-agonist. Furthermore, even with glycine and glutamate bound to the receptor, no change in neuronal activity occurs because the channel is blocked by physiological levels of magnesium ion. This channel block, dependent on use and voltage, is only removed by sufficient repeated depolarization of the membrane. There is now evidence that this removal of the channel block is produced by the tachykinins co-released with glutamate acting on their neurokinin receptors to depolarize the neuron. Transmission from C-fibers after brief acute mechanical or thermal stimuli appears to involve glutamate, which acts on the AMPA receptor to produce short-lasting excitations. Likewise, large A-fiber activation uses the same sort of mechanism, and repeated A-fiber stimulation never activates the NMDA receptor in normal conditions because these fibers do not contain peptides and so cannot remove the magnesium ion block of the channel. However, if a C-fiber stimulus is maintained or its frequency or intensity is increased, the release of peptides then contributes to transmission and further allows the NMDA receptor to become activated, with the resultant amplification of the response underlying many forms of central hyperalgesia (McMahon et al. 1993; Dickenson 1994a, 1997; Dray et al. 1994; Price et al. 1994). Increased release of both excitatory amino acids and peptides in inflammatory pains will facilitate these processes.

Developmental aspects of amino acid systems

In acute pains a continuum of central receptors is sequentially activated as the stimulus continues: the AMPA receptor is activated in the earliest events, followed by the peptide receptors and then the NMDA receptor, which seems to lie behind central hyperalgesia or hypersensitivity. Glutamate-NMDA activity takes on a further interesting dimension in the context of infant pain in view of its general role in development and given the plasticity of connections in the immature CNS. The receptor does not simply function as a signal mechanism in early life, but is required for development of normal connections and is a trophic factor (Carmignoto and Vicini 1992; Hofer et al. 1994). The AMPA receptor for glutamate, transmitting noxious and innocuous stimuli in a faithful manner in the adult (Dickenson 1997), alters in the spinal cord during development (Jakowec et al. 1995a,b), as does the metabotrophic receptor (Catania et al. 1994). For example, in the adult spinal cord, NMDA receptor binding is restricted to the substantia gelatinosa, but at P7 it is distributed throughout the entire spinal cord and so could induce more widespread excitatory influences. Restricted mature distribution of spinal NMDA receptors is not achieved in the rat until P28 (Gonzalez et al. 1993; Watanabe et al. 1994). In the immature hippocampus, where a similar overexpression of the receptor occurs, the excitatory events elicited by the receptor are much greater in amplitude and the channel is significantly less sensitive to magnesium ions and so more easily activated

(Morrisset et al. 1990). In the first week after birth in the rat, the NMDA-induced increases in intracellular calcium are greater than in the adult cord but gradually decline to adult levels; additionally, the affinity of NMDA for its receptor is highest at P1 (Hori and Kanda 1994). These observations suggest that NMDA-mediated central excitability evoked by C-fiber stimulation in the neonatal cord may well be more dramatic than in the adult because it is easier to activate and produces more functional activation. In addition, NMDA receptors may also play a role in establishing afferent fiber connections with neurons in the developing spinal cord (Mendelson 1994).

CENTRAL HYPERSENSITIVITY AND HYPERALGESIA

In addition to the peripheral changes that can lead to a persistent input into the CNS, central mechanisms can amplify activity within the spinal cord. The first report of central spinal hypersensitivity described how stimuli activating C-fibers lead to marked and prolonged increase in the flexion withdrawal reflex in spinal-decerebrate rats (Woolf 1983). Note again that low-threshold stimuli can produce this response in infants. The second observation was that the repetition of a constant-intensity C-fiber stimulus could induce wind-up and dramatically increase the number and duration of responses of certain dorsal horn neurons despite the lack of change in the input into the spinal cord (Dickenson 1995, 1997). Wind-up can increase these responses by up to 20-fold, and they continue even after the cessation of peripheral input. An NMDA receptor mechanism is needed for this amplification and prolongation of nociceptive activity because wind-up is sensitive to a wide range of NMDA receptor antagonists and channel blockers. This spinal event is thus thought to be crucial to central hypersensitivity or central hyperalgesia because the NMDA receptor switches a low level of pain-related activity to a high level without any change in the inputs arriving in the peripheral nerves (Dickenson 1994a, 1997; Dray et al. 1994; Price et al. 1994).

Studies with formalin provided the first direct evidence for the involvement of the NMDA receptor in the responses of cells to persistent but acute physiological stimuli (Haley et al. 1990). Formalin produces inflammation and leads to neuronal and behavioral responses consisting of an early acute response not involving tissue damage and a second phase that occurs 15 minutes later and lasts for up to 1 hour. This second phase results from peripheral inflammatory mediators activating C-fibers and subsequently dorsal horn nociceptive neurons. Importantly, the second phase, but not the first, is sensitive to NMDA block, indicating that "pathological pain" (inflammatory tissue damage) can be distinguished from nondamaging acute pain by sensitivity of the former to NMDA antagonism (Haley et al. 1990). It would appear that a relatively low level of incoming afferent activity, induced by acute inflammation or by nerve damage, is amplified centrally by the NMDA receptor. Similar NMDA-mediated nociceptive events have subsequently been reported in other animal models of persistent pains ranging from neuropathic (both central and peripheral lesions) to ischemic and inflammatory, and have been noted in clinical studies (Dickenson 1994a; Price et al. 1994; Dray et al. 1994; Eide et al. 1995). Importantly for clinical applications, ketamine at analgesic doses is an effective NMDA receptor-channel blocker, as noted in many of the studies listed above.

In general, the induction and maintenance of neuronal responses are dependent on NMDA processes. In one study, for example, nerve section triggered NMDA-mediated wind-up, which contributed to the subsequent pain behavior. Likewise, several studies on inflammation and models of neuropathic pain in rats confirmed the effectiveness of pretreatment (blocking induction) and post-treatment (blocking maintenance) (see Dickenson 1997). In clinical studies, ketamine has alleviated chronic pain (Eide et al. 1995). Thus, we can presume that the receptor not only sets up the enhanced pain transmission but also maintains this state, which is completely different from LTP in the brain, where only pretreatment with NMDA antagonists is effective, an indication that only the receptor participates in induction (Collingridge and Singer 1990). Many of these experiments have been performed in intact animals under full general anesthesia. Thus we can conclude that central hypersensitivity can still occur in humans during surgical procedures, even with administration of a general anesthetic, and that it contributes to postoperative pain states.

Peripheral tissue injury in newborn infants results in a fall in the flexor reflex threshold and a hyperalgesic state. In premature infants the cutaneous flexor reflex threshold in an area of local tissue damage created by repeated heel lances is half the value of that on the intact contralateral heel (Andrews and Fitzgerald 1994; Fitzgerald and Andrews 1998). The tenderness, akin to wind-up, is established for days and weeks in the presence of tissue damage.

In the adult this hyperalgesia is produced by the peripheral activation of C afferents that modify the functional response of the spinal cord to other inputs applied long after the conditioning input. The cellular mechanisms responsible for central sensitization in the adult are a focus of intense research, but we know little of these processes in the neonatal CNS. Importantly, we need to know how to control these enhanced pain states.

PAIN CONTROL

OPIOID ANALGESIA

The use of opium to relieve pain dates back centuries. The past two decades have witnessed a major step forward in our understanding of how and where opioids produce their actions. These remarkable advances can potentially lead to better treatment of pain that shows a poor response to opioids, especially for neuropathic pain, and to the production of new opioid drugs.

These advances received impetus from the discovery of the opioid receptors, which subsequently have been have isolated and cloned. Further functional studies have used numerous experimental approaches to explore the pharmacology of pain transmission and its control. Electrophysiological recordings of nociceptive neurons in intact animals and behavioral studies with intrathecal administration of opioids in several models of different pain states provide the means to study opioid receptor function (Dickenson 1994b).

Opioid receptors are synthesized in the cell bodies of small afferent fibers in DRG and are then transported within the nerves. The bulk of the receptors are located on the presynaptic terminals of C-fibers as they enter the spinal cord. The manufacture of opioid receptors in afferent sensory nerves means that such receptors can be vulnerable to pathological damage to a peripheral nerve. Thus, after nerve section (rhizotomy) a dramatic reduction occurs in opioid receptors at the spinal level, with about 70% lost to failure of transport. Less severe neuropathy may also lead to a decrease in functional receptors, although in some models partial nerve damage can produce an early increase in receptor number.

The peripheral receptors have no function in normal tissue but become accessible after inflammation, possibly due to inflammatory mediators and other agents at the sites of tissue damage, which cause leaks in the perineurium of the C-fibers. Consequently, peripheral effects of opioids, although somewhat weak, can be demonstrated in animals and humans after inflammation (Stein 1994). This peripheral action may be useful at inflammatory sites because it could avoid some of the central side effects of opioids. However, the predominant actions of opioids in producing analgesia occur in the CNS at spinal and supraspinal sites.

Opioid action is probably best understood in the spine. The spinal cord contains all the opioid receptors—the μ, δ, and κ receptors—and the recently discovered opioid-like receptor, ORL1. The μ receptor predominates, and there are reasonable amounts of δ receptors, but as yet we have not estimate of ORL1 receptors. Opioid receptors are present in the brain and the spinal cord from early fetal life in the rat and human, and display pre-

and postnatal maturational changes before achieving the final adult distribution (McDowell and Kitchen 1987; Sales et al. 1989; Attali et al. 1990; Kar and Quirion 1995; Rahman et al. 1998). Most studies investigating the development of opioid receptors have used homogenate binding, which provides information about the overall receptor density but not the localization and density of the receptors within the tissue (McDowell and Kitchen 1987; Attali et al. 1990). Different ligands, concentrations, and methods of expressing data make it difficult to compare data from different studies.

A recent study used quantitative autoradiography with tritiated ligands for μ, δ, and κ receptors. Investigations of the postnatal distribution and density of spinal opioid receptors revealed the presence of both μ-and κ-receptor binding sites from P0, and the first appearance of δ-receptor binding at P7. Thus, all three receptors are subject to postnatal modifications in density and localization over the first three weeks (Rahman et al. 1998).

Spinal opioid receptors are not only found on the afferents; about 30% are located postsynaptically on neurons within the dorsal horn of the spinal cord. However, the presynaptic opioid receptors on nociceptive fibers, which form the majority of the spinal opioid receptor population, are placed at the most strategic position for the control of sensory transmission. Activation of the presynaptic opioid receptors by opioids will lead to inhibition. Thus, at least in the case of μ and δ receptors, they will hyperpolarize the C-fiber terminals by opening potassium channels; this reduction in excitability means reduced release of several transmitters including glutamate, substance P, and other neurokinins, and CGRP. Consequently, the pain message is markedly attenuated as it enters the CNS (Dickenson 1994b). Any residual transmitter that is released into the spinal cord will have its excitatory actions inhibited by the actions of opioids at the postsynaptic sites.

Neonatal rat pups are capable of responding to nociceptive stimuli from early stages (Williams et al. 1990; Guy and Abbot 1992; Soyguder et al. 1994; Jennings and Fitzgerald 1996) and agonists acting at opioid receptors can mediate antinociceptive effects in young rat pups where the actions of μ- and κ-receptor agonists have mostly been investigated (see Johannesson and Becker 1973; Barr et al. 1986; Blass et al. 1993; McLaughlin and Dewey 1994; Abbott and Guy 1995). A recent behavioral study demonstrated morphine analgesia of the formalin response in neonatal rats and clearly showed the drug to be an effective analgesic as opposed to a sedative, even at early developmental stages (Abbot and Guy 1995). In keeping with this selective sensory action of the opioids, spinal morphine produced a greater inhibitory effect in rats on the electrically evoked C-fiber response or dorsal horn neurons and the hyperexcitability produced by wind-up when administered at P14 and P21 versus those inhibitions seen in the adult rat. Surprisingly, greater inhibitory effects of morphine on C-fiber responses were seen at P21 than at P14 despite the greater C-fiber-evoked responses at P21. This difference in inhibitions does not correlate with the lower density of μ receptors at P21 compared to P14 and suggests that μ receptor number is not the sole determinate of the actions of morphine in the developing rat, and that other systems may be developmentally regulated, which can influence the inhibitory effects of morphine. The potencies of opioids were significantly greater in the rat pups compared to adults (Rahman et al. 1998) (Fig. 1).

Aβ-fiber stimulation can evoke nociceptive behavioral responses in early life (Fitzgerald et al. 1988). Aβ-fibers occupy the superficial laminae of the dorsal horn alongside the C-fiber terminals for a relatively long period postnatally (Fitzgerald 1997) and may make contact with neurons destined to be nociceptive in later stages (Coggeshall et al. 1996). The electrophysiological study revealed a dose-related inhibition of the A-fiber-evoked response; these inhibitions were greater in the neonatal rat than in the adult rat spinal cord. Thus, even though A-fiber stimuli can evoke nociceptive responses in young rats, the lower selectivity of morphine for A- versus C-fiber responses compared to the adult may be beneficial for opioid control of evoked activity in early life. This response may result from the wider location of opioid receptors in the neonatal spinal cord (Rahman et al. 1998). Likewise, an in vitro study (Faber et al. 1997) has shown that morphine reduces A-fiber-evoked segmental spinal cord reflexes in the neonatal rat. DPDPE, the δ-receptor agonist, exhibited similar effects.

Some groups have shown that the density of opioid receptors, particularly μ and κ receptors, is greater in the brain and spinal cord at early stages (Attali et al. 1990; Kar and Quirion 1995; Rahman et al. 1998). Most in vitro studies on the cellular effects of opioids are performed using cells from very young animals, so it can be presumed that opioid receptors are functional at early stages (Faber et al. 1997). We could thus envisage that opioid receptor agonists would produce more widespread and dramatic receptor-mediated events in early life.

However, the developmental changes in the increased sensitivity of dorsal horn neurons to spinal morphine and DPDPE in the rat pups does not correlate with the density of μ- and δ-receptor binding sites in the spinal cord. The density of δ receptors in the spinal cord changes little during pre- and postnatal development (Attali et al. 1990; Rahman et al. 1998), and the affinity of DPDPE for the δ receptor remains constant during development (McDowell and Kitchen 1987). Thus, events beyond the receptor, linking the binding of a drug to the receptor and the initiation of the cellular inhibition, such as G-protein coupling and effector mechanisms, may be developmentally regulated. Many receptors act via an intracellular protein, a guanine

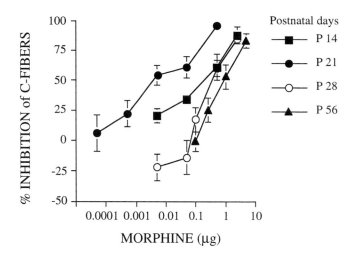

Fig. 1. A series of dose-response curves for spinal morphine in the rat at various stages of development from postnatal (P) day 14 to the adult (P56). Note that the analgesic effects (inhibition of C-fiber responses) are greater (lower doses are required) in early life as compared to the adult (P56).

nucleotide-binding (G) protein, and the opioids also act in this way. However, although G-protein coupling of opioid receptors diminishes with increasing age (Windh and Kuln 1995), G-protein activity is much greater in adult rats compared with P5 (Szucs and Coscia 1990); Milligan et al. (1987) have shown that concentrations of G_i and G_o are 100- to 1000-fold higher than those of μ and δ receptors in the brain of neonatal and adult rats. The findings from these studies would indicate that both levels and coupling of G proteins to opioid receptors in development are not responsible for the increased inhibitory effects of opioids.

NONOPIOID ANALGESIA

The spinal actions of opioids in the adult can be functionally altered by several pathological and pharmacological events such that the level of spinal analgesia can be changed in different pain states. Neuropathic pain has a reduced sensitivity to opioids, which indicates a loss of inhibitory function. Several pathological and physiological events may be involved, such as a loss of opioid receptors on afferent fibers following nerve section (Dickenson et al. 1994b). The degree of analgesia produced by morphine is controlled by the peptide cholecystokinin (CCK), which interferes with opioid inhibitory mechanisms in the normal spinal cord. After nerve damage, CCK levels rise and are at least partly responsible for resultant reduced opioid effects (Stanfa et al. 1994). CCK antagonists should at least partially restore opioid analgesia in neuropathic pain, Unfortunately, they are not yet available.

In addition, allodynia is relayed via large A-fiber pathways that lack opioid receptors. Furthermore, given the potential loss of opioid receptors after nerve damage, other conditions such as hyperalgesia may also respond poorly to opioids. Animal studies show that any loss or dysfunction of presynaptic opioid receptors can be partially overcome by increasing the dose of opioid (Dickenson 1994b), and human studies also indicate that this approach may be effective (Portenoy et al. 1990; Jadad et al. 1992). The simple augmentation of the morphine dose should be tried first, although side effects may confound this tactic. Another approach may be to use high-efficacy opioids such as alfentanyl or sufentanil, but data are lacking on this point. If opioids cannot produce the desired effects, different pharmacological approaches are possible, and in the case of the NMDA receptor many experimental drugs can effectively block the receptor, the channel, or associated sites. Some potential drugs are in development, but there clearly is a need for immediate testing of current agents. In fact, ketamine blocks the channel associated with the NMDA receptor and has current use in pain relief (Eide et al. 1995; Dickenson 1997), but it also has problematic side effects. Dextrophan and dextromethorphan are also antagonists at this site and are used in humans for their antitussive effects. Both not only reduce wind-up (Dickenson et al. 1991) but are effective in models of neuropathic pain after spinal application (Tal and Bennett 1993). However, the NMDA antagonists would only be effective in reducing hyperalgesia, not in abolishing the pain (Dickenson 1994a, 1995, 1997). These agents may be especially useful in allodynias that are sensitive to NMDA receptor antagonists but not to opioids. In fact, clinical trials showed that ketamine can reduce allodynias and hyperalgesias and relieve pain in circumstances where opioids had poor or restricted efficacy, such as postherpetic neuralgias (Eide et al. 1995).

One practical application of the poor opioid responsiveness of NMDA-mediated pains is that the co-administration of morphine with low doses of an NMDA antagonist should be beneficial in these pain states. This is indeed the case, and one study showed a synergy effect with this combination (Chapman and Dickenson 1992) while another study showed an additive effect in a different model of neuropathic pain (Yamamoto and Yaksh 1993). Furthermore, local spinal anesthetics synergize with spinal morphine, partly due to the ability of the former to indirectly reduce NMDA-mediated activity (Fraser et al. 1992). Few studies of children have examined whether agents such as ketamine can act as NMDA antagonists and thus as analgesics and whether such an effect can be achieved at subanesthetic doses. The psychotomimetic effects so prevalent in adults appear weaker in children, which may well arise from developmental changes in the receptor function and location in early life.

By contrast to nerve injury states, opioids appear to be more effective in the presence of peripheral inflammation than in a normal state. Peripheral hyperexcitability appears to set up central compensatory controls in the adult. Within 1–3 hours of inflammation, neurons with a high degree of NMDA wind-up become less active with regard to inhibitions, gamma-aminobutaric acid (GABA) controls and descending α_2 activity are increased, and the ability of morphine to inhibit nociception is also higher within 1–3 hours of the induction of inflammation in rats (Stanfa et al. 1992; Green and Dickenson 1997; Green et al. 1998). These increased effects of morphine after inflammation are thus due to two factors: the inflammation rapidly induces a new peripheral opioid site of action and there is an enhancement of the spinal effects of morphine.

Opioid receptors are not restricted to sensory pathways, and opioids will act at several other sites in the central and peripheral nervous systems that contribute to both the desirable analgesic effect and also the unwanted side effects of these drugs. Another important further mechanism of opioid analgesia involves many opioid receptors in the brain stem and midbrain. Opioids, by actions at sites including the periaqueductal gray, raphe nuclei, reticular formation, and locus cereleus, interact with noradrenergic and serotoninergic pathways to reduce spinal transmission via long descending pathways that run down to the spinal cord. These descending pathways mature slowly (Fitzgerald and Koltzenburg 1986), so it is possible that in early life morphine acts primarily in the spine, with this indirect supraspinal action fully developing only in the mature animal. We have incomplete knowledge of the exact mechanisms of supraspinal opioid analgesia, although they are important (Dickenson 1994b). First, noradrenaline and serotonin are key transmitters in the control of mood, anxiety, and stress. Second, antidepressants, which target these two transmitters and increase their synaptic levels by blocking reuptake, and agents that directly activate α_2 adrenoceptors, such as clonidine, are used to treat neuropathic pain. The dual actions of several drugs and the existence of these pathways provide a framework for understanding how states such as anxiety and depression can have not only psychological consequences but can also influence the level of pain perception and the responses to opioids. Fig. 2 shows the actions of the various excitatory and inhibitory transmitters described in this chapter.

The neonatal CNS proceeds through various functional stages before reaching maturity. Spinal opioid receptors play a major role in the modulation of nociception and show postnatal changes in their density and location within the lumbar spinal cord. Generally a greater density of receptors is

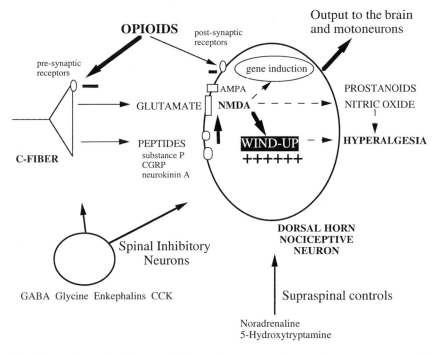

Fig. 2. A schematic diagram of the various transmitter and receptor systems, both excitatory and inhibitory, as described in the text, that interact at the level of the spinal cord. A C-fiber ending is shown terminating on a spinal cord neuron.

seen at the early postnatal ages for μ and κ receptors, with a peak in binding followed by a gradual decline toward adult levels. Delta-receptor binding is first seen at P7 in the spinal cord of rats, with no obvious changes in density with increasing postnatal age. Previous autoradiography and membrane homogenate binding studies for opioid receptors and other transmitter receptors have generally shown that receptor numbers tend to be greater early in life with a reduction in adulthood. Indeed, this pattern is seen with regard to most developmental aspects of anatomy. The very early stages of development involve a tremendous proliferation and differentiation of cells and an increase in the number of receptors. However, reductions occur later in development as neuronal activity, trophic factors, and neuronal markers such as receptors influence the formation of specific synapses. Neurons and axons that are not strengthened will die. Essentially an abundance of neurons and fibers is followed by cell death; for example, in the DRG large-scale cell death occurs just before birth in the rat and axon pruning occurs at around the same time (Coggeshall et al. 1994). We would thus assume that any receptors on these neurons would also be lost. Further, it is possible that postsynaptic receptors are also lost as a consequence of activity-related downregulation of receptors. Thus, the pattern of postnatal development of the density of μ and κ receptors, and indeed SP and NMDA receptors, seems appropriate in that receptor number decreases as neurons and fibers diminish with age.

LONG-TERM CONSEQUENCES OF PAIN AND ANALGESIA

It would seem that many different receptors, transmitters, and structures change with time, some in a phasic manner, some possibly in a linear manner, such that the functional activity in the spinal cord could well vary during the stages of life. Thus, the activity of the spinal cord and the messages sent to higher centers is dependent on the interplay of different transmitter systems that go through various stages of development. Thus, it could be argued that early painful experiences and even high doses of analgesics could act on a developing nervous system to alter connectivity and function and leave a permanent imprint upon sensory pathways that endures into adulthood.

The impact of pain and its alleviation in the newborn extends beyond the immediate recovery period, and it is essential to consider long-term sequelae. A feature of the developing nervous system is its plasticity, and alterations in normal activity patterns during development can permanently alter the pattern of connections within the CNS. It is well established, for example, that auditory or visual experiences during a critical period of early life determine future auditory and visual perception. Anatomical, neurochemical, and electrophysiological experiments in rats have identified significant neuroplasticity in peripheral and central sensory pathways following experimental nerve injury and target tissue damage. Such plasticity not only persists into adulthood but is likely to result in alterations in somatosensory perception (Chimelli and Scaravilli 1985; Killackey and Dawson 1989). Some of the key systems in the plasticity of the adult spinal cord following tissue injury or altered activity, such as the peptide and glutamate receptors, are overexpressed in the immature nervous system, so it is possible that they could be responsible for the long-term sequelae of early injury.

NMDA activation may be a mechanism through which further alterations in nociceptive processing occur as a result of the influx of calcium into neurons through the NMDA channel. This process may be the means by which genes can be activated in dorsal horn neurons a matter of minutes after noxious stimulation, either mechanical, thermal, or inflammatory (Wisden et al. 1990). In early life, these genes can be induced by not only noxious but also innocuous stimuli (Jennings and Fitzgerald 1996). Thus, there is potential for marked alterations in the mechanisms of processing and even the ultrastructure of neurons via gene expression. The physiological consequences of gene induction are still unclear. Many enzymes are calcium dependent, so any increase in intracellular calcium can increase their activity and cause neuronal depolarization. Nitric oxide synthase generates a gas, nitric oxide (NO), that acts as a freely diffusible transmitter in the vasculature and can also be released from neurons. The use of blockers of this enzyme reveals that NO is required for wind-up, inflammation-produced spinal neuronal responses, NMDA-elicited pain behavior, and neuropathic pain responses in animal models. However, as it appears to be released in response to NMDA-receptor activation, its mechanism of action could be to increase the release of C-fiber transmitters and so further enhance transmission into the spinal cord (Meller and Gebhart 1993). Nitric oxide production in early life again differs from the situation in the adult (Soyguder et al. 1994).

It has been suggested that once these central hypersensitivity states have been induced, they remain active in the absence of peripheral inputs (Coderre and Melzack 1992). However, both animal experiments and studies of human pain states show clear evidence that central changes are entirely dependent on peripheral inputs for maintenance (Dickenson and Sullivan 1987; Gracely et al. 1993). Thus, it would seem that the central pain hypersensitivity generators are continually triggered by afferent activity. This reliance of NMDA-mediated potentiation of transmission in the spinal cord on afferent inputs contrasts with long-term potentiation (LTP) in the hippocampus, a more persistent NMDA-dependent event, because LTP, once induced, persists in the absence of further inputs (Bashir and Collingridge 1992). In addition to potentiation, long-lasting depressive events evoked by NMDA-receptor activation can be observed in several regions of the brain (Kombain and Malenka 1994). These inhibitory controls may well be activated under normal conditions to control the level of excitability in the mature nervous system, but they develop slowly in the neonate. Thus, a local GABA control and also monoamines from descending pathways are important determinants of the level of activity transmitted through the spinal cord during inflammation (Stanfa et al. 1992; Green and Dickenson 1997; Green et al. 1998). Carrageenan-induced unilateral inflammation will increase the number of GABA-immunoreactive cells in the ipsilateral dorsal horn of rats, reaching a peak 4 days post-injection (Castro-Lopes et al. 1994). Sciatic neurectomy or administration of capsaicin can prevent this response, which suggests that GABA is upregulated in the dorsal horn by the increase in noxious input.

In the formalin model of inflammatory pain, intrathecal GABA-A and GABA-B agonists cause a dose-dependent suppression of nociceptive behavior in both the phase 1 and phase 2 response (Dirig and Yaksh 1995). Electrophysiological tests indicate that bicuculline, the GABA-A receptor antagonist, applied intrathecally after formalin prolongs the duration of the second peak. In addition, the antagonist causes a marked increase in the rate of neuronal firing of dorsal horn cells (Green and Dickenson 1997) and the duration of the formalin response. Block of GABA and glycine inhibitions in a normal rat induces allodynia (Yaksh 1989) and allows low-threshold inputs to activate nociceptive reflexes (Sivilotti and Woolf 1994) so that GABA controls both low-threshold mechanoreceptors and Aβ-afferents and high-threshold C-fiber inputs.

Neuropathic pain states also appear to be subject to GABAergic control. In the Bennett and Xie model (Bennett 1994), unilateral loose ligatures around the sciatic nerve induce an ipsilateral allodynia and hyperalgesia. Intrathecal bicuculline, administered postsurgically, causes an increase in the magnitude of the hyperalgesia (Yamamoto and Yaksh 1993). However, at later stages, there appears to be a loss of GABA control after nerve injury since spinal levels of GABA are reduced at 3 weeks postlesion (Castro-Lopes et al. 1993). Thus, a loss of spinal inhibitions may tip the balance toward excitations in neuropathic states, so that even if the peripheral activity is reduced after nerve injury there is a loss of compensatory central inhibitions.

The rearrangements that occur in spinal neuronal networks with development (Altman and Bayer 1984; Bicknell and Beal 1984; Fitzgerald 1987; Fitzgerald et al. 1993) involve both interneurons and descending pathways from the brain, destined to be inhibitory, which are slow to mature (Bicknell and Beal 1984). Thus, even though many receptors are functional and anatomical pathways are formed at early stages, their innervation by transmitters is likely to be delayed, such as with the descending controls (Fitzgerald and Koltzenburg 1986). Consequently, inhibitions may be lacking in early life. Several features of the neonatal spinal cord, such as the enhanced spatial range of afferent terminations, the low level of local and descending inhibitory controls, the wide distribution and high density of excitatory receptors such as those for SP and NMDA, and the increased NMDA-induced cellular activity, are likely to be major contributors to the increased excitability and decreased selectivity for modalities of stimuli that are such a feature of early life. Guy and Abbot (1992) have shown that the formalin response, an NMDA-dependent process, is slowly regulated during development, so that even an injection of saline to young pups disrupts behavior. In addition to the slow development of the interneurons that use GABA and

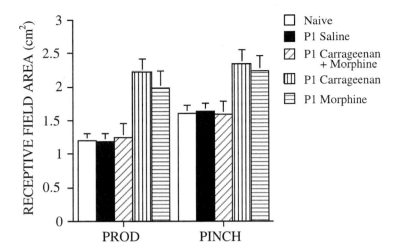

Fig. 3. Persistent changes in receptive field size are produced by exposure at day P0 to either morphine or carrageenan inflammation. The area of the receptive fields of spinal neurons in the adult is increased both for prod (non-noxious) and pinch (noxious) stimuli. Saline controls do not show this, nor do animals receiving morphine in the presence of pain (carrageenan + morphine).

glycine (both inhibitory neurotransmitters involved in local inhibitory processing in the adult spinal cord), these transmitters, if released, will act in the opposite direction in early life and will depolarize neonatal sensory neurons (Ben-Ari et al. 1994; Reichling et al. 1994; Strata and Cherubini 1994). Thus, chemical signaling molecules that function as excitatory transmitters in early life will become inhibitory in the adult. Some intrinsic inhibitory systems that would control the level of excitability in the adult may be slow to develop in the young so that pain transmission could be prolonged and enhanced as compared to the adult. Could these changes persist?

We have attempted to model the impact of pain and opioid analgesia in early life by administration of morphine in the presence of inflammation in young rat pups (Rahman et al. 1997). The results of behavioral tests showed that carrageenan inflammation at P1 produces a marked drop in threshold for withdrawal. In subsequent electrophysiological studies in these animals at adulthood, we observed a significant increase in the receptive field area responding to pinch and prod stimulation of the peripheral receptive field in the P1 carrageenan-treated animals (Fig. 3).

This result shows that even a relatively low-intensity noxious input in early life can cause a prolonged change to the CNS. It is known that inflammation produces various physiological changes in the peripheral and central nervous systems in the adult animal that are observable for several days, as discussed previously. If we assume that similar and perhaps even more dramatic plastic changes occur in the neonate, then the increase in afferent barrage may strengthen synapses that normally would not have survived. This process could explain the permanent expansion of the receptive field areas. Possibly a deviation from the normal "wiring" of the spinal cord has occurred. Indeed, a recent report has described heavier than normal staining in laminae I and II with wheat-germ agglutinin-HRP, a marker for small-diameter unmyelinated afferents, in 8-week-old adult rat spinal cords that at P1 received unilateral injection of the left hind paw with complete Freund's adjuvant, another model of inflammation (Ling and Ruda 1998). These findings suggest that neonatal persistent pain has resulted in alterations in the neural circuitry of spinal pain pathways that may relate to some of the clinical observations (Taddio et al. 1995). Increases in receptive field area have been purported to be a factor underlying central hyperexcitability. The expansion would result in greater overlap of receptive fields of nociceptive neurons, so that a given noxious stimulus to a certain area will activate a greater number of neurons than in the nonpathological situation leading to increased activity in the spinal cord and hyperalgesia. Of course, we cannot rule out the possibility that while the expansion of the receptive field areas may indeed activate a greater number of neurons in the dorsal horn, there could well be compensations to counteract any increased activity.

Somewhat surprisingly, a long-term increase in receptive field area to both pinch and prod stimuli was also seen for adult rats treated with morphine at P1. The proportional increases in the receptive field areas to pinch and prod stimuli, respectively, were of the same magnitude for rats treated with either carrageenan or morphine at P1. This finding is counterintuitive, as we would assume that these stimuli have opposing actions— an excitatory effect for inflammation and an inhibitory effect for morphine. However, the opioid systems play a trophic role in the developing nervous system, rather than acting solely as receptor ligands, so that opioids are involved in inhibition of dendritic growth (Hauser et al. 1989; Steine-Martin et al. 1991). This would suggest that administration of an opioid at early vulnerable stages of development could not only induce a potential change in neurons and synapses but also alter the balance between excitation and inhibition. Although these findings are difficult to reconcile, both treatments could potentially disrupt the normal function of the spinal cord and so result in the same outcome, although via opposing mechanisms.

After administration of morphine alone at P1, the potency of spinal morphine in the adult rat was decreased. A possible basis for this observation could be changes in the number or affinity of μ receptors or intracellular events mediated by μ receptors. This was not the case. However, changes in endogenous cholecystokinin could be involved, as we have shown that the dose-response curves can be shifted back toward the normal state by blocking one of the receptors for CCK. Inflammatory hyperalgesia at P1, either alone or in the presence of an effective dose of morphine, did not produce any changes in the neuropharmacology of adult rats' spinal opioid systems. The finding that early morphine, given without pain, caused persistent changes could be predicted from earlier studies. It has been suggested that exposure to morphine in early life can change opioid receptor numbers, analgesia, and tolerance in the adult animal (Johannesson and Becker 1973). Many of the studies used prolonged exposure and high doses of morphine, often to the mother, which may be more relevant for the study of street use than clinical practice. However, possibly permanent morphine tolerance can develop after early exposure to morphine. Thus, neonatal inflammation alone changes sensory processing and morphine alone changes sensory processing and opioid analgesia in later life. Most importantly, the administration of an effective dose of morphine at the time of inflammation produced no significant shift in the adult dose-response curve for morphine and also prevented the increase in receptive field area to pinch and prod stimulation. Therefore, these data would support the practice of providing adequate treatment of pain in young children, as no obvious changes in the adult CNS were seen. Undertreatment of infants and young children in pain produces not only physiological problems, but also psychological and social problems. Although it is prudent to be careful with powerful analgesics such as morphine, which have a much greater effect in the young, it would be unethical not to provide the best pain relief available, and the literature suggests that opioids in the presence of pain are unlikely to be detrimental.

CONCLUSIONS

Peripheral hyperalgesia can be produced by cooperative effects of several peripheral mediators, nerve injury pains can lead to multiple mechanisms of neuropathic pain, and central excitatory and inhibitory transmitter interactions lead to the eventual ascending message that finally generates both the sensory and affective nature of the response. The multitude of chemicals involved in these different events that together give rise to the final sensation of pain means that complexity is built into sensory transmission. The difficulty in understanding these events is balanced by the fact that a complex system offers more scope for establishing the basis for clinical observations on pain and offers more opportunities to develop new therapies. Importantly, even in the relatively immutable adult nervous system, the relative importance of these transmitters and their receptors can change in different pain states and with time, thus both excitatory and inhibitory events exhibit plasticity, and opioid controls also can vary. These systems change as a part of normal development and few, possibly none, of the transmitter systems implicated in pain and analgesia in the adult either behave in the same way or are located at the same sites in the young nervous system. Plasticity is very much a part of pain in the adult, and yet plasticity is a requirement for the normal development of the nervous system. We ignore this at our peril.

ACKNOWLEDGMENTS

The authors' work is supported by the Medical Research Council, European Community (Biomed BMH4-CT95-0172) and The Wellcome Trust (United Kingdom).

REFERENCES

Abbot FV, Guy ER. Effects of morphine, pentobarbital and amphetamine on formalin–induced behaviours in infant rats: sedation versus specific suppression of pain. *Pain* 1995; 62:303–312.

Anand KJS, McGrath PJ. *Pain in Neonates*. Amsterdam: Elsevier, 1993.

Andrews K, Fitzgerald M. The cutaneous withdrawal reflex in human neonates: sensitization, receptive fields, and the effects of contralateral stimulation. *Pain* 1994; 56:95–101.

Altman J, Bayer SA. The development of the rat spinal cord. *Adv Anat Embryol Cell Biol* 1984; 85:1–166.

Attali B, Saya D, Vogel Z. Pre- and postnatal development of opiate receptor subtypes in rat spinal cord. *Dev Brain Res* 1990; 53:97–102.

Barr GA, Paredes W, Erickson KL, Zukin RS. Kappa-opioid receptor mediated analgesia in the developing rat. *Dev Brain Res* 1986; 29:145–152.

Bashir ZI, Collingridge GL. Synaptic plasticity: long term potentiation in the hippocampus. *Curr Opin Neurobiol* 1992; 2:328–335.

Battaglia G, Rustioni A. Coexistence of glutamate and substance P in dorsal root ganglion cells of the rat and monkey. *J Comp Neurol* 1988; 277:302–312.

Ben-Ari Y, Tseeb V, Raggozzino D, Khazipov R, Gaiarsa JL. Gamma-aminobutyric acid (GABA): a fast excitatory transmitter which may regulate the development of hippocampal neurones in early postnatal life. *Prog Brain Res* 1994; 102:261–273.

Bennett GJ. Animal models of neuropathic pain In: Gebhart GF, Hammond DL, Jensen T (Eds). *Proceedings of 7th World Congress on Pain*. Progress in Pain Research and Management, Vol. 2. Seattle: IASP Press, 1994, pp 495–510.

Bennett GJ, Xie Y-K. A peripheral mononeuropathy in rat produces disorders of pain sensation like those seen in man. *Pain* 1988; 33:87–109.

Beyer JE, DeGood DE, Ashley LC, et al. Patterns of postoperative analgesic use with adults and children following cardiac surgery. *Pain* 1983; 17:71–81.

Bicknell HR, Beal JA. Axonal and dendritic development of substantia gelatinosa neurons in the lumbosacral spinal cord of the rat. *J Comp Neurol* 1984; 226:508–522.

Blass EM, Cramer CP, Fanselow, MS. The development of morphine induced antinociception in neonatal rats: a comparison of forepaw, hindpaw and tail retraction from a thermal stimulus. *Pharmacol Biochem Behav* 1993; 44:643–649.

Booker PD. Postoperative analgesia for neonates. *Anaesthesia* 1987; 42:343–345.

Carmignoto G, Vicini S. Activity dependent decrease in NMDA receptor responses during development of the visual cortex. *Science* 1992; 258:1007–1011.

Castro-Lopes JM, Tavares I, Coimbra A. GABA decreases in the spinal cord dorsal horn after peripheral neurectomy. *Brain Res* 1993; 620:287–291.

Castro-Lopes JM, Tavares I, Tolle TR Coimbra A. Carrageenan-induced inflammation of the hind foot provokes a rise of GABA-immunoreactive cells in the rat spinal cord that is prevented by peripheral neurectomy or neonatal capsaicin. *Pain* 1994:193–201.

Catania MV, Landwehrmeyer GB, Testa CM, et al. Metabotropic glutamate receptors are differentially regulated during development. *Neuroscience* 1994 61:481–495.

Chapman V, Dickenson AH. The combination of NMDA antagonism and morphine produces profound antinociception in the rat dorsal horn. *Brain Res* 1992; 573:321–323.

Chapman V, Charmarette H, Suzuki R, Rygh L,Dickenson AH. Effects of systemic carbamazepine and gabapentin on spinal neuronal responses in spinal nerve ligated rats. *Pain* 1998; 75:261–272.

Charlton CG, Helke CJ. Ontogeny of substance-P receptors in the rat spinal cord: quantitative changes in receptor number and differential expression in specific loci. *Dev Brain Res* 1986; 29:81–91.

Chimelli L, Scaravilli F. Secondary transneuronal degeneration:cortical changes induced by peripheral nerve section in neonatal rats. *Neurosci Lett* 1985; 57:57–63.

Coderre TJ, Melzack R. The contribution of excitatory amino-acids to central sensitization and persistent nociception after formalin-induced tissue injury. *J Neurosci* 1992; 12:3665–3670.

Coggeshall RE, Pover CM, Fitzgerald M. Dorsal root ganglion cell death and surviving cell numbers in relation to the development of sensory innervation in the rat hindlimb. *Dev Brain Res* 1994; 82:193–212.

Coggeshall RE, Jennings EA, Fitzgerald M. Evidence that large primary afferent fibers make synaptic contacts in lamina II of neonatal rats. *Dev Brain Res* 1996; 92:81–90.

Collingridge G, Singer W. Excitatory amino acid receptors and synaptic plasticity. *Trends Pharmacol Sci* 1990; 11:290–296.

Craig KD, Whitfield MF, Grunau RVE, Linton J, Hadjistavropoulous HD. Pain in the preterm neonate: behavioural and physiological indices. *Pain* 1993; 52:287–299.

Devor M, Wall PD, Catalan N. Systemic lidocaine silences ectopic neuroma and DRG discharge without blocking nerve conduction. *Pain* 1992; 48:261–268.

Dickenson AH. NMDA receptor antagonists as analgesics. In: Fields HL, Liebeskind JC (Eds). *Pharmacological Approaches to the Treatment of Chronic Pain: New Concepts and Critical Issues.* Progress in Pain Research and Management, Vol. 1. Seattle: IASP Press, 1994a; 173–187.

Dickenson AH. Where and how opioids act. In: Gebhart GF, Hammond DL, Jensen T (Eds). *Proceedings of the 7th World Congress on Pain*, Progress in Pain Research and Management, Vol. 2. Seattle: IASP Press, 1994b, pp 525–552.

Dickenson AH. Spinal cord pharmacology of pain. *Brit J Anaesth* 1995; 75:132–144.

Dickenson AH. Mechanisms of central hypersensitivity In: Dickenson AH, Besson JM (Eds). *The Pharmacology of Pain,* Handbook of Experimental Pharmacology, Vol. 130. Berlin: Springer-Verlag, 1997, pp 168–210.

Dickenson AH, Besson JM (Eds). *The Pharmacology of Pain,* Handbook of Experimental Pharmacology, Vol. 130. Berlin: Springer-Verlag, 1997.

Dickenson AH, Sullivan AF. Peripheral origins and central modulation of subcutaneous formalin-induced activity of rat dorsal horn neurones. *Neurosci Lett* 1987; 83:207–211.

Dickenson AH, Sullivan AF, Stanfa LC, McQuay H. Dextromethorphan and levorphanol on dorsal horn nociceptive neurones in the rat. *Neuropharmacology* 1991; 30:1303–1308.

Dickenson AH, Chapman V, Green M. The pharmacology of excitatory and inhibitory amino-acid mediated events in the transmission and modulation of pain in the spinal cord. *Gen Pharmacol* 1997; 28:633–638.

Dirig DM, Yaksh TL. Intrathecal Baclofen and Muscimol, but not Midazolam, are antinociceptive using the rat-formalin model. *J Pharmacol Exp Ther* 1995; 275:219–227.

Dray A. Peripheral mediators of pain. In : Dickenson AH, Besson JM (Eds). *The Pharmacology of Pain,* Handbook of Experimental Pharmacology, Vol. 130. Berlin: Springer-Verlag, 1997, pp 21–42.

Dray A, Urban L, Dickenson AH. Pharmacology of chronic pain. *Trends Pharm Sci* 1994; 15:190–197.

Dubner R, Ruda MA. Activity dependent neuronal plasticity following tissue injury and inflammation. *Trends Neurosci* 1992; 15:96–103.

Duggan AW, Hendrey IA, Morton CR, Hutchison WD, Zhao ZO. Cutaneous stimuli releasing immunoreactive substance P in the dorsal horn of the cat. *Brain Res* 1988; 451:261–273.

Eide PK, Stubhaug A, Oye I, Breivik H. Continuous subcutaneous administration of the N-methyl-D-aspartic acid (NMDA) receptor antagonist ketamine in the treatment of post-herpetic neuralgia. *Pain* 1995; 61:221–228.

Faber ESL, Chambers JP, Brugger F, Evans RH. Depression of A and C fibre-evoked segmental reflexes by morphine and clonidine in the in vitro spinal cord of the neonatal rat. *Br J Pharmacol* 1997; 120:1390–1396.

Fields HL, Rowbotham MC. Multiple mechanisms of neuropathic pain: a clinical perspective. In: Gebhart GF, Hammond DL, Jensen TS (Eds). *Proceedings of the 7th World Congress on Pain.* Progress in Pain Research and Management, Vol. 2. Seattle: IASP Press, 1994, pp 437–454.

Fitzgerald M. The postnatal development of cutaneous afferent fibre input and receptive field organization in the rat dorsal horn. *J Physiol* 1985; 364:1–18

Fitzgerald M. The prenatal growth of fine diameter afferents into the rat spinal cord–a transganglionic study. *J Comp Neurol* 1987; 261:98–104.

Fitzgerald M. Development of pain pathways and mechanisms. In: Anand KJS, Mcgrath PJ (Eds). *Pain in neonates.* Amsterdam: Elsevier, 1993, pp 19–37.

Fitzgerald M. Pain in infancy: some unanswered questions. *Pain Reviews* 1995; 2:77–91.

Fitzgerald M. Neonatal pharmacology of pain. In: Dickenson A, Besson J-M (Eds). *Handbook of Experimental Pharmacology,* The Pharmacology of Pain, Vol. 130. Berlin: Springer-Verlag, 1997, pp 447–460.

Fitzgerald M, Andrews K. Flexion reflex properties in the human infant: a measure of spinal sensory processing in the newborn. In: Finley GA, McGrath PJ (Eds). *Measurement of Pain in Infants and Children.* Progress in Pain Research and Management, Vol. 10. Seattle: IASP Press, 1998.

Fitzgerald M, Koltzenburg M. The functional development of descending inhibitory pathways in the dorsolateral funiculus of the newborn rat spinal cord. *Dev Brain Res* 1986; 24:261–270.

Fitzgerald M, Shaw A, Macintosh N. The postnatal development of the cutaneous flexor reflex: a comparative study in premature infants and newborn rat pups. *Dev Med Child Neurol* 1987; 30:520–526.

Fitzgerald M., Millard C, MacIntosh N. Hyperalgesia in premature infants. *Lancet* 1988; 8580:292.

Fitzgerald M, Millard C, MacIntosh N. Cutaneous hypersensitivity following peripheral tissue damage in newborn infants and its reversal with topical anaesthesia. *Pain* 1989; 39:31–36.

Fitzgerald M, Butcher T, Shortland P. Developmental changes in the laminar termination of A fibre cutaneous sensory afferents in the rat spinal cord dorsal horn. *J Comp Neurol* 1995; 348:225–233.

Fraser H, Chapman V, Dickenson AH. Spinal local anaesthetic actions on afferent evoked responses and wind-up of nociceptive neurones in the rat spinal cord: combination with morphine produces marked potentiation of antinociception. *Pain* 1992; 49:33–41.

Goedert M, Stoeckel K, Otten U. Biological importance of the retrograde axonal transport of nerve growth factor in sensory neurons. *Proc Natl Acad Sci USA* 1981; 78:5895–5898.

Gold MS, Reichling DB, Shuster MJ, Levine JD. Hyperalgesic agents increase a tetrodoxin-resistant Na+ current in nociceptors. *Proc Natl Acad Sci USA* 1996; 93:1108–1112.

Gonzalez DL, Fuchs JL, Droge MH. Distribution of NMDA receptor binding in developing mouse spinal cord. *Neurosci Lett* 1993; 151:134–137.

Gracely R, Lynch SA, Bennett GJ. Painful neuropathy: altered central processing maintained dynamically by peripheral input. *Pain* 1993; 52:251–253.

Green M, Dickenson AH. GABA receptor control of the amplitude and duration of the neuronal responses to formalin in the rat spinal cord. *Eur J Pain* 1997;1:95–104.

Green M, Lyons L, Dickenson AH. α_2 adrenoceptor antagonists enhance responses of dorsal horn neurones to formalin induced inflammation. *Eur J Pharm* 1998; 347:201–204.

Grunau RVE, Whitfield MF, Petrie JH, Fryer EL. Early pain experience: child and family factors as precursors somatization: a prospective study of extremely premature and fullterm children. *Pain* 1994a; 56:353–359.

Grunau RVE, Whitfield MF, Petrie JH. Pain sensitivity and temperament in extremely low birthweight premature toddlers and preterm and fullterm controls. *Pain* 1994b; 58:341–346.

Guy ER, Abbott FV. The behavioural response to formalin pain in preweanling rats. *Pain* 1992; 51:81–90.

Haley JE, Sullivan AF, Dickenson AH. Evidence for spinal N-methyl-D-aspartate receptor involvement in prolonged chemical nociception in the rat. *Brain Res* 1990; 518:218–222.

Hauser KF, McLaughlin PJ, Zagon IS. Endogenous opioid systems and the regulation of dendritic growth and spine formation. *J Comp Neurol* 1989; 281:13–22.

Hofer M, Constantine-Paton M. Regulation of N-methyl-D-aspartate (NMDA) receptor function during the rearrangement of developing neuronal connections. *Prog Brain Res* 1994; 102:277–285.

Hokfelt T, Zhang X, Wiesenfeld-Hallin Z. Messenger plasticity in primary sensory neurones following axotomy and its functional implications. *Trends Neurosci* 1994; 17:22–30.

Hori Y, Kanda K. Developmental alterations in NMDA receptor-mediated $[Ca2+]_i$ elevation in substantia gelatinosa neurons of neonatal rat spinal cord. *Dev Brain Res* 1994; 80:141–148.

Jadad AR, Carroll D, Glynn CJ, Moore RA, McQuay HJ. Morphine responsiveness of chronic pain: double-blind randomized crossover study with patient-controlled analgesia. *Lancet* 1992; 339:1367–1371.

Jakowec MW, Fox AJ, Martin CJ, Kalb RG. Quantitative and qualitative changes in AMPA receptor expression during spinal cord development. *Neuroscience* 1995a; 67:893–907.

Jakowec MW, Yen L, Kalb RG. In situ hybridization analysis of AMPA receptor subunit gene expression in the developing rat spinal cord. *Neuroscience* 1995b; 67:909–920.

Jennings E, Fitzgerald M. C-fos can be induced in the neonatal rat spinal cord by both noxious and innocuous stimulation. *Pain* 1996; 68:301–306.

Johannesson T, Becker BA. Morphine analgesia in rats at various ages. *Acta Pharmacol et Toxicol* 1973; 33:429–441.

Johnston CC, Stevens B, Craig, KD, Grunau RVE. Developmental changes in pain expression in premature, full-term, two and four month old infants. *Pain* 1993; 52:201–208.

Johnston CC, Stevens BJ, Yang F, Horton L. Differential response to pain by very premature neonates. *Pain* 1995; 61:471–479.

Kajander KC, Bennett GJ. Onset of a painful peripheral neuropathy in rat: a partial and differential deafferentation and spontaneous discharge in Aβ and Aδ primary afferent neurons. *J Neurophysiol* 1992; 68:734–744.

Kar S, Quirion R. Neuropeptide receptors in developing and adult rat spinal cord: an in vitro quantitative autoradiography study of calcitonin gene-related peptide, neurokinins, μ-opioid, galanin, somatostatin, neurotensin and vasoactive intestinal polypeptide receptors. *J Comp Neurol* 1995; 354:253–281.

Killackey HP, Dawson DR. Expansion of the central hindpaw representation following fetal forelimb removal in the rat. *Eur J Neurosci* 1989; 1:210–221.

Kim SH, Chung JM. An experimental model for peripheral neuropathy produced by segmental spinal nerve ligation in the rat. *Pain* 1992; 50:355–363.

Kombain SB, Malenka RC. Simultaneous LTP of non-NMDA- and LTD of NMDA-receptor-mediated responses in the nucleus accumbens. *Nature* 1994; 368:242–246.

Laird JMA, Bennett GJ. An electrophysiological study of dorsal horn neurons in the spinal cord of rats with an experimental peripheral neuropathy. *J Neurophysiol* 1993; 69:1–14.

Lekan HA, Carlton SM, Coggeshall RE. Sprouting of Aβ fibers into lamina II of the rat dorsal horn in peripheral neuropathy. *Neurosci Lett* 1996; 208:147–150.

Levine JD, Fields HL, Basbaum AI. Peptides and the primary afferent nociceptor. *J Neurosci* 1993; 13:2273–2286.

Ling QD, Ruda MA. Neonatal persistent pain alters spinal neural circuitry. *Soc Neurosci Abs* 1998; 24:386.

Marshall RE. Strarron WC. More JA, Boxman SB. Circumcision: effects on new born behavior. *Infant Behav Dev* 1980; 3:1–14.

Marti E, Gibson SJ, Polak JM, et al. Ontogeny of peptide and amine-containing neurones in motor, sensory, and autonomic regions of rat and human spinal cord, dorsal root ganglia, and rat skin. *J Comp Neurol* 1987; 266:332–359.

McDowell J, Kitchen I. Development of opioid systems: peptides, receptors and pharmacology. *Brain Res Rev* 1987; 12:397–421.

McLaughlin CR, Dewey WL. A comparison of the antinociceptive effects of opioid agonists in neonatal and adult rats in phasic and tonic nociceptive tests. *Pharmacol Biochem Behav* 1994; 49:1017–1023.

McMahon SB, Bennett DLH. Growth factors and pain. In: Dickenson AH, Besson JM (Eds). *The Pharmacology of Pain,* Handbook of Experimental Pharmacology, Vol. 130. Berlin: Springer-Verlag, 1997, pp 135–165.

McMahon SB, Lewin GR, Wall PD. Central excitability triggered by noxious inputs. *Curr Opin Neurobiol* 1993; 3:602–610.

McQuay H, Dickenson AH. Implications of central nervous system plasticity for pain management. *Anaesthesiology* 1990; 45:101–102.

McQuay H, Carroll D, Jadad AR, Wiffen P, Moore A. Anticonvulsant drugs for management of pain: a systematic review. *BMJ* 1995; 311:1047–1052.

McQuay HJ, Tramer M, Nye BA, et al. A systematic review of antidepressants in neuropathic pain, *Pain* 1996, 68:217–227.

Meller ST, Gebhart GF. Nitric oxide (NO) and nociceptive processing in the spinal cord. *Pain* 1993; 52:127–136.

Mendelson B. Chronic embryonic MK-801 exposure disrupts the somatotopic organization of cutaneous nerve projections in the chick spinal cord. *Dev Brain Res* 1994; 82:152–166.

Milligan G, Streaty RA, Gierschik P, Spiegel AM, Klee WA. Development of opioid receptors and GTP–binding regulatory proteins in neonatal rat brain. *J Biol Chem* 1987; 262:8626–8630.

Morrisett RA, Mott DD, Lewis DV, Wilson WA, Swartzwelder HS. Reduced sensitivity of the N-methyl-D-aspartate component of synaptic transmission to magnesium in hippocampal slices from immature rats. *Dev Brain Res* 1990; 56:257–262.

Na HS, Leem JW, Chung JM. Abnormalities of mechanoreceptors in a rat model of neuropathic pain: possible involvement in mediating mechanical allodynia. *J Neurophysiol* 1993; 70:522–528.

Otsuka M, Yoshioka K. Neurotransmitter functions of mammalian tachykinins. *Physiol Rev* 1993; 73:229–303.

Palecek J, Paleckova V, Dougherty PM, Carlton SM, Willis WD. Responses of spinothalamic tract cells to mechanical and thermal stimulation of skin in rats with experimental peripheral neuropathy. *J Neurophysiol* 1992; 67:1562–1573.

Portenoy RK, Foley KM, Inturrisi CE. The nature of opioid responsiveness and its implications for neuropathic pain: new hypotheses derived from studies of opioid infusions. *Pain* 1990; 43:273–286.

Price DD, Mao J, Mayer DJ. Central neural mechanisms of normal and abnormal pain states In: Fields HL, Liebeskind JC (Eds). *Pharmacological Approaches to the Treatment of Chronic Pain: New Concepts and Critical Issues.* Progress in Pain Research and Management, Vol. 1. Seattle: IASP Press, 1994, pp 61–84.

Rahman W, Fitzgerald M, Aynsley-Green A, Dickenson AH. The effects of neonatal exposure to inflammation and/or morphine on neuronal responses and morphine analgesia in adult rats. In: Jensen T, Turner JA, Wiesenfeld-Hallin Z (Eds). *Proceedings of the 8th World Congress of Pain,* Progress in Pain Research and Management, Vol. 8. Seattle: IASP Press, 1997, pp 783–794.

Rahman W, Dashwood MR, Fitzgerald M, Aynsley-Green A, Dickenson AH. Postnatal development of multiple opioid receptors in the spinal cord and development of spinal morphine analgesia. *Dev Brain Res* 1998; 108:239–254.

Reichling DB, Kyrozis A, Wang J, McDermott AB. Mechanisms of GABA and glycine depolarization-induced calcium transients in rat dorsal horn neurons. *J Physiol* 1994; 476:411–421.

Reynolds M, Fitzgerald M. Long term sensory hyperinnervation following neonatal skin wounds. *J Comp Neurol* 1995; 358:487–498.

Sales N, Charnay Y, Zajac J-M, Dubois P-M, Roques BP. Ontogeny of μ and δ opioid receptors and neutral endopeptidase in human spinal cord: an autoradiographic study, *J Chem Neuroanat* 1989; 2:179–188.

Schechter NL. The undertreatment of pain in children. *Ped Clin North Am* 1989; 36:781–794

Seltzer Z, Dubner R, Shir Y. A novel behavioral model of neuropathic pain disorders produced in rats by partial sciatic nerve injury. *Pain* 1990, 43:205–218.

Sivilotti L, Woolf C. The contribution of GABA$_A$ and glycine receptors to central sensitization: disinhibition and touch: evoked allodynia in the spinal cord. *J Neurophysiol* 1994; 72:169–179.

Soyguder Z, Schmidt HHHW, Morris R. Postnatal development of nitric oxide synthase type I expression in the lumbar spinal cord of the rat: a comparison of c-fos in response to peripheral application of mustard oil. *Neurosci Lett* 1994; 180:188–192.

Stanfa LC, Sullivan AF, Dickenson AH. Alterations in neuronal excitability and the potency of spinal mu, delta and kappa opioids after carrageenan-induced inflammation. *Pain* 1992; 50:345–354.

Stanfa LC, Dickenson AH, Xu X-J, Wiesenfeld-Hallin Z. Cholecystokinin and morphine analgesia: variations on a theme, *Trends in Pharm Sci* 1994; 15:65–66.

Stein C. Interaction of immune-competent cells and nociceptors. In: Gebhart GF, Hammond DL, Jensen T (Eds). *Proceedings of the 7th World Congress on Pain,* Progress in Pain Research and Management, Vol. 2. Seattle: IASP Press, 1994, pp 285–297.

Steine-Martin A, Gurwell JA, Hauser KF. Morphine alters astrocyte growth in primary cultures of mouse glial cells: evidence for a direct effect of opiates on neural maturation. *Dev Brain Res* 1991; 60:1–7.

Stevens BJ, Johnston CC, Horton L. Factors that influence the behavioural pain responses of premature infants. *Pain* 1994; 59:101–109.

Strata F, Cherubini E. Transient expression of a novel type of GABA response in rat CA3 hippocampal neurones during development. *J Physiol* 1994; 480:493–503.

Szucs M, Coscia CJ. Evidence for delta opioid binding and GTP regulatory proteins in 5-day old rat brain membranes. *J Neurochem* 1990; 54:1419–1425.

Taddio A, Goldback M, Ipp M, Stevens B, Koren G. Effect of neonatal circumcision on pain responses during vaccination in boys. *Lancet* 1995; 344:291–292.

Takaishi K, Eisele JH, Carstens E. Behavioral and electrophysiological assessment of hyperalgesia and changes in dorsal horn responses following partial sciatic nerve ligation in rats. *Pain* 1996; 66:297–306.

Tal M, Bennett GJ. Dextrophan relieves neuropathic heat-evoked hyperalgesia in the rat. *Neurosci Letts* 1993; 151:107–110.

Todd AJ, Spike RC. The localization of classical transmitters and neuropeptides within neurons in laminae I–III of the mammalian spinal dorsal horn. *Prog Neurobiol* 1993; 41:609–645.

Wall PD, Devor M. Sensory afferent impulses originate from dorsal root ganglia as well as from the periphery in normal and nerve injured rats. *Pain* 1983; 17:321–339.

Watanabe M, Mishina M, Inoue Y. Distinct spatiotemporal distributions of the N-methyl D-aspartate receptor channel subunit mRNAs in the mouse cervical cord. *J Comp Neurol* 1994; 345:314–319.

Williams SG, Evan G, Hunt SP. Changing patterns of c-fos induction in spinal neurons following thermal cutaneous stimulation in the rat. *Neuroscience* 1990; 36:73–81.

Windh RT, Kuhn CM. Increased sensitivity to mu opiate antinociception in the neonatal rat despite weaker receptor-guanyl nucleotide protein coupling. *J Pharmacol Exp Ther* 1995; 273:1353–1360.

Wisden W, Errington ML, Williams S, et al. Differential expression of immediate early genes in the hippocampus and spinal cord. *Neuron* 1990; 4:603–614.

Woolf CJ. Evidence for a central component of post-injury pain hypersensitivity. *Nature* 1983; 306:686–688.

Woolf CJ. A new strategy for the treatment of inflammatory pain. *Drugs* 1994; (Suppl)5:1–9.

Woolf CJ, Doubell T. The pathophysiology of chronic pain—increased sensitivity to low threshold Ab-fibre inputs. *Curr Opin Neurobiol* 1994; 4:525–534.

Yaksh TL. Behavioural and autonomic correlates of the tactile evoked allodynia produced by spinal glycine inhibition: effects of modulatory receptor systems and excitatory amino acid antagonists. *Pain* 1989; 37:111–123.

Yaksh TL, Malmberg AB. Interaction of spinal modulatory systems. In: Fields HL, Liebeskind JC (Eds). *Pharmacological Approaches to the Treatment of Chronic Pain: New Concepts and Critical Issues,* Progress in Pain Research and Management, Vol. 1. Seattle: IASP Press, 1994, pp 151–171.

Yamamoto T, Yaksh TL. Effects of intrathecal strychnine and bicuculline on nerve compression-induced thermal hyperalgesia and selective antagonism by MK-801. *Pain* 1993; 54:79–84.

Zeltser R, Seltzer Z. A practical guide for the use of animal models in the study of neuropathic pain. In: Boivie J, Hansson P, Lindblom U (Eds). *Touch, Temperature and Pain in Health and Disease: Mechanisms and Assessments,* Progress in Pain Research and Management, Vol. 3. Seattle: IASP Press, 1994, pp 295–338.

Correspondence to: Professor A.H. Dickenson, PhD, Department of Pharmacology, University College, Gower Street, London WC1E 6BT, United Kingdom. Tel/Fax: 44-171-419-3742; email: anthony.dickenson@ucl.ac.uk.

Chronic and Recurrent Pain in Children and Adolescents, Progress in Pain Research and Management, Vol. 13, edited by Patrick J. McGrath and G. Allen Finley, IASP Press, Seattle, © 1999.

3

Consequences of Early Experience: Lessons for Rodent Models of Newborn Pain

Heather MacIntosh Schellinck[a] and K.J.S. Anand[b]

[a]Department of Psychology, Dalhousie University, Halifax, Nova Scotia, Canada; and
[b]Departments of Pediatrics, Anesthesia, and Anatomy, University of Arkansas for Medical Sciences, Little Rock, Arkansas, USA

The mechanisms associated with the processing of painful stimuli in the newborn are unlike those found in the adult animal. The nervous, endocrine, and immune systems are maturing, and the neonatal brain is in a constant state of functional and structural reorganization. Neonatal plasticity has been demonstrated in the somatosensory system (Charleton and Helke 1986; Marti et al. 1987; Catania et al. 1994; Crair and Malenka 1995; Jakowec et al. 1995a,b) and throughout the brain (Kolb 1995; Rabinowicz et al. 1996). The plasticity associated with the developing brain reflects changes that result not only from normal maturation but also from ever-changing experiential factors. An enriched environment may lead to a positive outcome (Wallace et al. 1992; Knudsen 1998), while early pain or stress may result in irrevo-cable damage (Kumazawa 1998; Winberg 1998).

This chapter investigates how the experience of early pain influences behaviors and physiology later in life. Some of the behavioral changes associated with such processes have been documented in humans (Johnston et al. 1993; Grunau et al. 1994, in press; Gunnar et al. 1995; Taddio et al. 1997). Nonetheless, because of the invasive procedures required in this work, it is impossible to implement the necessary experimental manipulations in humans. Consequently, much of our understanding of the early development and continuing influence of pain mechanisms must come from investiga-tions with rodents. This chapter briefly addresses the appropriateness of the rat as a model for studying these processes. It then describes the changing nature of behavioral responses to pain in neonatal rats and delineates the mechanisms underlying these responses. It concludes with an examination of the literature that describes the consequences for the adult animal of stressful experiences in the neonate. The effects of prenatal stress (Kehoe and Shoemaker 1991; McLaughlin et al. 1997; Zagon et al. 1998), while of undoubted interest and potential relevance to behavioral and physiological changes in the adult, will not be addressed in this chapter; however, one should note that prenatal stress in conjunction with postnatal manipulations modulates physiological, behavioral, and immune responses in adult rats (Poltyrev et al. 1996; Smythe et al. 1996; Kay et al. 1998). Thus, knowledge of the gestational history of an animal is a prerequisite if we are to fully understand the outcome of postnatal experimental manipulations.

THE RAT AS A MODEL OF THE HUMAN PAIN EXPERIENCE

The rat provides a particularly good model for examining both the short- and long-term effects of pain in humans. The development of pain pathways and mechanisms has been extensively characterized in pre- and postnatal rats (see review by Fitzgerald 1997). Moreover, it appears that the sequence of events in the development of the pain system of newborn rat pups and humans follows a parallel course (Fitzgerald and Anand 1993). It is gener- ally agreed that the stage of central nervous system (CNS) development of a 7-day-old rat is equivalent to that of a full-term human neonate, a 14-day- old rat corresponds to an infant of 1 year, and a 21-day-old rat is compa- rable to a 2-year-old child (Fitzgerald and Anand 1993). The plasticity that characterizes the developing human brain has also been found in neonatal rats (Wilson 1995; Kim et al. 1996).

The pain systems of newborn rat pups and human infants have several similarities. For example, the development of primary C- and A-fiber affer- ents follows a similar course in both species (Fitzgerald and Anand 1993); moreover, exaggerated cutaneous reflexes occur in both the newborn rat and human (Stelzner 1971; Issler and Stephens 1983; Fitzgerald and Gibson 1984), as does sensitization caused by noxious repeated stimulation (Fitzgerald et al. 1988). Large receptive fields of dorsal horn cells have been characterized in both rats and infants, which may reflect the immaturity of central inhibitory control systems, a hypothesis that has been confirmed in rats (Fitzgerald and Koltzenburg 1986). Studies of the chemistry of develop- ing pathways have found neurotransmitters such as substance P (SP), soma- tostatin, enkephalin, calcitonin gene-related peptide (CGRP), and vasoactive intestinal polypeptide (VIP) in the spinal cords of the developing rat and human (Marti et al. 1987). The functioning of the neurotransmitter systems is not well understood, although several neurotransmitter receptors are known to be present during early development (Charleton and Helke 1986; Jakowec et al. 1986a,b; Gonzalez et al. 1993).

INCREASED PAIN SENSITIVITY IN RAT PUPS

BEHAVIORAL EVIDENCE

Neonatal rat pups show an enhanced sensitivity to somatosensory stimuli compared with older juveniles and adults, and it is believed that humans show comparable responses. For example, studies of the physiological responses to surgical procedures have revealed that higher plasma concentrations of anesthetic are needed to induce analgesia in human neonates than in older age groups (Yaster 1987; Greeley and de Bruijn 1988; Chay et al. 1992). Also, hormonal, metabolic, and cardiovascular responses to surgery may increase in preterm and full-term infants (Anand et al. 1985; Anand 1990).

The developmental pattern of behavioral responses to noxious stimuli has been studied in rat pups, including extensive investigations of their response to formalin injections. Following formalin injection, rat pups tested at days 1, 3, 6, 10, 15, and 20 all responded with limb flexion and shaking and licking of the injected paw; nonetheless, the intensity and duration of the responses decreased with increasing age, and limb flexion was consistently found only in pups younger than 10 days (Guy and Abbott 1992). Consistent behaviors could only be produced in 20-day-old animals after the dose of formalin was increased from 1% to 2.5%. Nonspecific responses such as limb flexion following saline injection, decreased sleep, squirming, kicking, jerking, and whole-body convulsions decreased as the rat pups developed (Guy and Abbott 1992). Using the same behavioral measures, Teng and Abbott (1998) examined the responses to different formalin concentrations in day 3 (0.3%, 0.6%, and 0.9%), day 15 (0.5%, 1.0%, and 2.0%), and day 25 rats (2.5%, 5.9%, and 10.0%). When pain behaviors were plotted against formalin concentration, a similar logarithmic concentration-effect relationship across ages was found, but the sensitivity shifted in that the thresholds for inflammatory pain increased 2.5-fold from 3 to 15 days of age, and a further 4-fold from 15 to 25 days. The 25-day-old pups showed a sensitivity response similar to that of adults over the 40-minute test period.

Lower thresholds to mechanical stimuli, i.e., testing of the dorsal flexor reflex with calibrated von Frey hairs, have also been demonstrated in newborn rat pups compared with older pups or adults (Fitzgerald et al. 1988).

The reflex threshold was found to increase over 4 weeks until it approached adult values. Responses to thermal stimulation have also been tested by measuring the response latency for limb or tail withdrawal from either a hotplate or heated water bath (Blass et al. 1993; Falcon et al. 1996; Hu et al. 1997). In both tests, sensitivity decreased with increasing age, with the maximum response developing between 7 and 12 days. Regardless of the stimulation used, the evidence is overwhelming that the neonate is more sensitive to pain than is an adult animal, which further justifies our concern that negative experiences may profoundly influence the development of the brain at this time.

UNDERLYING MECHANISMS OF PAIN SENSITIVITY

Multiple characteristics of the pain system may underlie the increased sensitivity found in neonates (Anand, in press). This period of sensitivity parallels the development of spinothalamic and thalamocortical connections, which follow the general pattern of an earlier maturation of excitatory than inhibitory mechanisms (Dani et al. 1991). Low pain thresholds may be a result of the activity of immature inhibitory interneurons within the dorsal horn and the lack of descending inhibitory controls from supraspinal centers (Fitzgerald and Anand 1993). In addition, the changes in expression of both excitatory and inhibitory neurotransmitters and their receptors may contribute to decreasing sensitivity with maturation (Marti et al. 1987; Charleton and Helke 1986; Jakowec et al. 1986a,b; Gonzalez et al. 1993). Other contributing factors are the development of inhibitory interneurons and the withdrawal of the A-fiber terminals from the substantia gelatinosa (Pignatelli et al. 1989).

LONG-TERM EFFECTS OF NEONATAL EXPERIENCE

It has been well established that events experienced at a very early age may profoundly influence an animal's behavioral and physiological responses to stimuli in later life (Denenberg 1975; Hofer 1994). For example, a seemingly innocuous stimulus such as an odor cue can have a dramatic impact on adult behavior. One-day-old rat pups are capable of learning a negative association for a neutral odor that is paired with an illness-inducing chemical, so that after a single exposure, they will avoid the odor as an adult. Olfactory conditioning in young animals is not necessarily aversive; rat pups that have been exposed to a particular scent during suckling will as adults preferentially mate with an individual scented with the same odor (Fillion and Blass 1986). Nonetheless, physiological responses to early experiences have generally been studied in the context of negative events; for example, the effect of isolation treatments in neonatal rats on their subsequent response to stress has been investigated. Effects range from alterations in dopamine transmission (Sorg and Kalivas 1993) to changes in long-term potentiation (Bronzino et al. 1996).

Few experimental studies have specifically assessed the long-term effects of repetitive pain in neonates upon subsequent adult physiology and behavior (Anand et al., in press). Researchers have used several paradigms to investigate the lasting influences of both psychosocial and physical stressors in neonatal and juvenile rat pups. The focus has been on the consequences of exposing young animals to differential housing conditions, early handling, maternal isolation, and endotoxins. Pain is irrevocably associated with stress, and an examination of these studies should be helpful in illustrating the influence of early experience on adult life. In many respects, the conditions of these paradigms mirror the maternal separation, physical handling, and environmental stress experienced by the premature infant in neonatal care.

EFFECTS OF HOUSING ON RESPONSE TO STRESS

The long-term effects of differential housing of rats, i.e., housing the animals individually versus in small groups, are unclear. Research has shown that adult rats that were isolated after weaning are more fearful in open field tests and also show enhanced freezing (i.e., immobility) and more frequent urination and defecation compared with group-housed controls. Conversely, other reports indicate that open field activity is enhanced and defecation is reduced in isolated versus grouped animals (reviewed by Holson et al. 1988). The physiological data are also inconsistent; some studies found no changes in plasma corticosteroid levels, whereas others reported increased or decreased adrenocortical responses. Variations in rearing techniques, e.g., degree of isolation with regard to olfactory, visual, and auditory contact, may be responsible for these different results (Holson et al. 1988). Many experiments have studied the long-term effects of pain in neonates before weaning, when housing in isolation is not an option. If these animals are to be tested following weaning, the decision to house these animals individually or in groups could influence the outcome of the experiment. As social isolation may induce physiological and behavioral abnormalities, group housing should be considered.

EFFECTS OF POSTNATAL HANDLING ON RESPONSES TO STRESS

The long-term effects of early handling of rat pups have been extensively studied, most specifically in the context of the effect on the hypothalamic-pituitary-adrenal axis (HPA) (Meaney et al. 1991, 1993, 1996a,b). The postnatal handling of rat pups involves removing the animals from their home cages, placing them together in small containers, and returning them to their cages 15–20 minutes later (Denenberg 1975). Thus, the paradigm also involves maternal separation, albeit for a limited time. Nonetheless, this handling is not considered to represent a significant period of maternal deprivation because nursing mothers are frequently away from their pups for up to 20 minutes during the normal rearing process (Liu et al. 1997).

Early behavioral studies revealed that, as adults, rats handled postnatally for 10 or 20 days compared with unhandled controls showed a decrease in fearfulness in novel environments as manifested by decreased freezing and increased exploration (Levine et al. 1967). This response was attributed to a decrease in pituitary adrenocorticotropic hormone (ACTH) and secretion of adrenal corticosterone and a faster return to corticosterone basal levels after the stressful stimuli were terminated (Levine 1967). Numerous studies conducted by Meaney and his colleagues (reviewed in Meaney et al. 1996a) have convincingly demonstrated that early handling results in alterations in HPA activity in response to stress in adult animals. They have shown that handling increases type II glucocorticoid receptors in the frontal cortex and hippocampus and have suggested that the differences in stress-induced corticosterone result from enhanced sensitivity to glucocorticoid negative feedback (Meaney et al. 1996b). This hypothesis was confirmed by their report of an increase in hippocampal glucocorticoid receptor expression as a result of early handling. Activation of thyroid hormones appears to play a role in the changes in glucocorticoid receptor density (Meaney et al. 1987).

The role of mother–pup interactions in mediating the effects of postnatal handling has been often hypothesized. Liu et al. (1997) recently examined the behavior of mothers of handled and nonhandled pups and found that mothers of handled pups showed increased levels of licking and grooming of pups and more arch-backed nursing than did mothers of nonhandled pups. Most significantly, the authors then examined the relationship between naturally occurring differences in maternal care and responses of their offspring as adults. As adults, rats that had received more licking and grooming from their mothers showed significantly reduced plasma ACTH and corticosterone responses following 20 minutes of restraint stress; they also showed increased hippocampal glucocorticoid receptor mRNA expression. In general, the results of these studies demonstrate the plasticity of the developing HPA axis in neonates and reflect the importance of early experience in determining later responses to stress.

Early experience of pain is often more repetitive and chronic compared with the stress produced in the early handling paradigm described above. Interestingly, it appears that early handling could reduce the long-term effects of an intermittent chronic stressor. Bhatngar et al. (1995) have examined this possibility by exposing handled and nonhandled rat pups to 21 consecutive days of cold (4°C). On day 1, there was no difference in plasma ACTH responses between the handled and nonhandled animals, yet by day 22 the handled animals had lower levels than found initially. The authors suggested that the handled animals were able to adapt more easily to a repeated but intermittent stressor. Nonetheless, this adaptation effect did not generalize to a novel stressor. When the animals were subjected to 20 minutes of restraint stress, plasma ACTH responses were higher in the previously stressed but handled rats. This result suggests that the neuroendocrine system was negatively affected by chronic stress. It is not clear whether this finding would generalize to other forms of chronic stress or to novel stressors (Meaney et al. 1996a); nonetheless, it may have significant implications for our understanding of individual variations in the adult response to early pain.

Most of the research on the long-term changes to early handling has centered around changes in the HPA axis. Nonetheless, it is clear that postnatal stress may initiate changes in other neural systems including the opioid (Kehoe and Blass 1986) and mesolimbic dopamine systems (Cahib et al. 1993). The stress-induced analgesia produced in adults can also be demonstrated in neonatal rats. Exposure to a mildly stressful situation such as that produced by handling or group housing away from the mother produces a marked analgesia in rat pups, as manifested by slightly increased paw withdrawal reflexes (Kehoe and Blass 1986). Kehoe and Blass confirmed the role of opioid systems in this response when they determined that the analgesic effect was blocked by pretreatment with the opioid antagonist naltrexone. Moreover, the authors showed that the opioid mediation of separation distress is immediately reversed in the presence of an anesthetized female and significantly reduced in the presence of home bedding. Follow-up studies revealed that the opioid-mediated effect during isolation conditions was due to a release of enkephalin and beta-endorphin levels in the midbrain (Shoemaker and Kehoe 1995). These opioid-dependent changes may produce permanent effects on pain sensitivity. Pieretti et al. (1991) found that mice that were removed from the nest from days 2 to 19 and group housed for 10 minutes per day had significantly higher latencies in both tail-flick and hotplate tests when tested at 25 and 45 days of age. These effects were eliminated by naloxone pretreatment and they enhanced the analgesic effect of morphine.

Neonatal stress consisting of 20 minutes of isolation daily has also decreased the development of hippocampal oxytocin receptors in rat pups. This effect was limited to a reduction in receptor binding at day 8, and the change did not last into adulthood (Noonan et al. 1994). Unfortunately, the study did not address the possibility that the behavior of these individuals as adults might be altered. These results warrant further investigation in light of the recent finding that postnatal oxytocin injections cause increased nociceptive thresholds in male and female rats (Uvnas-Moberg et al. 1998). This study determined that when tested at day 60, rats injected with oxytocin 10 days after birth had a prolonged tail-flick latency compared with controls. The authors suggested that the changes observed in the adults may be a result of permanent changes in oxytocin receptors, although oxytocin may also have influenced the endogenous opioid system (Petersson et al. 1996).

EFFECTS OF EXTENDED MATERNAL SEPARATION ON RESPONSE TO STRESS

In general, long-term maternal separation leads to qualitatively different responses to stress than those seen as a result of early handling (Kuhn et al. 1990; Meaney et al. 1996a). They appear to involve the development of exaggerated HPA responses as well as changes in hormone and neurotransmitter release (Kuhn et al. 1990). Moreover, isolation stress enhances and prolongs long-term potentiation in the hippocampus in freely moving juvenile rats (Kehoe et al. 1995). While the relevance of this response is unclear, these findings emphasize the neuroplasticity of the developing system and suggest that the hippocampus is dramatically influenced by repeated isolation stress.

The definition of "long-term isolation" varies, both with regard to the amount of separation time per day and the number of days of separation (Ogawa et al. 1994; Kehoe et al. 1996a). Plotsky and Meaney (1993) examined the response to stress in pups that were isolated from their mothers for 0–360 minutes. They determined that pups isolated from days 2–14 for 180–360 minutes per day showed a significant increase in plasma corticosterone levels both during and after the separation. This response is the converse of that found in animals handled for short periods of time. Results of a dexamethasone suppression test in these adult animals indicated that the efficiency of glucocorticoid negative feedback was reduced, and circulating levels of corticosteroids were detected 9 hours after administration. This response was not found in handled or nonhandled control groups. Thus, it would appear that repeated periods of maternal separation result in exaggerated responses to subsequent stress. The authors point out that inadequate early maternal contact could lead to an increased vulnerability to stress and subsequent pathology in adults.

Abnormal behavioral and pharmacological responses have also been observed in adult rats isolated as neonates for as short a period as 1 hour. Kehoe and her colleagues (1998) found that 60 minutes of isolation a day from postnatal days 2 to 9 resulted in a reduction in activity in adults following restraint stress. An examination of the response to a psychostimulant also revealed that previously isolated animals demonstrated increased activity as a result of an amphetamine injection compared to nonisolated controls. These results are consistent with a similar finding of increased activity in juvenile rats following a similar amphetamine challenge (Kehoe et al. 1996b). In Kehoe's investigation, the increased behavioral response was accompanied by an elevation of dopamine levels in the ventral striatum. The origin of this exaggerated dopamine response is unknown; however, it may be linked to perturbations of the dopamine receptor systems as a result of the experimental procedure (Guisado et al. 1980). Indeed, evidence indicates that dopamine release is enhanced in rat pups at the time of isolation stress (Kehoe et al. 1996a). This early experience may contribute to sensitization in adult animals as a result of long-lasting changes in the dopaminergic mesolimbocortical pathways associated with reward (Zimmerberg and Shartrand 1992).

Investigations of the influence of periodic maternal separation on activity and dopamine levels in adult animals have not always produced consistent results. For example, Cahib et al. (1993) reported that isolated mouse pups showed increased exploration and less fearfulness in an elevated plus (+) maze and reduced responsiveness to a psychostimulant. Moreover, compared with nonhandled controls, the isolated animals showed no increase in dopamine levels in response to restraint stress. In this experiment, the amount of isolation stress was minimal; moreover, the animals were maintained at nest temperature during their stress sessions. Both factors may have contributed to the anomalous results. The issue of temperature control is essential in understanding the subsequent effects of early stress. Rat pups maintained at room temperature have significant growth delays, exhibit less activity, and as adults are more sensitive to an amphetamine challenge compared with subjects maintained at nest temperature (Zimmerberg and Shartrand 1992). Clearly, temperature-dependent effects must be considered in attempts to understand the effect of separation on the adult animal. Apparent differences in individual adult behaviors could be a result of injudicious control of temperature variables in the maternal separation paradigm.

EARLY ACTIVATION OF THE IMMUNE SYSTEM
AND RESPONSES TO STRESS

Thus far, we have emphasized the relationship between early experience and later responses to stressful situations as a result of alterations in function of the HPA axis. The effects of both early handling and maternal separation have also been described in the context of changes in reactivity of the immune system in adults. In most cases early handling enhances antibody responses (Solomon et al. 1968; Neveu et al. 1993; Laban et al. 1995), whereas extended maternal deprivation leads to a suppressed immune response (Michaut et al. 1981; Ackerman et al. 1988; von Hoersten et al. 1993). Inconsistencies found in these investigations may be due to sex or strain differences. For example, female rats that were handled and gentled showed a decreased susceptibility to autoimmune disease compared with handled males, which showed an enhanced immune response following exposure to autoantibodies (Laban et al. 1995). The implication that males and females and animals of different strains are affected differently by early experiences requires further investigation if we are to understand their behavior as adults. Failure to consider such factors can only hinder our goal of understanding the influence of experience on adult behavior.

EFFECTS OF ENDOTOXIN EXPOSURE ON RESPONSE TO STRESS

The effects of activation of the immune system during development upon the physiology and behavior of the adult animal are not well understood. In adults, the immediate response to endotoxins involves a release of cytokines (Besedovsky and del Ray 1996). Cytokines activate the HPA axis, initially stimulate the release of thyroid-stimulating hormone, growth hormone, and prolactin, suppress gonadotrophins and sex hormones, and alter brain mechanisms. Cytokines are present in the neonatal period (Lipodollva and Holan 1990; Montgomery and Dallman 1991), and their activation could cause hormonal and metabolic responses, with a potentially significant effect on the adult animal. Illness at an early age may well permanently modify the response to stress in adult animals. Del Ray et al. (1996) found that adult mice exposed to interleukin-1 as neonates showed a reduction in ACTH-like immunoreactivity following acute cold and restraint stress.

Several studies of the effects of perturbations in early life upon the development of the HPA response have also examined the effect of early illness on the adult response to environmental stimuli. Rats exposed to endotoxins as neonates exhibit marked alterations in their later response to physical and social stimuli (Shanks et al. 1995; Granger et al. 1996). Administration of *Salmonella enteritidis* to pups in doses that produced serious illness but not death stimulated an HPA response to restraint stress in adults comparable to that found after prolonged maternal separation. The animals had significantly greater ACTH and corticosterone responses than did controls, decreased negative feedback to glucocorticoids, and reduced glucocorticoid receptor density throughout the brain. Exactly how the neonatal endotoxin exposure alters the HPA response to stress is not known; the authors suggest that disruption in the expression of glucocorticoid receptors may be involved.

Investigators have also examined the influence of endotoxin exposure in neonates on later social behavior. Exposing mice selectively bred for high and low aggressiveness to *Escherichia coli* as neonates has been shown to alter their later social interactions (Granger et al. 1996). Compared with littermate controls, mice from both strains were more socially reactive, showing greater startle responses and more jumping and kicking in response to the introduction of an unfamiliar conspecific. Thus, early activation of the immune system affects later social interactions and alters adult responses to physical stress. Only the highly aggressive line of mice showed decreased mobility and a decrease in attack frequency. The authors suggest that these variations in social interactions could be a result of differential sensitivity to the endotoxin exposure as neonates.

The results of this study raise the issue of genetic susceptibility to early stress as a mediating factor in determining immune responses in later life. Recently, Shanks and Kusnecov (1998) found that restraint stress caused an enhanced immune response in one strain of inbred mice (BALB/cByJ) but not in another strain (C57BL/6J). These findings and those of Shanks et al. (1995) emphasize the need for further investigation into the interactive nature of the genetic background and the developing immune and endocrine systems in response to illness and other early life stressors.

EFFECTS OF ACUTE OR CHRONIC PAIN ON ADULT RESPONSES

The effects of neonatal pain in modifying an individual's experience as an adult have remained largely unexplored in both animals and humans, yet there is increasing evidence that the experience of pain at the peak of plasticity of the developing nervous system may result in permanent alterations in the connections within the CNS. For example, Reynolds and Fitzgerald (1995) determined that neonatal skin wounds in rat pups cause a marked hyperinnervation of the injured area that remains evident for at least 3 months after the wound has healed. Moreover, there appears to be a critical period for a maximum response; both the duration and magnitude of the neural sprouting response were maximal in adult animals that had been wounded on the day of birth. Both A- and C-fibers contribute to this response, and sprouting has been determined to be the result of unspecified neurotrophic factors (Reynolds et al. 1997). In Chapter 2 of this volume, Dickenson and Rahman cite further evidence of the dramatic influence of early pain in altering responses in adults. Perhaps most significant is their description of evidence that carrageenan inflammation induced in day 1 rat pups results in long-term expansion in the receptive field area of the neurons of adult animals. This finding demonstrates that even a rather low-intensity stimulus is sufficient to cause permanent changes in the CNS of adults. The mechanisms by which these changes are mediated have yet to be investigated.

An extensive analysis of the behavior of adult rats lends further support to the hypothesis that repetitive pain experience in neonates may result in long-term changes (Anand et al., in press). Rat pups subjected to one needle prick in each paw each day during postnatal days 0–7 showed an increase in defensive withdrawal behavior and a reluctance to explore an open field as adults in comparison with control animals that had received similar tactile stimulation. In addition, the experimental animals demonstrated a greater preference for alcohol and remembered an encounter with a conspecific 2 hours previously. The authors hypothesize that increased anxiety and hypervigilance could cause these behaviors, although the mechanisms responsible for the response are unclear. These animals showed no stress-induced changes in HPA axis responsiveness; the corticosterone and ACTH responses of experimental animals to a puff of air did not differ significantly from controls. A more severe stressor, such as that produced by restraint, could possibly discriminate between the experimental and control animals. An analysis of the neural activation in the somatosensory cortex as measured by early gene response revealed lower fos protein expression in animals that were subjected to pain rather than tactile stimulation. This seemingly anomalous result may reflect the higher levels of exploratory and escape behavior seen in the control group. The experimental animals showed responses more reflective of fear conditioning, i.e., freezing, shrieking, and autotomy (self-mutilation). Consequently, it would seem appropriate to examine the role of the amygdala and its cortical and subcortical projections to assess their possible involvement in behavioral responses to early repetitive pain.

CONCLUSIONS

To investigate the hypothesis that exposure to early pain and stress alters brain development, this chapter has focused on the effects of early

experience on the response to pain in rats. We have described the role of early handling, maternal separation, endotoxin exposure, and acute and chronic stress. Experience during the perinatal period has a dramatic impact on the expression of hormonal and immunological responses in adult rats. Recent research has confirmed that these physiological perturbations also predicate behavioral changes (Zarahia et al. 1996; Kehoe et al. 1998; Anand et al., in press).

Hebb (1949) postulated that the response to pain is a complex perceptual process influenced by both specific and nonspecific early experiences. Researchers have investigated this premise by developing models of clinical pain using newborn rat pups that involve recording pain-related behaviors at different postnatal ages. Neuronal activation from painful stimulation has been studied using various neurophysiological, neurobiological, and behavioral methods. Further research on the influence of early pain and stress on the genes regulating neuronal plasticity will help to probe the mechanisms of such long-term effects on development in the sensory cortex, thalamus, and hypothalamus. Differential effects of inflammatory pain, increasing pain intensity, and repetitive pain must also be tested. We propose that robust correlations between adult behavioral patterns, HPA responses, and the expression of specific receptor populations (opioid, serotonin, and SP) will generate mechanistic hypotheses for the neurobiological basis of behavior following neonatal pain and stress. Such data will have important implications for understanding the behavior and health-care problems of many children born prematurely who will be approaching adolescence and adulthood in the next decade.

ACKNOWLEDGMENTS

We would like to thank Patrick J. McGrath for his financial support in the production of this manuscript. Jennifer Stapleton provided invaluable assistance in locating numerous references for this review.

REFERENCES

Ackerman SH. Keller SE, Schleifer SJ, et al. Premature maternal separation and lymphocyte function. *Brain Behav Immun* 1988; 2:161–165.

Anand KJS. Neonatal stress responses to anesthesia and surgery. *Clin Perinatol* 1990; 17:207–214.

Anand KJS. Effects of perinatal pain. *Brain Res Rev,* in press.

Anand KJS, Brown MJ, Causon RC, et al. Can the human neonate mount an endocrine and metabolic response to surgery? *J Pediatr Surg* 1985; 20:41–48.

Anand KJS, Coskun V, Thrivikraman KV, Nemeroff CB, Plotsky PM. Long-term behavioral effects of repetitive pain in neonatal rat pups. *Physiol Behav,* in press.

Besedovsky HO, del Ray A. Immune-neuro-endocrine interactions: facts and hypotheses. *Endocr Rev* 1996; 17:64–102.

Bhatngar S, Mitchell JB, Betito K, et al. Effects of chronic intermittent cold stress on pituitary adrenocortical and sympathetic adrenomedullary functioning. *Physiol Behav* 1995; 57:633–639.

Blass EM, Cramer CP, Fanselow MS. The development of morphine-induced antinociception in neonatal rats: a comparison of forepaw, hindpaw, and tail retraction from a thermal stimulus. *Pharm Biochem Behav* 1993; 44:643–649.

Bronzino JD, Kehoe P, Austin-Lafrance RJ, Rushmore RJ, Kurdian J. Neonatal isolation alters LTP in freely moving juvenile rats: sex differences. *Brain Res Bull* 1996; 41:175–183.

Cahib S, Puglisi-Allegra S, D'Amato FR. Effects of postnatal stress on dopamine mesolimbic system responses to aversive experiences in adult life. *Brain Res* 1993; 604:232–239.

Catania MV, Landwehrmeyer GB, Testa CM, et al. Metabotropic glutamate receptors are differentially regulated during development. *Neuroscience* 1994; 61:481–495.

Charleton CG, Helke CJ. Ontogeny of substance-P receptors in the rat spinal cord: quantitative changes in receptor number and differential expression in specific loci. *Dev Brain Res* 1986; 29:81–91.

Chay PCW, Duffy BJ, Walker JS. Pharmacokinetic-pharmacodynamic relationships of morphine in neonates. *Clin Pharmacol Ther* 1992; 51:334–342.

Crair MC, Malenka RC. A critical period for long-term potentiation at thalamocortical synapses. *Nature* 1995; 375:325–328.

del Ray A, Furukawa H, Monge-Arditi G, et al. Alterations in the pituitary-adrenal axis of adult mice following neonatal exposure to interleukin-1. *Brain Behav Immun* 1996; 10:235–248.

Dani JW, Armstrong DM, Benowitz, LI. Mapping the development of the rat brain by GAP-43 immunocytochemistry. *Neuroscience* 1991; 40:277–287.

Denenberg VH. Effects of exposure to stressors in early life upon later behavioral and biological processes. In: Levin L (Ed). *Society, Stress, and Disease.* New York: Oxford University Press, 1975, pp 268–281.

Falcon M, Guendelman, D, Stolberg A, Frenk H, Urca G. Development of thermal nociception in rats. *Pain* 1996; 67:203–208.

Fillion T, Blass EM. Infantile experience with suckling odors determines adult sexual behavior in male rats. *Science* 1986; 231:729–731.

Fitzgerald M. Development of pain pathways and mechanisms. In: Anand KJS, McGrath PJ (Eds). *Handbook of Experimental Pharmacology: The Pharmacology of Pain.* Berlin: Springer-Verlag, 1997, pp 447–460.

Fitzgerald M, Anand KJS. The developmental neuroanatomy and neurophysiology of pain. In: Schechter N, Berde C, Yaster M (Eds). *Pain Management in Infants, Children and Adolescents.* Baltimore, MD: Williams and Williams, 1993, pp 11–32.

Fitzgerald M, Gibson S. The postnatal physiological and neurochemical development of peripheral sensory C-fibres. *Neuroscience* 1984; 13:933–944.

Fitzgerald M, Koltzenburg M. The functional development of descending inhibitory pathways in the dorsolateral funiculus of the newborn rat spinal cord. *Dev Brain Res* 1986; 24:261–270.

Fitzgerald M, Shaw A, MacIntosh N. The postnatal development of the cutaneous flexor reflex: a comparative study in premature infants and newborn rat pups. *Dev Med Child Neurol* 1988; 30:520–526.

Gonzalez DL, Fuchs JL, Droge MH. Distribution of NMDA receptor binding in developing mouse spinal cord. *Neurosci Lett* 1993; 151:134–137.

Granger DA, Hood KE, Ikeda SC, Reed CL, Block ML. Neonatal endotoxin exposure alters the development of social behavior and the hypothalamic-pituitary-adrenal axis in selectively bred mice. *Brain Behav Immun* 1996; 10:249–259.

Greeley WJ, de Bruijn NP. Changes in sufentanil pharmacokinetics within the neonatal period. *Anesth Analg* 1988; 67:86–90.

Grunau RVE, Whitfield MF, Petrie JH. Pain sensitivity and temperament in extremely low birthweight premature toddlers and preterm and full-term controls. *Pain* 1994; 58:341–346.

Grunau RVE, Whitfield MF, Petrie JH. Children's judgements about pain at age 8–10 years: Do extremely low birthweight (<1000 gm) children differ from full birth weight peers? *Pain,* in press.

Guisado E. Fernandez-Tome P, Garzon J, Del Rio J. Increased dopamine receptor binding in the striatum of rats after long-term isolation. *Eur J Pharmacol* 1980; 65:463–464.

Gunnar MR, Porter FL, Wolf CM, Rigatuso J, Larson MC. Neonatal stress reactivity: predictions to later emotional temperament. *Pediatrics* 1995; 66:1–13.

Guy ER, Abbott FV. The behavioral response to formalin in preweanling rats. *Pain* 1992; 51:81–90.

Hebb DO. *The Organization of Behavior.* New York: John Wiley and Sons, 1949.

Hofer M. Early relationships as regulators of infant physiology and behavior. *J Paediatr Suppl* 1994; 397:9–18.

Holson RA, Scallet AC, Ali SF, Sullivan P, Gough B. Adrenocortical, beta-endorphin and behavioral responses to graded stressors in differentially reared rats. *Physiol Behav* 1988; 42:125–130.

Hu D, Hu R, Berde CB. Neurologic evaluation of infant and adult rats before and after sciatic nerve blockade. *Anesthesiol* 1997; 86:957–965.

Issler H, Stephens JA. The maturation of cutaneous reflexes studied in the upper limb in man. *J Physiol* 1983; 335:643–654.

Jakowec MW, Fox AJ, Martin LJ, Kalb RG. Quantitative and qualitative changes in AMPA receptor expression during spinal cord development. *Neuroscience* 1995a; 67:893–907.

Jakowec MW, Yen L, Kalb RE. In situ hybridization analysis of AMPA receptor subunit gene expression in the developing rat spinal cord. *Neuroscience* 1995b; 67:909–920.

Johnston CC, Stevens B, Craig KD, Grunau RVE. Developmental changes in pain expression in premature, full-term, two-and four-month-old infants. *Pain* 1993; 52:201–208.

Kay G, Tarcic N, Poltyrev T, Weinstock M. Prenatal stress depresses immune function in rats. *Physiol Behav* 1998: 63:397–402.

Kehoe P, Blass EM. Opioid- mediation of separation distress in 10-day-old rats; reversal of stress with maternal stimuli. *Dev Psychobiol* 1986; 19:385–398.

Kehoe P, Hoffman JH, Austin-Lafrance RJ, Bronzino JD. Neonatal isolation enhances hippocampal dentate gyrus response to tetanization in freely moving juvenile male rats. *Exp Neurol* 1995; 136:89–97.

Kehoe P, Clash K, Skipsey K, Shoemaker WJ. Brain dopamine response in isolated 10-day-old rats: Assessment using D2 binding and dopamine turnover. *Pharm Biochem Behav* 1996a; 53:41–49.

Kehoe P, Shoemaker WJ, Triano L, Hoffman J, Arons C. Repeated isolation in the neonatal rat produces alterations in behavior and ventral striatal dopamine release in the juvenile following amphetamine challenge. *Behav Neurosci* 1996b; 110:1435–1444.

Kehoe P, Shoemaker WJ, Triano L, Callahan M, Rappolt G. Adult rats stressed as neonates show exaggerated behavioral responses to both pharmacological and environmental challenges. *Behav Neurosci* 1998; 112: 116–125.

Kim JJ, Foy MR, Thompson RF. Behavioral stress modifies hippocampal plasticity through N-methyl-D-aspartate receptor activation. *Proc Natl Acad Sci USA* 1996; 93:4750–4753.

Knudsen EI. Capacity for plasticity in the adult owl auditory system expanded by juvenile experience. *Science* 1998; 279:1531–1533.

Kolb B. *Brain Plasticity and Behavior.* New Jersey: Lawrence Erlbaum Associates, 1995.

Kuhn CM, Pauk J, Schanberg SM. Endocrine responses to mother–infant separation in developing rats. *Dev Psychobiol* 1990; 23:395–410.

Kumazawa T. Primitivism and plasticity of pain–implication of polymodal receptors. *Neurosci Res* 1998; 32:9–31.

Laban O, Dimitrijevic M, von Hoersten S, Markovic BM, Jankovic BD. Experimental allergic encephalomyelitis in adult DA rats subjected to neonatal handling or gentling. *Brain Res* 1995; 676:133–140.

Levine S. Maternal and environmental influences on the adrenocortical response to stress in weanling rats. *Science* 1967; 156:258–259.

Levine S, Haltmeyer GC, Karas G, Dennenberg VH. Physiological and behavioral effects of infantile stimulation. *Physiol Behav* 1967; 2:55–59.

Lipodollva M, Holan V. Expression of genes for interleukin-1 alpha and tumor necrosis factor-alpha in newborn mice. *Immunology* 1990; 70:136–137.

Liu D, Diorio J, Tannenbaum B, et al. Maternal care, hippocampal glucocorticoid receptors, and hypothalmaic-pituitary-adrenal responses to stress. *Science* 1997; 277:1659–1662.

Marti E, Gibson SJ, Polak JM, et al. Ontogeny of peptide and amino-containing neurons in motor, sensory, and autonomic regions of rat and human spinal cord. *J Comp Neurol* 1987; 266: 332–359.

McLaughlin PH, Tobias SW, Lang CM, et al. Opioid receptor blockade during prenatal like modifies postnatal behavioral development. *Pharmacol Biochem Behav* 1997; 58:1075–1082.

Meaney MJ, Aitken DH, Sapolsky RM. Thyroid hormones influence the development of hippocampal glucocorticoid receptors in the rat: a mechanism for the effects of postnatal handling on the development of the adrenocortical stress response. *Neuroendocrinology* 1987; 45:278–283.

Meaney MJ, Mitchell JB, Aitken DH, et al. The effects of neonatal handling on the development of the adrenocortical response to stress: implications for neuropathology and cognitive deficits in later life. *Psychoneuroendocrinology* 1991; 16:85–103.

Meaney MJ, et al. Individual differences in the hypothalamic-pituitary-adrenal stress response and the hypothalamic CRF system. *Ann N Y Acad Sci* 1993; 697:70–85.

Meaney MJ, Bhatngar S, Larocque S, et al. Early environment and the development of individual differences in the hypothalamic-pituitary-adrenal stress response. In: Pfeffer CR (Ed). *Severe Stress and Mental Disturbance in Children.* Washington, DC: American Psychiatric Press, 1996a, pp 85–127.

Meaney MJ, Diorio J, Francis D, et al. Early environmental regulation of forebrain glucocorticoid receptor gene expression: implications for adrenocortical responses to stress. *Dev Neurosci* 1996b; 18:49–72.

Michaut RJ, Dechambre RP, Doumero S. Influence of early maternal deprivation on adult humoral response in mice. *Physiol Behav* 1981; 26:189–191.

Montgomery RA, Dallman MJ. Analysis of cytokine gene expression during fetal thymic ontogeny using the polymerase chain reaction. *J Immunol* 1991; 147:554–560.

Neveu PJ, Puglisi-Allegra S, Damato FR, Cabib S. Influence of early life events on immune reactivity in adult mice. *Dev Psychobiol* 1993; 27:205–213.

Noonan LR, Caldwell JD, Li L, et al. Neonatal stress transiently alters the development of hippocampal oxytocin receptors. *Dev Brain Res* 1994; 80:115–120.

Ogawa T, Mikuni M, Kuroda Y, Muneoka K, Moria KJ, et al. Periodic maternal deprivation alters stress response in adult offspring: potentiates the negative feedback regulation of restraint stress-induced adrenocortical response and reduces the frequencies of open field-induced behaviors. *Pharmacol Biochem Behav* 1994; 49:961–967.

Petersson M, Alster P, Lundeberg T, Uvnas-Moberg K. Oxytocin increases nociceptive thresholds in a long-term perspective in female and male rats. *Physiol Behav* 1996; 212:87–90.

Pieretti S, d'Amore A, Loizzo A. Long-term changes induced by developmental handling on pain threshold: effects of morphine and naloxone. *Behav Neurosci* 1991; 105:215–218.

Pignatellli D, Ribero-da-Silva A, Coimbra A. Postnatal maturation of primary afferent terminations in the substantia gelatinosa of the rat spinal cord: an electron microscopic study. *Brain Res* 1989; 491:33–441.

Plotsky PM, Meancy MJ. Early postnatal experience alters hypothalmic corticotropin-releasing factor (CRF) mRNA, median eminence CRF content and stress-induced release in adult rats.

Mol Brain Res 1993; 18:195–200.

Poltyrev T, Keshet GI, Kay G, Weinstock M. Role of experimental conditions in determining differences in exploratory behavior of prenatally stressed rats. *Dev Psychobiol* 1996; 453–462.

Rabinowicz T, de Courten-Myers GM, Petetot JM, Xi G, de los Reyes E. Human cortex development: estimates of neuronal numbers indicate major loss late during gestation. *J Neuropathol Exp Neurol* 1996; 55:320–328.

Reynolds M, Fitzgerald M. Long term sensory hyperinnervation following neonatal skin wounds. *J Comp Neurol* 1995; 358:487–498.

Reynolds M, Alvares D, Middleton J, Fitzgeral M. Neonatally wounded skin induces NGF-independent sensory neurite outgrowth in vitro. *Dev Brain Res* 1997; 102:275–283.

Shanks N, Kusnecov AW. Differential immune reactivity to stress in BALB/cByJ and C57BL/6J mice: in vivo dependence on macrophages. *Physiol Behav* 1998; 65:95–103.

Shanks N, Larocque S, Meaney MJ. Neonatal endotoxin exposure alters the development of the hyothalamic-pituitary-adrenal axis: early illness and later responsivity to stress. *J Neurosci* 1995; 15:376–384.

Shoemaker W, Kehoe P. Effect of isolation conditions on brain regional enkephalin and beta-endorphin levels and vocalizations in 10-day-old rat pups. *Behav Neurosci* 1995; 109:117–122.

Smythe JW, McCormick CM, Meaney MJ. Median eminence corticotrophin-releasing hormone content following prenatal stress and neonatal handling. *Brain Res Bull* 1996; 40:195–199.

Solomon GF, Levine S, Kraft JK. Early experience and immunity. *Nature* 1968; 220:821–822.

Sorg BA, Kalivas PW. Effects of cocaine and footshock stress on extracellular dopamine levels in the medial prefrontal cortex. *Neuroscience* 1993; 53:695–703.

Stelzner DJ. The normal postnatal development of synaptic end-feet in the lumbosacral spinal cord and of responses in the hindlimbs of the albino rat. *Exp Neurol* 1971; 31:337–357.

Taddio A, Katz J, Ilersich AL, Koren G. Effect of neonatal circumcision on pain response during subsequent routine vaccination. *Lancet* 1997; 349:599–603.

Teng CJ, Abbott FV. The formalin test: a dose-response analysis at three development stages. *Pain* 1998; 76:337–347.

Uvnas-Moberg K, Alster P, Petersson M, et al. Postnatal oxytocin injections cause sustained weight gain and increased nociceptive thresholds in male and female rats. *Pediatr Res* 1998; 43:344–348.

von Hoersten S, Dimitrijevic M, Markovic M, Jankovic BD. Effect of early experience on behavior and immune response in the rat. *Physiol Behav* 1993; 54:931–940.

Wallace CS, Kilman VL, Withers GS, Greenough WT. Increases in dendritic length in occipital cortex after 4 days of differential housing in weanling rats. *Behav Neural Biol* 1992; 58:64–68.

Winberg J. Do neonatal pain and stress program the brain's response to future stimuli? *Acta Paediatr* 1998; 87:723–725.

Wilson DA. NMDA receptors mediate expression of one form of functional plasticity induced by olfactory deprivation. *Brain Res* 1995; 677:238–242.

Yaster M. The dose response of fentanyl in neonatal anesthesia. *Anesthesiology* 1987; 66, 433–435.

Zagon IS, Tobias SW, Hytrek SD, McLaughlin PJ. Opioid receptor blockade throughout prenatal life confers long-term insensitivity to morphine and alters mu opioid receptors. *Pharmacol Biochem Behav* 1998; 59:201–207.

Zarahia MD, Kulczycki J, Shanks N, Meaney MJ, Anisman H. The effects of early postnatal stimulation on Morris water-maze acquisition in adult mice: genetic and maternal factors. *Psychopharmacology* 1996; 128:227–239.

Zimmerberg B, Shartrand AM. Temperature-dependent effects of maternal separation on growth, activity, and amphetamine sensitivity in the rat. *Dev Psychobiol* 1992; 25:213–226.

Correspondence to: Heather M. Schellinck, Department of Psychology, Dalhousie University, Halifax, Nova Scotia, Canada, B3H 4J1. Email: heathers@is.dal.ca.

Chronic and Recurrent Pain in Children and Adolescents, Progress in Pain Research and Management, Vol. 13, edited by Patrick J. McGrath and G. Allen Finley, IASP Press, Seattle, © 1999.

4

Effects of Early Pain Experience: The Human Literature

Anna Taddio

Departments of Pharmacy and Paediatrics, Division of Clinical Pharmacology and Toxicology, The Hospital for Sick Children, and Faculty of Pharmacy, University of Toronto, Toronto, Ontario, Canada

Studies of the development of pain pathways suggest that the functional capability for nociception is present in neonates (see reviews by Anand et al. 1989; Fitzgerald 1993). Studies in the neurophysiology of pain have demonstrated the remarkable plasticity of dorsal horn neurons. Acute pain, if untreated, contributes to an increase in the excitability of the central nervous system (CNS), which prolongs pain and creates a memory of pain. Animal studies have demonstrated that early experience with pain may alter the development of pain pathways and integration of pain signals (see Chapter 3). These findings have raised concerns about the possible effects of untreated pain in infancy and have led to increasing research in this area.

Scientists studying the long-term effects of pain in young infants have followed two avenues of clinical research. The first has been to investigate the effect of a single surgical procedure on clinical outcomes and future pain behavior. The second has been to study the effect of prolonged hospitalization (which is associated with repeated painful procedures) on both clinical outcomes (mainly neurological development) and pain behavior. This chapter will include a summary of the findings of these studies and suggest directions for future studies.

EFFECTS OF SURGERY

Studies of adults undergoing surgery have demonstrated the profound pathophysiological effects of pain. Surgical trauma triggers the release of stress hormones (e.g., catecholamines, glucagon, corticosteroids, and growth hormone), which stimulate the breakdown of protein, fat, and carbohydrate stores. If sufficiently severe or prolonged, the stress response may cause complications such as cardiac dysrhythmia, pulmonary insufficiency, impaired immune function, or thromboembolism that may lead to increased mortality (Anand et al. 1989).

Anand and colleagues have investigated the effects of anesthesia in preterm and full-term neonates undergoing different surgical procedures. They reported statistically significant reductions in stress responses and improvements in postoperative recovery in three separate randomized controlled trials (Anand et al. 1987, 1988, 1992). In a landmark study (1992), they demonstrated that clinical outcome was influenced by anesthesia regimen. Forty-five full-term neonates undergoing cardiac surgery to repair complex congenital cardiac defects were randomized either to intraoperative anesthesia with high-dose sufentanil and postoperative analgesia with continuous opioid infusions, or to halothane and morphine followed by intermittent morphine and diazepam. All infants underwent cardiopulmonary bypass and hypothermic circulatory arrest during surgery. Infants given deep anesthesia (i.e., sufentanil) had a significantly reduced stress response. In addition, the incidence of sepsis ($P = 0.03$), disseminated intravascular coagulation ($P = 0.03$), and persistent metabolic acidosis ($P < 0.01$) was lower in the infants in the deep anesthesia group compared to the other group. No postoperative deaths occurred among the 30 infants in the deep anesthesia group, compared to 4 of the 15 infants in the other group ($P < 0.01$). Neonates who survived postoperatively had less extreme hormonal and metabolic changes than those who died. This was the first study to demonstrate the vulnerability of neonates to surgically induced stress and pain and to indicate that inadequate anesthesia in neonates could be a direct cause of death.

Pain from a single early physical insult may also have long-term effects on infant behavior. Richards et al. (1976) proposed that male neonatal circumcision could have long-term behavioral consequences. They cited studies demonstrating changes in infant sleeping patterns, fussiness, crying, and arousal level during the hours immediately after the procedure as evidence of short-term adverse effects of circumcision. They also hypothesized that circumcision may contribute to the gender differences observed in studies of taste (although no mechanism was proposed) and maternal handling of infants that were conducted in countries where boys are routinely circumcised. These studies, however, provide only indirect evidence for the long-term effects of circumcision, and the authors recommended further research.

In a randomized controlled trial of EMLA cream (eutectic mixture of local anesthetics; lidocaine-prilocaine 5%, Astra Pharmaceutical Products,

Inc.) for pain management during routine 4- and 6-month immunizations, we observed that pain scores were higher in boys (Taddio et al. 1994). We hypothesized that their exaggerated pain responses were related to the acute pain they had experienced during circumcision. We performed a post hoc analysis to compare the pain responses of circumcised and uncircumcised male infants who had received either diphtheria-pertussis-tetanus (DPT) alone ($n = 42$) or DPT followed by *Haemophilus influenzae* type b conjugate (HIB) ($n = 18$). During DPT, visual analogue scale (VAS) pain scores were higher in the circumcised group than the uncircumcised group (4.0 vs. 2.6 cm, $P = 0.03$). During HIB inoculation, circumcised infants had higher behavioral pain scores (8 vs. 6, $P = 0.01$) and cried longer (53 vs. 19 seconds, $P = 0.02$) (Taddio et al. 1995).

Because of the retrospective nature of our analysis and the small sample size, we could not make any definite conclusions. We therefore set out to prospectively evaluate whether neonatal circumcision affects infant pain response to routine vaccination 4–6 months after surgery. We also investigated whether vaccination response could be attenuated by pretreatment of neonatal circumcision pain with EMLA. We studied three groups of male infants (total sample size = 87): uncircumcised infants, and infants who had been randomly assigned EMLA or placebo in a previous clinical trial to assess the efficacy of EMLA cream as pretreatment for pain during neonatal circumcision (Taddio et al. 1997b). Immunization was performed at each infant's own physician's clinic (total number of participating clinics = 64). Boys circumcised with placebo were found to have significantly ($P < 0.05$) increased pain scores compared to uncircumcised boys, as measured by facial action (136.9% vs. 77.5%), proportion of time crying (53.8% vs. 24.7%), and VAS scores (5.1 vs. 3.1 cm). Among the circumcised group, VAS scores were significantly higher in infants circumcised with placebo than in those circumcised with EMLA (5.1 vs. 3.3 cm; $P < 0.05$). All outcome measures showed a significant linear trend of increasing pain scores, from uncircumcised infants to those circumcised with EMLA to those circumcised with placebo (Taddio et al. 1997a). We postulated that circumcision may induce long-lasting changes in infant pain behavior because of alterations in the infant's central neural processing of painful stimuli. The involvement of the CNS is supported by the fact that the changes were observed months after the surgery, when the site would have healed, and that the site of vaccination differed from the site of surgery. The specific mechanisms by which long-lasting central neuronal changes occur are not well elucidated, but previous studies have demonstrated that the N-methyl-D-aspartic acid (NMDA) receptor ion-channel complex, excitatory amino acids (glutamate), and C-fiber neuropeptides (substance P) are involved (Woolf and Thompson

1991; Coderre et al. 1993).

EMLA cream provided only a 50% reduction in pain response during circumcision (Taddio et al. 1997b); thus, even infants treated with EMLA experienced some pain during surgery. We speculate that EMLA may not have sufficiently blocked afferent input during the circumcision and the days that followed to prevent central sensitization. Several recent studies have demonstrated improved analgesia when using combinations of interventions such as EMLA combined with dorsal penile nerve block (Serour et al. 1998) or sucrose (Mohan et al. 1998). Combinations of analgesics are probably more effective in preventing long-term changes.

The data suggest that the pain of circumcision is *remembered* by infants, that is, there is a physiological (and implicit) memory of the event. Our conclusions are limited by issues related to study design. For instance, infants were only partially randomized to the three study groups (i.e., circumcised infants were randomized to pretreatment with EMLA or placebo). It is possible that an unidentified variable may account for the correlation between pain response and circumcision status. Differences between circumcised and uncircumcised infants in their experiences with pain outside the bounds of this study were ruled out as a confounding variable. Moreover, infant factors such as age, weight, temperament, ingestion of acetaminophen, time of last feeding, and time of last sleep before vaccination did not correlate significantly with pain response.

EFFECTS OF PROLONGED HOSPITALIZATION

PHYSIOLOGICAL CHANGES IN PAIN BEHAVIOR

Studies have investigated the development and responsiveness of the neonatal flexion reflex in hospitalized preterm neonates. The flexion reflex consists of the withdrawal of a limb from a painful stimulus. It is believed to be a sensitive index of nociceptive function in neonates (Fitzgerald et al. 1989). In one study, 103 neonates whose postconceptional age was 27.5–39.5 weeks were observed following application of graded von Frey hairs to the lateral plantar surface of the foot (Fitzgerald et al. 1988). Infants of younger postconceptional age had lower thresholds than did older infants, and demonstrated an increase in the reflex response (i.e., hypersensitivity) with repeated stimulation. This behavior was visible until a postconceptional age of 32 weeks, when a pattern of habituation began to appear (i.e., no response) (Fitzgerald et al. 1988). In another study, Andrews and Fitzgerald (1994) observed the flexion reflex responses of 50 infants (postconceptional age 23–43 weeks), and reported similar results. Pain threshold increased with increasing postconceptional age and culminated at 35 weeks. Repeated stimulation resulted in decreasing thresholds for infants at up to 35 weeks postconceptional age.

In a landmark study, Fitzgerald and colleagues (1989) investigated the effect of repeated heel lancing (a procedure commonly used to draw blood samples from infants) on the threshold for the flexion response in preterm infants. Seventeen premature neonates (27–32 weeks postmenstrual age) who were scheduled to receive medically indicated heel lances were assigned to three groups: those who received no analgesia or placebo ($n = 4$), those given a placebo ($n = 6$), and those treated with EMLA ($n = 7$). A double-blind design was used in the latter two groups. For the purposes of the study, heel lances (usually performed every 4 hours or at multiples of 4 hours) were restricted to one foot. For infants in the EMLA- and placebo-treated groups, the study cream was applied every 4 hours, whether heel lancing was performed or not. Flexor reflex thresholds were evaluated for the lanced foot as well as the unlanced foot over a 1–4-week period. For babies treated with placebo or nothing, the threshold for the flexor reflex in the lanced foot was less than half the value of the unlanced foot. The mean threshold for the reflex in the lanced foot of the EMLA-treated group was not significantly different from the control threshold from the unlanced foot, but was significantly higher than that of the lanced foot of the placebo or no-analgesia groups. Thus, repeated heel lancing led to hypersensitivity (or tenderness) in the injured heel, but this could be prevented by repeated application of EMLA prior to heel lancing. This was the first study to demonstrate a chronic pain response (i.e., peripheral hypersensitivity) in neonates following peripheral tissue injury and inflammation. The changes observed in the flexor reflex response may be attributable to developmental changes in the neonate in both peripheral and central nociceptive pathways. The plasticity in flexion reflex threshold may result from cutaneous hyperinnervation of the injured tissue (Reynolds et al. 1995); hypersensitivity may also result from changes in the excitability of the central spinal cord neurons. Moreover, the interneurons in the dorsal horn of the spinal cord and descending inhibitory pathways are thought to develop in late gestation in the human fetus; they inhibit inputs to dorsal horn neurons, thus reducing the size of receptive fields (Fitzgerald 1993).

Johnston and Stevens (1996) tested the hypothesis that prolonged hospitalization, which is associated with repeated painful interventions, could affect infant pain behavior. In a cross-sectional study, they compared the responses to heel lancing of two groups of infants of the same postconceptual age: 53 newborn infants of 32 weeks gestation and 36 infants of 28 weeks gestation delivered 4 weeks earlier. It appears that the data were analyzed post hoc from infants recruited for other studies. The two groups of infants differed significantly in their responses to heel lancing. The earlier-born infants showed significantly less behavioral activity (i.e., brow bulge, eyes squeezed shut) but greater physiological changes (lower oxygen saturation values, higher heart rates) during the procedure than did later-born infants. The factors that significantly ($P < 0.05$) affected behavioral response were the number of painful procedures and Apgar score (a numerical expression of the infant's condition) at delivery. For physiological responses, gestational age at delivery and birth weight were significant predictors. The investigators concluded that infants born more prematurely had greater behavioral and physiological "immaturity," due to past painful experiences and birth factors, respectively. Future studies should evaluate whether the magnitude of the differences in response increases as the age difference increases and whether consistent administration of analgesia prevents these changes.

A previous study reported the developmental changes in response to heel lancing for the same earlier-born infant group (Johnston et al. 1996). Increases in facial action were observed over an 8-week follow-up period. The study did not measure changes in heart rate or oxygen desaturation. The frequency of invasive procedures was not significantly related to pain response (Johnston et al. 1996).

Although Johnston and Stevens (1996) suggested that previous pain experience could affect infant pain behavior later on, they could draw no definite conclusions due to the observational nature of their study. Further research will be necessary to discern differences due to postnatal adaptation.

CONDITIONED ANXIETY AFTER REPEATED PAIN

Children rapidly develop conditioned anxiety responses to painful procedures and associated objects (Katz et al. 1980; Milgrom et al. 1995; Berggren et al. 1997). In addition, most children do not become used to repeated procedures over time (Katz et al. 1980; Fearon et al. 1996), although their anxiety can increase. Level of fear influences pain experience during a painful event (Broome 1986; McGrath and de Veber 1986; Broome et al. 1990). In children, there is also a significant relationship between coping behaviors and pain perceptions during medical procedures (Kuttner 1989; Broome et al. 1990). Coping behavior may serve as a "gating" mechanism to decrease pain (Hester 1979). In neonates and young infants, rocking, patting, and offering a pacifier for the infant to suck have been used as strategies to decrease pain (Kuttner 1989).

Anticipatory fear has been reported in infants, and researchers believe that some type of memory for prior stimuli must be present (Loeser 1990). The age at which apprehensive behavior develops is not well studied. Some researchers suggest that this behavior begins after the first 6–12 months of life (Levy 1960; Craig et al. 1984, 1988; Taddio et al. 1994, 1997a); however, these studies have not typically included infants that were hospitalized and subjected to repeated painful procedures in the first weeks of life.

Derrickson et al. (1993) investigated the effects of using a conditioning stimulus to signal painful medical procedures versus "safe" periods on the affective behavior of a 9-month-old prematurely delivered infant. They observed that when a visual and auditory stimulus was consistently used to signal an impending painful event, the infant displayed more positive behaviors (e.g., smiling) during nonpainful events (e.g., bathing, caregiver proximity).

Anecdotal reports of conditioning have also been published. In a letter to the editor, Langland and Langland (1988) spoke of "an aversion to human contacts" in premature infants due to the association between human contact and pain. They cited their own premature infant as an example. Brereton (1991) similarly described crying *before* intravenous cannulation in postsurgical neonates aged 2–3 weeks who had learned the steps involved in the procedure. McGrath and Craig (1989) referred to "breathholding" by hospitalized neonates subjected to repeated aversive procedures when approached by any person.

Conditioning may play a role in the altered pain behavior of hospitalized premature infants over time. It is possible also that interventions intended for repeated use to soothe infants and decrease pain response (such as pacifiers and sucrose solutions) may lose their effect over time if associated with aversive stimuli. Moreover, physiological instability associated with conditioning may increase the vulnerability of infants to adverse events. The effects of conditioning clearly warrant further study.

CLINICAL AND NEUROBEHAVIORAL OUTCOMES

Many studies have documented long-term deficits in cognitive and psychomotor skills for children born prematurely (cited in Horwood et al. 1998). Significant predictors of outcome include birth weight and neonatal complications such as cerebral ultrasonographic abnormalities (intraventricular hemorrhage, periventricular leukomalacia), septicemia, apnea of prematurity, chronic lung disease, and necrotizing enterocolitis (Taylor et al. 1998). Some of the long-term adverse sequelae of preterm birth may be at least partially explained by the aversive postnatal environment.

The frequency of invasive procedures in a neonatal intensive care unit is very high. A recent study of 54 neonates (gestational ages 23–41 weeks, birth weight 0.56–4.42 kg) recorded a total of 3283 procedures (Barker and Rutter 1995). Heel lancing was the most prevalent procedure (56%), followed by endotracheal suctioning (26%) and intravenous cannula insertion (8%). Seventy-four percent of the procedures were performed in infants of less than 31 weeks' gestation. One female infant (gestational age 23 weeks, birth weight 0.56 kg) experienced 488 procedures.

The same physiological responses that occur during painful procedures (e.g., variations in blood pressure, heart rate, intracranial pressure, and hypoxemia) are important predictors of medical complications such as intraventricular hemorrhage (Abdel-Rahman and Rosenberg 1994). Several studies have been conducted to determine the effects of cumulative stress and pain associated with prolonged hospitalization on infant outcomes. The results have demonstrated that infants who received care aimed at minimizing pain and stress had significantly better clinical and neurobehavioral outcomes than infants who received standard care.

Several studies have assessed the effects of developmental care, a specific care-giving approach for hospitalized preterm infants that aims to decrease stress and pain (Als et al. 1986, 1994; Becker et al. 1991, 1993; Mouradian and Als 1994; Buehler et al. 1995; Fleisher et al. 1995; Stevens et al. 1996; Ariagno et al. 1997; Westrup et al. 1997). Developmental care is an individualized approach based on formal observation and evaluation of infant behaviors before, during, and after various care-giving procedures. Infant behaviors are conceptualized as "stress" or "regulatory" and are interpreted as infant "vulnerabilities" or "strengths," respectively. A care plan is designed and implemented to alter the physical environment and care-giving procedures in order to avoid stress, promote infant stability and competence in self-regulation, and better coincide with infant maturity and natural sleep and wake cycles. Formal observations are repeated at predetermined intervals, and care plans are altered accordingly. Developmental care may include the following techniques: optimal positioning of the infant (e.g., prone or on one side, using supports as necessary), scheduling sleep and feeding to be in synchrony with the infant's sleep and wake cycles, manipulations (e.g., touching and the reduction of unnecessary procedures), and aids to self-regulation (e.g., non-nutritive sucking) (Als et al. 1986).

Studies of developmental care were reviewed and are summarized in Table I. Most trials used a phase-lag (i.e., before and after) study design. The first study, by Als et al. (1986), showed that infants who received individualized care plans with minimization of inappropriate sensory input had a reduction in the number of days of supplemental oxygen and ventilation and in the number of days before bottle-feeding. Neurodevelopmental outcome, as measured by blinded testers at up to 9 months postconceptional age using the Bayley Scales of Infant Development, was significantly better in the experimental group. Several other small studies of similar design also reported clinical benefits with this approach (Becker et al. 1991, 1993; Stevens et al. 1996, Westrup et al. 1997). In a retrospective before and after study, Mouradian and Als (1994) demonstrated that infants who received developmental care had improved behavioral and specific motor system functioning.

The effectiveness of developmental care has also been evaluated in randomized controlled trials. Als et al. (1994) observed the most impressive results, reporting fewer days to bottle feeding (59 vs. 104 days, $P = 0.05$), fewer days of supplemental oxygen (57 vs. 139 days, $P = 0.05$), and fewer days in hospital (87 vs. 151 days, $P = 0.04$) for infants randomized to developmental care compared to a control group. The developmental care group had fewer medical complications such as severe bronchopulmonary dysplasia and intraventricular hemorrhage. Neurodevelopmental outcome at 9 months was significantly improved in the study group: the Mental Developmental Index and Psychomotor Developmental Index scores of the Bayley Scales of Infant Development were 118 vs. 94, and 101 vs. 84, respectively (Als et al. 1994). Buehler et al. (1995) and Fleisher et al. (1995) found no differences in medical outcomes, although both groups demonstrated improved developmental outcomes during follow-up. Ariagno and colleagues (1997) found no differences in either sleep parameters (determined at 36 weeks and 3 months) or neurological outcome (assessed at 24 months) in infants randomized to developmental care or a control group. These results were criticized by Als (1998), who suggested that the negative findings may be at least partially due to a biased subsample available for follow-up.

Als (1998) reported preliminary findings from a multicenter randomized controlled trial of developmental care that included 94 infants born at less than 28 weeks gestation. Significantly better weight gain, growth parameters, and developmental outcome were observed in the developmental care group compared to the control group; in addition, the developmental care group had a reduction in hospitalization stay and cost (data and statistical significance not reported).

Although the concept of developmental care has increased awareness of infant pain and stress, the benefits of this approach are uncertain due to limitations in study designs (Garland 1995; Lacy 1995; Ohlsson 1995; Saigal 1995). For instance, phase-lag study designs do not allow us to discern differences caused by the intervention or changes that occur over time. Lack of blinding may also contribute to differences between groups due to caregiver bias. Studies of developmental care have typically used narrow

Table I
Summary of studies of developmental care

Reference	Study Design	Sample Size	GA (wk)	BW (g)	Outcome Measures	Significant Findings
Als 1998	M, RCT	94	<28	NR	NR	Weight gain, growth parameters, hospital stay/cost, developmental outcome, parental distress/depression
Als et al. 1994	RCT	20 DC; 18 CTR	27.1 vs. 26.5	872 vs. 862	Growth parameters (weight gain, head circumference, height), oxygen days, ventilator days, gavage feeding, hospital days/cost, age at discharge, morbidity (IVH, pneumothorax, BPD, ROP), neurodevelopment	Oral feeding, oxygen days, BPD, IVH, hospital days, age at discharge, hospital charges, 3 out of 6 APIB system scores, BMPDI
Buehler et al. 1995	RCT	12 DC; 12 CTR	32.2 vs. 32.1	1732 vs. 1707	Weight gain, oxygen days, pulmonary score (MDPI), gavage feeding, morbidity (AOP, ROP, IVH, NEC, RDS), hospital days, age at discharge, behavioral outcome (APIB, Prechtl), EEG	4 out of 6 APIB system scores, Prechtl, EEG
Fleisher et al. 1995	RCT	17 DC; 18 CTR	26.5 vs. 26.1	893 vs. 815	Ventilator days, gavage feeding, hospital days/cost, age at discharge, morbidity score (NMI), APIB	Ventilator days, gavage feeding, hospital stay >42 wk PCA, 4 out of 6 APIB system scores
Ariagno et al. 1997*	RCT	14 DC; 14 CTR	26.4 vs. 26.1	884 vs. 812	Sleep developmental measures, neurodevelopment	

Study	Design	N	GA	BW	Variables measured	APIB / outcome variables
Als et al. 1986	P, B&A	8 DC; 8 CTR	26.6 vs. 26.3	879 vs. 831	Growth parameters (height, weight, head circumference), morbidity (IVH, PDA, RDS, pneumothorax, BPD), gavage feeding, oxygen days, ventilator days, hospital days, neurodevelopment	Ventilator days, oxygen days, oral feeding, BMPDI, 2 out of 6 APIB system scores, behavior regulation
Becker et al. 1991, 1993	P, B&A	24 DC; 21 CTR	29 vs. 28.4	1209 vs. 1199	Morbidity score (NMS), IVH, respiratory status, weight gain, gavage feeding, hospital days, NBAS, motor activity, sleep/wake, O_2 saturation	Morbidity score, hospital days, ventilator days, gavage feeding, O_2 saturation, NBAS score
Stevens et al. 1996; Petryshen et al. 1997	P, B&A	63 DC; 61 CTR	28.6 vs. 28.4	1140 vs. 1078	Oxygen days, ventilator days, weight, head circumference, hospital days, hospital costs	Physiological stability score, head circumference
Westrup et al. 1997	P, B&A	21 DC; 21 CTR	28.6 vs. 28.5	1095 vs. 1116	Ventilator days, oxygen days, ventilation requirements, mortality, morbidity (IVH, NEC, BPD, ROP), weight gain, gavage feeding, age at discharge	Age at discharge
Mouradion et al. 1994	R, B&A	20 DC; 20 CTR		1460 vs. 1550	APIB	Subset of variables of APIB

Abbreviations: AOP = apnea of prematurity; APIB = Assessment of Preterm Infants' Behavior; B&A = before and after study using different patients; BMPDI = Bayley Mental and Psychomotor Developmental Index; BPD = bronchopulmonary dysplasia; BW = birth weight; CTR = controls; DC = developmental care; GA = gestational age; IVH = intraventricular hemorrhage; M = multicenter; MDPI = mean daily pulmonary index; NBAS = Neonatal Behavioral Assessment Scale; NEC = necrotizing enterocolitis; NMI = Neonatal Medical Index; NMS = neonatal morbidity scale; NR = not reported; P = prospective; PCA = post-conceptional age; PDA = patent ductus arteriosus; R = retrospective; RCT = randomized controlled trial; RDS = respiratory distress syndrome; ROP = retinopathy of prematurity.
*Follow-up study of patients who participated in Fleischer et al.'s (1995) study.

inclusion/exclusion criteria, which prevents extrapolation of results to all preterm neonates. In addition, most studies predate the widespread use of pharmacological interventions such as antenatal steroids and postnatal surfactant, which may significantly reduce infants' ventilatory requirements and enhance their well-being. All the studies reviewed utilized fairly small sample sizes, and although no significant demographic differences between treatment groups were reported at study entry, entry characteristics consistently favored the intervention groups. Moreover, differences in outcomes between treatment groups cannot be attributed specifically to pain.

CHILDHOOD BEHAVIORS

Another avenue of research has focused on the effect on childhood behaviors of prolonged hospitalization in a neonatal intensive care unit. One study prospectively examined the differences in pain-related behavior between children at 4.5 years of age who had a normal infancy and those who experienced prolonged neonatal intensive care (Grunau et al. 1994a). The former group included infants of extremely low birth weight (ELBW; <1000 g) who were being monitored by the hospital neonatal follow-up program. The full-term infants were recruited from community health centers. Seventy-two children participated (36 per group). The ELBW group had higher somatic complaints of unknown origin than did full-term children ($P = 0.008$). Familial factors were significantly associated with somatization. The number of weeks in a neonatal intensive care unit was a significant predictor of somatization scores. In another prospective study investigating long-term behavioral sequelae of prematurity, Schothorst and van Engeland (1996) compared 177 children born prematurely (<1500 g) and free of serious physical or mental handicaps with 276 control children obtained from the general population. Preterm children had more learning and social difficulties, and preterm girls had a higher rate of somatic complaints. In both studies, somatization data were obtained from the parents and may have been biased.

Another prospective study evaluated parents' ratings of pain sensitivity in their 18-month-old infants (Grunau et al. 1994b). Infants were divided into four groups according to birth weight: 480–800 g ($n = 49$), 801–1000 g ($n = 75$), 1500–2499 g ($n = 42$), and >2500 g ($n = 29$). Both groups of ELBW infants were rated by their parents to be significantly less reactive to everyday pain compared to infants in the other groups. Temperament was also significantly associated with pain sensitivity ratings, except in the lowest birth weight category. Parenting style, on the other hand, was not related to pain sensitivity. The investigators speculated that pain behavior may be related to prior painful experiences. These conclusions are limited by the observational nature of the study, in that the observed differences may be due to factors that were not measured. Also, the researchers did not measure pain behavior but relied on parental ratings of the infants' pain sensitivity; it is not clear how sensitivity ratings correlate with actual pain intensity in infants.

A recent study evaluated the association between 8- to 10-year-old children's prior nociceptive experiences and their interpretations of pain-producing situations (Grunau et al. 1998). Two groups of children were asked to judge the pain intensity and affect depicted by pictures of medical and recreational situations, scenes of daily living, and psychosocial situations. One group consisted of children born prematurely ($n = 47$, mean birth weight 808 g), and the other of children born full-term ($n = 37$, mean birth weight 3487 g). There were no differences between groups in "overall" perception of pain. However, the prematurely born children rated the intensity of medical pain significantly higher than psychosocial pain ($P = 0.004$), whereas the full-term group found no difference in pain intensity between the two settings. For the ELBW infants, the number of days spent in the neonatal intensive care unit was significantly correlated with pain affect ratings for recreational ($r = 0.3$, $P < 0.04$) and daily living settings ($r = 0.37$, $P < 0.01$). Unlike the previous study by the same group, somatization (measured by the Personality Inventory for Children) did not differ between groups.

Together, these data suggest that prolonged hospitalization may be associated with differences in childhood behaviors. It has not been determined, however, whether these changes are specific to pain. Hospitalized infants experience not only repeated painful procedures, but medical complications associated with preterm delivery and hospitalization, changes in sleep patterns and nutrient intake, and altered family and environmental conditions. All of these factors may be important contributors to the observed results.

CLINICAL AND BEHAVIORAL IMPORTANCE OF EARLY PAIN AND RECOMMENDATIONS FOR FUTURE STUDIES

The cumulative evidence from studies on the long-term consequences of neonatal pain suggests that untreated infant pain can lead to alterations in clinical outcomes and pain behaviors. This evidence runs counter to the myth that untreated pain in infancy has no long-lasting consequences. Based on the data, it is clear that emphasis must be placed on preventing pain in infants, preventing preterm delivery where possible, and avoiding any un-necessary painful procedures (e.g., circumcision). If painful procedures are necessary, the least painful method should be chosen. For example, veni-puncture caused less pain than did heel lancing in full-term infants (Shah et al. 1997; Larsson et al. 1998) and should be the preferred method of blood sampling for this population. Other strategies for reducing pain include us-ing non-invasive monitoring devices, clustering painful procedures, obtain-ing permanent central vessel access (for infants who require repeated vascu-lar access), using skilled personnel to perform invasive procedures, and employing general comfort measures.

Analgesics should be administered to minimize pain. Surgical pain should be managed with general and regional anesthetic techniques using opioids and local anesthetics. Local anesthetics may be infiltrated superficially for painful cutaneous procedures. Procedural pain should be treated with opio-ids, local anesthetics, or sucrose solutions. For more specific recommenda-tions, see reviews by Kart et al. (1997), Stevens et al. (1997), Taddio et al. (1998).

A much-needed area of research is to determine the safety and efficacy of consistent analgesia with opioids and propacetamol (a precursor of ac-etaminophen, available in an injectable formulation) during intensive care. Data from randomized controlled trials demonstrate that opioids blunt infant stress and pain responses during ventilation and routine medical procedures (Pokela 1994; Orsini et al. 1996; Anand et al. 1998). However, the incidence of adverse clinical outcomes such as intraventricular hemorrhage or other medical complications of prematurity have not been proven to be decreased by opioid administration (Quinn et al. 1992, 1993; Orsini et al. 1996, Anand et al. 1998). It is important to note the limitations of infant analgesia studies such as these. In general, their small sample sizes limit their power to detect statistically significant differences, and analgesics may have been adminis-tered after the "critical" period when hemorrhage is most likely and only for brief periods of time.

Only one study has demonstrated improved neurological outcome in ventilated premature neonates treated with opioid infusions (Anand et al. 1998). Sixty-seven prematurely born infants randomized to morphine, midazolam, or dextrose infusions in the neonatal period were examined for neurological and other clinical outcomes. Satisfactory neurological outcome was defined as survival beyond 28 days of age, absence of severe intraven-tricular hemorrhage, and absence of periventricular leukomalacia. The fre-quency of satisfactory neurological outcome differed significantly among groups and was 96%, 68%, and 76% for the morphine, midazolam, and dex-trose groups, respectively ($P = 0.03$). Secondary clinical outcomes, however, including number of days of ventilation, incidence of pneumothorax, duration of hospital stay, weight gain, and neurobehavioral assessment scores (at 36 weeks gestation) did not differ among the groups. The infants randomized to the dextrose and midazolam groups were on average (although not statistically significantly) younger, weighed less, were sicker (as defined by the Clinical Risk Index for Babies, or CRIB score), and had a lower ratio of female to male infants compared to the morphine group. All of these trends favor a worse outcome.

There are concerns that opioids may have detrimental effects on ventilation requirements, on feeding, and on the developing brain. Recent research has begun to address these issues. One study investigated the neurological outcomes of 95 5–6-year-old prematurely born children who had been randomly allocated to morphine or nonmorphine treatment in the neonatal period; the results showed no significant differences in neurological and behavioral outcome between groups (MacGregor et al. 1998).

In summarizing the evidence for the long-term effects of pain in infants we have reviewed investigations of both the direct and indirect (or inferred) effects of pain. However, we know little about the actual experience of pain in infants or about developmental changes due to pain, so this chapter may have overlooked studies where the investigators did not attribute observed effects at least in part to pain. Nevertheless, the cumulative data suggest that pain may have long-lasting effects on infants and therefore should be prevented.

REFERENCES

Abdel-Rahman AM, Rosenberg AA. Prevention of intraventricular hemorrhage in the premature infant. *Clin Perinatol* 1994; 21(3):505–521.

Als H. Developmental care in the newborn intensive care unit. *Curr Opin Pediatr* 1998; 10:138–142.

Als H, Lawhon G, Duffy FH, et al. Individualized developmental care for the very low-birth-weight preterm infant. *JAMA* 1994; 272:853–858.

Als H, Lawhon G, Brown E, et al. Individualized behavioral and environmental care for the very low birth weight preterm infant at high risk for bronchopulmonary dysplasia: neonatal intensive care unit and developmental outcome. *Pediatrics* 1986; 78:1123–1132.

Anand KJS, Sippell WG, Aynsley-Green A. Randomised trial of fentanyl anaesthesia in preterm babies undergoing surgery: effects on the stress response. *Lancet* 1987; 1:243–248.

Anand KJS, Sippell WG, Schofield NM, Aynsley-Green A. Does halothane anaesthesia decrease the metabolic and endocrine stress responses of newborn infants undergoing operation? *BMJ* 1988; 296:668–672.

Anand KJS, Phil D, Carr DB. The neuroanatomy, neurophysiology, and neurochemistry of pain, stress, and analgesia in newborns and children. *Pediatr Clin North Am* 1989; 36:795–822.

Anand KJS, Phil D, Hickey PR. Halothane-morphine compared with high-dose sufentanil for anesthesia and postoperative analgesia in neonatal cardiac surgery. *N Engl J Med* 1992;

326:1–9.

Anand KJS, McIntosh N, Lagercrantz H, et al. Analgesia and sedation in preterm neonates who require ventilatory support: results from the N.O.P.A.I.N. trial. *Arch Pediatr Adolesc Med* 1999; 153:331–338.

Andrews K, Fitzgerald M. The cutaneous withdrawal reflex in human neonates: sensitization, receptive fields, and the effects of contralateral stimulation. *Pain* 1994; 56:95–101.

Ariagno RL, Thoman EB, Boeddiker MA, et al. Developmental care does not alter sleep and development of premature infants. *Pediatrics* 1997; 100(6):e9.

Barker DP, Rutter N. Exposure to invasive procedures in neonatal intensive care unit admissions. *Arch Dis Child* 1995; 72:F47–F48.

Becker PT, Grunwald PC, Moorman J, Stuhr S. Outcomes of developmentally supportive nursing care for very low birth weight infants. *Nurs Res* 1991; 40:150–155.

Becker PT, Grunwald PC, Moorman J, Stuhr S. Effects of developmental care on behavioral organization in very-low-birth-weight infants. *Nurs Res* 1993; 42:214–220.

Berggren BM, Bogdanov O, Hakeberg M. Dental anxiety among adolescents in St. Petersburg Russia. *Eur J Oral Sci* 1997; 105(2):117–122.

Brereton RJ. Letter to editor. *J Pediatr Surg* 1991; 26(10):1262.

Broome ME. The relationship between children's fears and behavior during a painful event. *Children's Health Care* 1986; 14(3):142–145.

Broome ME, Bates TA, Lillis PP, McGahee TW. Children's medical fears, coping behaviors, and pain perceptions during a lumbar puncture. *Oncol Nurs Forum* 1990; 17(3):361–367.

Buehler DM, Als H, Duffy FH, McAnulty GB, Liederman J. Effectiveness of individualized developmental care for low-risk preterm infants: behavioral and electrophysiologic evidence. *Pediatrics* 1995; 96:923–932.

Coderre TJ, Katz J, Vaccarino AL, Melzack R. Contribution of central neuroplasticity to pathological pain: review of clinical and experimental evidence. *Pain* 1993; 52:259–285.

Craig KD, McMahon RJ, Morison JD, Zaskow C. Developmental changes in infant pain expression during immunization injections. *Soc Sci Med* 1984; 19:1331–1337.

Craig KD, Grunau RVE, Branson SM. Age-related aspects of pain: pain in children. In: Dubner R, Gebhart GF, Bond MR (Eds). *Pain Research and Clinical Management.* Amsterdam: Elsevier, 1988, pp. 317–328.

Derrickson JG, Neef NA, Cataldo MF. Effects of signaling invasive procedures on a hospitalized infants' affective behaviors. *J Appl Behav Anal* 1993; 26(1):133–134.

Fearon I, McGrath PJ, Achat H. 'Booboos': the study of everyday pain among young children. *Pain* 1996; 68:55–62.

Fitzgerald M. Development of pain pathways and mechanisms. In: Anand KJS, McGrath PJ (Eds). *Pain in Neonates.* Amsterdam: Elsevier, 1993, pp 19–37.

Fitzgerald M, Shaw A, MacIntosh N. Postnatal development of the cutaneous flexor reflex: comparative study of preterm infants and newborn rat pups. *Develop Med Child Neurol* 1988; 30:520–526.

Fitzgerald M, Millard C, McIntosh N. Cutaneous hypersensitivity following peripheral tissue damage in newborn infants and its reversal with topical anaesthesia. *Pain* 1989; 39:31–36.

Fleisher BE, VandenBerg K, Constantinou J, et al. Individualized developmental care for very-low-birth-weight premature infants. *Clin Pediatr* 1995; 34:523–529.

Garland JS. Developmental care for very low-birth-weight infants. *JAMA* 1995; 273:1575.

Grunau RVE, Whitfield MF, Petrie JH, Fryer EL. Early pain experience, child and family factors, as precursors of somatization: a prospective study of extremely premature and fullterm children. *Pain* 1994a; 56:353–359.

Grunau RVE, Whitfield MF, Petrie JH. Pain sensitivity and temperament in extremely low-birth-weight premature toddlers and preterm and full-term controls. *Pain* 1994b; 58:341–346.

Grunau RVE, Whitfield MF, Petrie J. Children's judgements about pain at age 8–10 years: do extremely low birthweight (<1000 g) children differ from full birthweight peers? *J Child Psychol Psychiatry* 1996; 39(4):587–594.

Hester NKO. The preoperational child's reaction to immunization. *Nurs Res* 1979; 28(4):250–255.

Horwood LJ, Mogridge N, Darlow BA. Cognitive, educational, and behavioural outcomes at 7 to 8 years in a national very low birthweight cohort. *Arch Dis Child Fetal Neonatal Ed* 1998; 79:F12–F20.

Johnston CC, Stevens BJ. Experience in a neonatal intensive care unit affects pain response. *Pediatrics* 1996; 98:925–930.

Johnston CC, Stevens B, Yang F, Horton L. Developmental changes in response to heelstick in preterm infants: a prospective cohort study. *Dev Med Child Neurol* 1996; 38:438–445.

Kart T, Christrup LL, Rasmussen M. Recommended use of morphine in neonates, infants and children based on a literature review: part 2. Clinical use. *Paediatr Anaesth* 1997; 7:93–101.

Katz ER, Kellerman J, Siegel SE. Behavioral distress in children with cancer undergoing medical procedures: developmental considerations. *J Consult Clin Psychol* 1980; 48(3):356–365.

Kuttner L. Management of young children's acute pain and anxiety during invasive medical procedures. *Pediatrician* 1989; 16:39–44.

Lacy JB. Developmental care for very low-birth-weight infants. *JAMA* 1995; 273:1575–1576.

Langland JT, Langland PI. Letter to the editor. *N Engl J Med* 1988; 318(21):1398–1399.

Larsson BA, Tannfeldt G, Lagercrantz H, Olsson GL. Venipuncture is more effective and less painful than heel lancing for blood tests in neonates. *Pediatrics* 1998; 101:882–886.

Levy DM. The infant's earliest memory of inoculation: a contribution to public health procedures. *J Gen Psychol* 1960; 96:3–46.

Loeser JD. Pain in children. In: Tyler DC, Krane EJ (Eds). *Advances in Pain Research and Therapy: Pediatric Pain*, Vol. 15. Raven Press: New York, 1990, pp 1–4.

MacGregor R, Evans D, Sugden D, Gaussen T, Levene M. Outcome at 5–6 years of prematurely born children who received morphine as neonates. *Arch Dis Child Fetal Neonat Ed* 1998; 79:F40–F43.

McGrath PA, de Veber LL. The management of acute pain evoked by medical procedures in children with cancer. *J Pain Symptom Manage* 1986; 1(3):145–150.

McGrath PJ, Craig K. Developmental and psychological factors in children's pain. *Pediatr Clin North Am* 1989; 36(4):823–836.

Milgrom P, Mancl L, King B, Weinstein P. Origins of childhood dental fear. *Behav Res Ther* 1995; 33(3):313–319.

Mohan CG, Risucci DA, Casimir M, Gulrajani-LaCorte M. Comparison of analgesics in ameliorating the pain of circumcision. *J Perinatol* 1998; 18(1):13–19.

Mouradian LE, Als H. The influence of neonatal intensive care unit caregiving practices on motor functioning of preterm infants. *Am J Occu Ther* 1994; 48(6):527–533.

Ohlsson A. Developmental care for very low-birth-weight infants. *JAMA* 1995; 273:1576.

Orsini AJ, Leef KH, Costarino A, Dettorre MD, Stefano JL. Routine use of fentanyl infusions for pain and stress reduction in infants with respiratory distress syndrome. *J Pediatr* 1996; 129:140–145.

Petryshen P, Stevens B, Hawkins J, Stewart M. Comparing nursing costs for preterm infants receiving conventional vs. developmental care. *Nurse Economics* 1997; 15(3):138–150.

Pokela M-L. Pain relief can reduce hypoxemia in distress neonates during routine treatment procedures. *Pediatrics* 1994; 93:379–383.

Quinn MW, Otoo F, Rushforth JA, et al. Effect of morphine and pancuronium on the stress response in ventilated preterm infants. *Early Hum Dev* 1992; 30:241–248.

Quinn MW, Wild J, Dean HG, et al. Randomised double-blind controlled trial of effect of morphine on catecholamine concentrations in ventilated preterm babies. *Lancet* 1993; 342:324–327.

Reynolds ML, Fitzgerald M. Long-term sensory hyperinnervation following neonatal skin wounds. *J Comp Neurol* 1995; 358:487–498.

Richards MPM, Bernal JF, Brackbill Y. Early behavioral differences: gender or circumcision? *Dev Psychobiol* 1976; 9:89–95.

Saigal S. Developmental care for very low-birth-weight infants. *JAMA* 1995; 273:1576–1577.

Schothorst PF, van Engeland H. Long-term behavioral sequelae of prematurity. *J Am Acad Child Adolesc Psychiatry* 1996; 35(2):175–183.

Serour F, Mandelberg A, Zabeeda D, Mori J, Ezra S. Efficacy of EMLA cream prior to dorsal penile nerve block for circumcision in children. *Acta Anaesthesiol Scand* 1998; 42(20):260–263.

Shah V, Taddio A, Bennett S, Speidel BD. Neonatal pain response to heelstick versus venepuncture- randomized controlled trial. *Arc Dis Child Fetal Neonatal Ed* 1997; 77:F143–F144.

Stevens B, Petryshen P, Hawkins J, Smith B, Taylor P. Developmental versus conventional care: a comparison of clinical outcomes for very low birth weight infants. *Can J Nurs Res* 1996; 28(4):97–113.

Stevens B, Taddio A, Ohlsson A, Einarson TR. The efficacy of sucrose for relieving procedural pain in neonates—a systematic review and meta-analysis. *Acta Paediatr* 1997; 86:837–842.

Taddio A, Nulman I, Goldbach M, Ipp M, Koren G. Use of lidocaine-prilocaine cream for vaccination pain in infants. *J Pediatr* 1994; 124:643–648.

Taddio A, Goldbach M, Ipp M, Stevens B, Koren G. Effect of neonatal circumcision on pain response during vaccination in boys. *Lancet* 1995; 345:291–292.

Taddio A, Katz J, Ilersich AL, Koren G. Effect of neonatal circumcision on pain response during subsequent routine vaccination. *Lancet* 19 97a; 349:599–603.

Taddio A, Stevens B, Craig K, et al. Efficacy and safety of lidocaine-prilocaine cream for pain during circumcision. *N Engl J Med* 1997b; 336:1197–1201.

Taddio A, Ohlsson A, Einarson TR, Stevens B, Koren G. A systematic review of lidocaine-prilocaine cream (EMLA) in the treatment of acute pain in neonates. *Pediatrics* 1998; 101(2):e1.

Taylor HG, Klein N, Schatschneider C, Hack M. Predictors of early school age outcomes in very low birth weight children. *Dev Behav Pediatr* 1998; 19(4):235–243.

Westrup M, Klegerg A, Wallin L, et al. Evaluation of the newborn individualized developmental care and assessment program (NIDCAP) in a Swedish setting. *Perinatal Neonatal Med* 1997; 2:366–375.

Woolf CJ, Thompson SWN. The induction and maintenance of central sensitization is dependent on N-methyl-D-aspartic acid receptor activation; implications for the treatment of post-injury pain hypersensitivity states. *Pain* 1991; 44:293–299.

Correspondence to: Anna Taddio, MSc, PhD, Department of Pharmacy, The Hospital for Sick Children, 555 University Avenue, Toronto, Ontario, Canada M5G 1X8.

Chronic and Recurrent Pain in Children and Adolescents, Progress in Pain Research and Management, Vol. 13, edited by Patrick J. McGrath and G. Allen Finley, IASP Press, Seattle, © 1999.

5

Neuropathic Pain in Children

Gunnar L. Olsson

Department of Pediatric Anesthesia, Astrid Lindgren Children's Hospital, Karolinska Hospital, Stockholm, Sweden

Neuropathic pain is not uncommon in children, although the etiology is often different in children than it is in adults. Until recently, neuropathic pain in children has not been closely studied. Most epidemiological studies investigating pediatric pain have addressed specific pain conditions, e.g., headache and recurrent abdominal pain (Goodman and McGrath 1991). Diabetic neuropathy, herpes zoster, and stroke are rare in the pediatric population, whereas other types of pain, e.g., complex regional pain syndrome, type I (CRPS-I, also known as reflex sympathetic dystrophy) are more common. In adults, neuropathic pain is often diagnosed according to etiology, whereas the origin of neuropathic pain in children is often unknown and the diagnosis is determined by typical symptomatology and careful analysis of the pain. Neuropathic pain is often mixed with other types of pain due to combined trauma of skeletal or soft tissue with trauma to the nervous system, e.g., from injury or invasive cancer growth. Neuropathic pain can also develop secondary to longstanding pain states. Longstanding pain must thus be evaluated carefully for components of neuropathic pain, and a thorough pain analysis should always be included in cases of longstanding pain.

OVERVIEW OF TREATMENT

CASE REPORT OF LONGSTANDING ABDOMINAL PAIN IN A 13-YEAR-OLD BOY

Pain in the upper right quadrant of the abdomen started in the spring of 1995. The patient was extensively investigated for organic disease. High transaminase levels detected in September 1995 could have been due to acetaminophen (paracetamol) intoxication, but this could not be verified.

Child psychiatrists and psychologists were consulted. A magnetic resonance imaging (MRI) scan revealed suspected thickening of the gallbladder. The patient had a cholecystectomy in November 1995 on very vague indications. The pain was not relieved, and in May 1996 he was hospitalized with excruciating pain. Intravenous opioids failed to provide pain relief, and he was referred to the pain treatment unit in our hospital. He had a complicated psychosocial history. After conception the father had been absent, and there had been problems in school. At admission to our hospital in June 1996, the boy had spontaneous continuous pain deep in the abdomen localized in the upper right quadrant, periods of cramp-like attacks in smooth muscle, and a constant allodynia of the skin of the upper right quadrant of the abdomen. On examining his records, gastroenterologists found no liver disease and did not believe there had ever been any problem with his gallbladder. Intravenous ketamine in a subanesthetic dose relieved his pain for the first time in many months. The effect lasted 9 hours. The next day he received an infusion of adenosine at 60 $\mu g \cdot kg^{-1} \cdot min^{-1}$ for 60 minutes. The allodynia that he had suffered for many months disappeared and did not return. We spent a long time explaining the function of the central nervous system in the transmission of pain signals and in reassuring the boy that there was nothing wrong in his abdomen but that his experience of pain was due to an erroneous transmission of signals to his brain, which is not uncommon. After four additional ketamine injections the pain did not reoccur, and he has remained pain free. Was this a case of psychological conversion syndrome cured by placebo effects and psychological reassurance? Was it a case of abdominal neuropathic pain of unknown origin?

MULTIDISCIPLINARY TREATMENT PROTOCOL

In Stockholm, pediatric surgery is concentrated in one hospital. There is little private care. Most children with pain are referred to the pediatric surgeons or pediatric orthopedic surgeon at the pain treatment unit of Astrid Lindgren Children's Hospital at the Karolinska Hospital. Children are referred by pediatric surgeons, pediatric orthopedic surgeons, rheumatologists, and pediatricians. Also, more and more parents are directly contacting the clinic, although this is often disadvantageous because it is important that the patient's orthopedic or rheumatological status be thoroughly investigated. A pain treatment team meets every second week to discuss complex cases. The team includes a specialist in pain medicine, a pediatric orthopedic surgeon, a rheumatologist, a psychiatrist, a psychologist, and a physiotherapist. Neurologists, pediatricians, and a neurosurgeon are invited when appropriate. This multidisciplinary approach leads to an early focus on pain transmission disorders as causes for the patients' symptoms and avoids unwanted delay in treatment and unnecessary investigations and surgery.

TYPES OF PAIN

Pain has traditionally been classified as nociceptive, neuropathic, or psychogenic. Neuropathic pain includes abnormalities in the pain transmission system, which often go unrecognized by physicians. If the orthopedic surgeon finds no abnormalities in the foot, or the pediatric surgeon can detect no abdominal pathology, they often believe that the pain is psychogenic. The specialist in pain medicine (now a recognized specialty in Sweden) can be an intermediary between the surgeon and the psychologist or psychiatrist and must cooperate closely with both.

Pain is a complaint in many types of psychosomatic disorders, but psychogenic pain is probably not very common in children. Sexual child abuse and extreme social stress situations can give rise to conversion syndromes, which can manifest as CRPS-I and may respond to pharmacological treatment or a sympathetic block. Of course, major stress factors must be addressed, but psychological intervention alone seldom relieves the pain. Special psychological profiles have been proposed for various longstanding pain states, as discussed for CRPS-I below.

Nociceptive pain is usually simpler to understand. However, even in a trauma situation, central nervous system (CNS) mechanisms are initiated and transmission is modulated in a way that has many features in common with neuropathic pain.

Thus, cases of longstanding pain demand a multidisciplinary approach. Simple classification as psychogenic, neuropathic, or nociceptive pain is insufficient. A team of experienced physicians and paramedical staff (including physical therapists, psychologists, and play therapists) is of utmost importance. The patient may have several pain syndromes at the same time. For example, a child with cancer may have nociceptive pain from a bone metastasis, tumor growth in a nerve plexus, and considerable psychological stress. These different aspects must be evaluated separately to provide the best care.

SYMPTOMS OF NEUROPATHIC PAIN

The term "neuropathic pain" indicates pathology in the nervous system, such as trauma to nervous tissue or diabetic polyneuropathy (Table I). Symptoms are different from nociceptive pain and include dysesthesia or allodynia.

Table I
Classification of neuropathic pain

Central pain
  Stroke
  Spinal cord injury

Peripheral neuropathic pain
  Polyneuropathies,
    Metabolic, e.g., diabetes
    Toxic
  Nerve trauma
    Mononeuropathies, entrapment
  Neuralgia
    Cranial
      Trigeminal
      Glossopharyngeal
    Postherpetic
  Post-amputation, phantom limb pain

Sympathetic nervous system
  Complex regional pain syndrome, type II (causalgia)
  Complex regional pain syndrome, type I (reflex sympathetic dystrophy)

Neuropathic pain without identified lesion in the nervous system
  Complex regional pain syndrome, type I (reflex sympathetic dystrophy)
  Failure of normal sensory inhibition

The pain is often disproportionate to objective findings. However, pain states with similar symptoms are also classified as neuropathic, even where no pathology of nervous tissue can be identified (Bennet 1994). Classification is thus dependent on symptomatology and not always on identified nervous system pathology.

In many neuropathic pain states, pain sensation is spontaneous (as opposed to evoked by touching) and continuous. It is very common for a child with CRPS-I to smile and talk to the doctor without seeming to be in severe pain, and still rate pain as 80 on VAS scale of 1–100. Pain can be burning, throbbing, or may feel like needles or electrical shocks. Stimulation may cause unexpected and prolonged pain.

Dysesthesia often exists in neuropathic pain states and means that stimulation is experienced in an abnormal way, and may feel "different" or "strange," and often "tingling" and "uncomfortable." Touching healed scars often produces dysesthesia. Stimulation of low-threshold mechanoreceptors (LTM receptors) is transmitted to the CNS, where a modulation gives rise to the sensation.

Allodynia is defined as pain evoked by non-noxious stimulation of normal (non-inflamed/sensitized) tissue. Dynamic allodynia can be elicited by stimulation with a soft brush; the signal is transmitted by LTM receptors. Static allodynia can be provoked with a moderately stiff von Frey hair; the signal is thought to be transmitted by sensitized C-fibers. Allodynia must be distinguished from the normal secondary hyperesthesia found close to a traumatized or inflamed area.

Hyperalgesia is often erroneously used as a synonym for allodynia, but hyperalgesia implies that more pain is evoked than expected from the magnitude of the stimulus. Primary hyperalgesia occurs after trauma. Inflammation leads to release of bradykinin, prostaglandins, potassium, and many other algogenic substances that decrease the threshold for nociceptive A-delta and C-fibers. Secondary hyperalgesia due to central sensitization occurs outside the area of inflammatory response. In hyperalgesia, touch can evoke pain by stimulating LTM receptors. Torebjörk et al. (1992) stimulated a nerve at the ankle to create a sensation of touch on the dorsum of the foot, clearly stimulating LTM-fibers. They then applied capsaicin (a selective C-fiber receptor stimulator) a short distance from the site on the foot where touch had been felt; stimulation of the same nerve fibers was now experienced as pain. Thus signals from LTM fibers were processed abnormally in the spinal cord and transmitted to the cortex as a pain message. When the effect of capsaicin wore off, the stimulation again produced a sensation of touch. This experiment clearly demonstrates how central processing can change normal nonpainful stimulation into pain.

Hyperpathia is a term given to abnormal pain evoked in an area with an increased threshold for sensory detection (Merskey and Bogduk 1994). The pain is often felt after a significant delay, and "after-sensations" often occur.

LOCALIZATION OF DIFFERENT TYPES OF PAIN

Nociceptive pain is localized to the site of injury, although there can be referred pain and pain in the area adjacent to the trauma (secondary hyperalgesia). Neuropathic pain, however, usually has a different localization. With a specific lesion of the nervous system, pain could be localized to the area corresponding to a single nerve, or to dermatomes for more central lesions. In other types of neuropathic pain, such as CRPS-I, the localization follows neither anatomic structures nor an area corresponding to any known organization of the nervous system. Often the entire distal part of an extremity is involved.

MECHANISMS IN NEUROPATHIC PAIN

Knowledge of the mechanisms of neuropathic pain has increased enormously during recent decades. Much research has been performed on lesions of the sciatic nerve in rats in order to create models for studying neuropathic pain. However, clinicians can become confused when such factors as the diets fed to the rats influence the results. For example, some soy formulas that include proteins with GABA-like activity can cause different nociceptive reactions than seen in rats fed other diets.

Many different mechanisms have been suggested for the etiology of neuropathic pain, and certainly much is still not understood. Children with CRPS-I, the most common childhood neuropathic pain syndrome, often have no known lesion in the nervous system, although an unrecognized trauma such as a viral infection may have caused hidden damage (Marshall Devor, personal communication). Neuropathic pain may involve distorted information processing in the spinal cord (Jänig 1996). An important mechanism may be that input from LTM receptors reaches the spinal cord and gains access to pain transmission systems. Dynamic allodynia is transmitted at least partially in A-beta fibers, and in the CNS, a wind-up phenomenon leads to pain. There could also be an abnormal nociceptor sensitization, where the allodynia is elicited by puncture stimulation with von Frey hairs. Other proposed explanations involving the peripheral nervous system include ectopic discharge from the dorsal root ganglion (DRG), primary afferent axons, or synapses, or inflammation of nerve trunks. Sensitization via the sympathetic nervous system has also been suggested, and hypersensitivity to circulating noradrenaline could be a factor in sympathetically maintained pain (SMP). Altered central processing and central hyperexcitability are probably also involved. Changes in receptor sensitivity, genetic changes in dorsal horn neurons, and neuroanatomical reorganization can lead to central sensitization and wind-up (Walker and Cousins 1997). In some cases of trauma to nervous tissue, inflammation of the nerve trunk and sensory input from n. nervorum could explain neuropathic pain.

DIAGNOSIS OF NEUROPATHIC PAIN

The diagnosis is based on history and typical neuropathic symptoms. First, clinical examination should include skin temperature measurement and reaction to cold and heat stimulation, as tested with a metal object cooled or heated in water. A simple sensory evaluation should always be performed including a soft brush to diagnose dynamic allodynia and a set of von Frey hairs to look for static allodynia and sensory disturbances such as sensory loss and hypo- or hyperesthesia. Differences between extremities in sensory and pain thresholds are easily revealed. Color changes and edema should be noted. Motor impairment is common in neuropathic pain states, and a simple test of motor function should be performed.

CRPS-I now has quite clear diagnostic criteria, and when a known lesion is correlated with the results of sensory testing there are few diagnostic problems. In cases with normal quantitative sensory testing (QST) (Gruener and Dyck 1994) and no known lesion, diagnosis is more difficult. Ochoa (1993) proposed that CRPS-I is a psychological disturbance and should not be handled by neurophysiologists. However, there is little evidence for this (Lynch 1992), and pain clinicians must take on the challenge of helping these patients. When symptoms are typical of neuropathic pain and other causative factors are excluded, patients should be treated as having a pain transmission syndrome.

QST often reveals sensory abnormalities, including changes in thresholds for temperature sensation and temperature pain. Areas of hyposensitivity can often be seen in the patient who exhibits allodynia. In children with CRPS-I, these sensory abnormalities are usually normalized after a successful sympathetic block. A 12-year-old girl with CRPS-I treated in the pain unit still had substantial sensory disturbances revealed by QST 2 weeks after a guanethidine block had provided complete pain relief. A week later her pain reoccurred. QST could thus perhaps serve both as a diagnostic and prognostic tool in the evaluation of children with CRPS-I. The pain treatment unit at Astrid Lindgren Children's Hospital is evaluating the validity of QST in children with CRPS-I.

Other laboratory tests include nerve conduction studies and tests of autonomic function. Resting skin temperature is easily performed; standardized measurement points should be used. At the patient's first visit to the pain clinic, we measure skin temperature bilaterally over the plantar surface of the big toe, dorsal mid-metatarsal, distal tibia, and distal femur in cases of lower extremity pain. Resting sweat output and sweating elicited by axon reflex could also be measured (Chelimsky et al. 1995). Tests of sympathetic nervous system function include evaluation of sympathetic reflex vasoconstriction. Blood flow can be studied with laser-Doppler flowmetry (Kurvers et al. 1995) or photoelectrical pulse plethysmography. Sympathetic dysfunction in a painful extremity could be studied by various techniques. The veno-arteriolar reflex is studied by measuring skin blood flow bilaterally before and after lowering the extremities below the heart level. Activation of the sympathetic nervous system can also be achieved by performing sudden deep breaths (inspiratory gasp), performing mental arithmetic, or immersing the feet in cold water (cold pressor test) (Birklein et al. 1998). Differences in the response (measured as changes in the skin blood flow) between the extremities indicate sympathetic involvement and could aid clinicians in deciding whether to perform a sympathetic blockade. Sympathetic skin response can also be studied by measuring skin conductance (Schondorf 1993). In cases without recognized nerve tissue damage, great effort must be taken to exclude other organic disease that may explain the pain.

Many children with longstanding pain do not fit into the traditional classification of neuropathic pain. For example, rheumatologists treat many children with multiple pains arising in the tendons and connective tissue who show no clinical or laboratory signs of inflammation. Treatment with NSAIDs and other analgesics is often unsuccessful. Patients may be diagnosed with entesopathy, fibromyalgia, or chronic fatigue syndrome. We often see children with pain in the extremities that is similar to CRPS-I, but without dysautonomy (temperature or color changes, sudomotor disturbances, or edema) this diagnosis cannot be made (see Table II). Back pain and abdominal pain often seem unrelated to organic disease after meticulous investigations. Sometimes there is allodynia or dysesthesia, and often multifocal localization. Neurologists working with pain patients may lose interest if they find no neurological disease or sensory abnormalities. These children are frequently referred to pediatric psychiatrists or psychologists, but usually no causative factor is revealed and the pain is not alleviated. I view these pain syndromes as neuropathic pain, possibly explained by decreased normal sensory inhibition at the spinal level. Treatment should be similar to that of CRPS-I patients who do not respond to sympathetic block.

CENTRAL PAIN

Stroke due to arteriosclerotic disease is common in the elderly but is not seen in children. Hypoxia during the perinatal period often leads to cerebral hypoxia and leucomalacia; we do not know whether these conditions are linked to pain syndromes. Children with cerebral palsy are often incapable of communicating their pain, but their facial expressions would indicate that pain is often present. Stroke due to ischemic disease occurs most commonly in childhood due to nonarteriosclerotic cardiac disease such as ventricular septal defects or rheumatic heart disease. A recently published review of pediatric ischemic stroke made no comment on central pain syndromes as complications of stroke (Ferrera et al. 1997).

Cerebral aqueduct stenosis and Chiari type I malformation have been associated with pain syndromes in children (Yglesias et al. 1996; Gallagher and Trounce 1998). Lesions in the spinal cord could be complicated by neuropathic pain, as in adults. Uncommon disorders such as familial idiopathic intracranial hypertension could be associated with spinal and radicular pain in children (Santinelli et al. 1998).

PERIPHERAL NEUROPATHIC PAIN

POLYNEUROPATHY

Polyneuropathies due to metabolic or toxic disorders are not common in childhood. However, even in children with type I diabetes a subclinical neuropathy can usually be revealed (Meh and Denislic 1998). Neuropathies with excruciating pain can be observed after administration of certain anticancer drugs, such as vincristine (Weintraub et al. 1996). Immunosuppressive treatment after transplantation is also associated with neuropathies.

NERVE TRAUMA

As in adults, neuropathic pain is seen in children after nerve trauma. We have little information on incidence, which is possibly lower than in adults. An occasional nerve trauma in neonates is avulsion of the brachial plexus during delivery. Surgical repair is usually performed around the age of 3 months. Whether this nerve trauma is associated with later development of significant neuropathic pain is not known. A study of 1486 patients with obstetrical palsy, including late follow-up of function, mentioned nothing about pain (Gilbert 1995). In a series of 16 radial mononeuropathies seen at the electromyography laboratory at the Children's Hospital in Boston, clinical assessment revealed weakness and sensory loss but not pain (Escolar and Jones 1996).

CRANIAL NEURALGIA

Well-defined neuralgias in adults, such as trigeminal and glossopharyngeal, are not common in children. A series of 336 cases of trigeminal neuralgias included no patient below the age of 12 years (Heyck 1981), whereas the youngest patient undergoing microvascular decompression for trigeminal neuralgia in a study of 1166 patients was 5 years old (Barker et al. 1996).

POSTHERPETIC NEURALGIA

Chicken pox occurs in childhood and is caused by a herpes virus. The virus remains inactive in the dorsal root ganglion, and in later life herpes zoster can be a sign of reactivation of the virus. The incidence of herpes zoster correlates directly with increasing age. The higher risk of viral reactivation is attributed to an age-associated decline in immune function (Arvin 1996). The risk is especially high in immunodeficient patients, and in children immunodeficiency is the main risk factor. In a series of 21 children with herpes zoster, only three patients experienced mild to moderate pain sensations in the acute phase and at 8 weeks after onset no patient had postherpetic neuralgia (Kakourou et al. 1998).

PHANTOM LIMB PAIN

Recently several publications have examined phantom limb pain in children (Krane and Heller 1995; Melzack et al. 1997; Dangel 1998; Wilkins et al. 1998). Krane and Heller, in their retrospective study, found that the incidence of phantom sensations in amputees was 100% and that phantom pain occurred in 92%, according to a questionnaire a median of 2.5 years after amputation. The most common descriptors of pain were "sharp," "tingling," "stabbing," and "uncomfortable." Onset generally occurred within the first week after amputation, and by the time of follow-up phantom pain had resolved in 35%. On examining the charts and case records of these patients, the authors found that phantom sensations were recorded for only 50% of patients during their hospital stay, perhaps showing that clinicians should pay specific attention to this problem. Wilkins and colleagues, in a similar retrospective study, found a lower incidence of phantom pain. This series included more cases of congenital limb deficiency ($n = 27$), and in this group the incidence of phantom pain was 4% compared to 49% in the group of surgery/trauma patients ($n = 33$). Patients with phantom pain often experienced other forms of pain, and phantom pain was related to stump pain. The time between amputation and follow-up was longer in the study of Wilkins et al., which also may account for a lower incidence. Both studies had a considerable number of nonrespondents, and a prospective multicenter study to evaluate different prophylactic strategies and treatments is desirable. Pain before amputation predisposes to a higher incidence of phantom pain, and in nonemergency cases a preoperative epidural block could reduce the incidence of phantom limb pain (Bach et al. 1988). Melzack and colleagues (1997) reported that 20% of patients with congenital limb deficiency, experienced phantom limb sensations. During 1998, our pain unit treated three cases of traumatic lower extremity amputations in 14–15-year-old adolescents. We administered epidural regional anesthesia for at least a week postoperatively, and then gave amitriptyline (in one case gabapentine where the mother refused amitriptyline). Opioids, NSAIDs, acetaminophen, tramadol, and transcutaneous electrical nerve stimulation (TENS) were used liberally, and so far these patients have experienced no major problems with phantom limb pain.

COMPLEX REGIONAL PAIN SYNDROME, TYPE I

Pain involving the sympathetic nervous system has long been recognized in adults. CRPS-I is not a medical entity based on a defined cause. It is a symptom complex that may result from any one of multiple causes, through any variety of pathophysiological mechanisms, to yield a common but nonspecific clinical profile (Ochoa 1995). Recently, new criteria for the diagnosis of CRPS-I have been presented (Table II) (Stanton-Hicks et al. 1995).

CRPS-I pain usually involves a distal part of one extremity, although involvement of multiple extremities and cases of migratory pain have been described (Barrera et al. 1992; Schiffenbauer and Fagien 1993). Of about 150 cases seen in our pain treatment clinic, three have involved more than one extremity.

Motor impairment is common in CRPS-I and could be a secondary guarding phenomenon due to the pain elicited by moving the limb. However, functional paresis is often seen. The child is often totally unable to move the foot or the toes. This motor disability usually disappears immediately after a successful guanethidine block. Sometimes weakness persists for weeks after the pain has disappeared, and is usually attributed to the muscle wasting seen after long immobilization. A neglect-like syndrome has been proposed for the motor disturbances in CRPS-I, which involve supraspinal mechanisms in the CNS orienting system (Galer et al. 1995). Dystonia and myoclonus are other motor phenomenon seen in CRPS-I.

Table II
Diagnostic criteria for complex regional pain syndrome, type I
(reflex sympathetic dystrophy)

1)	A syndrome that develops after an initiating noxious event
2)	Spontaneous pain or allodynia/hyperalgesia occurs that is not limited to the territory of a single peripheral nerve and is disproportionate to the inciting event
3)	There is or has been evidence of edema, skin blood flow abnormality, or abnormal sudomotor activity in the region of the pain since the inciting event
4)	This diagnosis is excluded by existence of conditions that would otherwise account for the degree of pain and dysfunction

DIFFERENCES BETWEEN ADULTS AND CHILDREN

The first criterion for CRPS-I does not fit the pediatric population. A history of trauma is uncommon, and when reported it is usually minor. CRPS-I is most common in girls (female to male ratio 4:1) aged 9–15 years, most commonly 11–12 years. There are just a few case reports in younger children. In studying musculoskeletal pain in children, Mikkelsson et al. (1998) found that boys had a lower risk for persistence of pain than did girls and that the risk for the persistence of pain increased 1.2 times per age year. There are usually fewer dystrophic changes in children, perhaps due to a shorter time before successful intervention. The autonomic dysfunction varies: temperature differences are most common. Usually the affected foot is colder than the contralateral (a skin temperature difference of 1°C is necessary to define temperature disturbance). Temperatures vary, however, and sometimes the affected extremity is warmer. The three stages of CRPS-I are usually not seen in children. The first stage is characterized by burning pain and an increased temperature. In children the limb is more often cold from the beginning, and the pain is less often characterized as burning. The lower extremity is more often affected, in contrast to adults. Color changes are common in children, and often there is discrete edema. In adults, early treatment has been advocated, while the duration of disease seems to be of little importance in the success of treatments in children (Wilder 1996).

Inactivity often leads to wasting of the calf muscles. Radiography may show osteoporosis (Lloyd-Thomas and Lauder 1995), although atrophic changes are less common in children.

PAIN SENSATION

Patients often report spontaneous pain that is scored high on a VAS. Localization in a foot could include the entire foot and preclude any possibility for weight bearing. Pain can be more localized, allowing a limping walk. More often there is just a dull aching, sometimes combined with varying types of dysesthesia, rather than burning pain. Pain is often continuous with no pain-free intervals. In a few cases pain occurs in more than one location. Sometimes there is no spontaneous pain, but there is allodynia and inability to bear weight.

PSYCHOLOGICAL PROFILE

Patients with CRPS may suffer from enhanced anxiety, be emotionally rather unstable, and display a tendency for depression associated with a marked self-esteem problem (Egle and Hoffman 1990). A recent life event may have created stress (Geertzen et al. 1994). Ochoa (1993) recommended that we "accept the real and relatively common eventuality that a patient may have a legitimate health disorder centered in the psyche, and that it may masquerade a nerve or muscle disease." He criticizes the use of the term "neuropathic pain" for cases without recognized neurological findings, and uses the expression "undiagnosed psychogenic pseudoneuropathy." This view has been questioned by others; Ciccone et al. (1997), studying adults with CRPS-I and other longstanding pain states, found a high incidence of sexual and other abuse in childhood but found no difference in incidence when compared to patients with other pain syndromes. The authors concluded that "the burden of proof would appear to be upon those who advocate the non-organic hypothesis to provide credible evidence of psychological involvement in the etiology of RSD." It has often been suggested that certain personality traits predispose development of sympathetically related pain syndromes. Lynch (1992), reviewing the literature, could find no valid evidence to substantiate this claim. As in most diseases, and certainly when dealing with subjective experiences such as pain, psychological factors are involved. We have had cases of sexual abuse associated with CRPS-I in our pediatric pain clinic. Such cases should be classified as a conversion syndrome. However, few patients with histories of sexual abuse develop CRPS-I, and in most CRPS-I cases no major psychological factors are revealed. Thus it is a syndrome of abnormal sensory transmission with mainly unknown etiology. In an ongoing study, we are comparing life stress factors in a series of CRPS-I patients to a normal population of the same age and gender. We believe that there could be a connection between stress and pain where there is involvement of the sympathetic nervous system. We and others have found that the syndrome often affects children who place high demands on themselves, often working hard to get high grades in school and competing in sports (Lloyd-Thomas 1995). Sherry and Weisman (1988) found that most of the children with reflex neurovascular dystrophy in their study were described as especially bright, but less than 20% had superior intelligence test scores. Negative life experiences, such as the death of a family member or bullying in school, could also be involved.

DIAGNOSIS

If a patient shows typical symptoms for CRPS-I, we prefer early sympathetic block for both diagnostic and therapeutic reasons. The physical examination should measure skin temperature and thresholds for sensation and pain, and should test for allodynia with von Frey hairs. In less typical cases, especially when signs of dysautonomy are absent and an ongoing nociceptive, organic diagnosis cannot be fully excluded, analgesic tests are of value, both as a diagnostic tool and for future treatment.

Oral NSAID test. When orthopedic or inflammatory disease is not excluded, we perform an oral diclofenac test. The child is given a protocol for pain assessment. For 3 days the patient assesses pain three times a day and records the worst pain of the day using a VAS. Thereafter diclofenac is given divided in three doses at 2 mg·kg^{-1}·d^{-1}. This protocol continues for 10 days. In neuropathic pain syndromes there is typically no pain relief. If there is substantial pain relief, an organic diagnosis must be sought more vigorously and diclofenac therapy can be used for a longer time.

Opioid test. Previously we have found that children with CRPS-I get very little pain relief from intravenous morphine administration (Olsson 1994). Now we perform a standardized alfentanil test. A normal full analgesic dose (7 µg/kg) is divided into three syringes, and another two syringes containing saline are prepared. Under a randomized and double-blinded protocol, a syringe is given every 4 minutes, with pain assessment by a VAS between doses. At the end naloxone is given. Children with neuropathic pain usually are not affected at all by alfentanil, whereas nociceptive pain decreases with alfentanil and returns after naloxone. Adverse effects such as respiratory depression, sedation, and nausea are seldom seen in neuropathic patients, but are more common with ongoing nociception.

Phentolamine test. Although the first reported phentolamine test was performed at our clinic (Olsson et al. 1990), and all cases with a positive test had a good effect from a sympathetic block, we now seldom use it. We find that many of cases with a negative phentolamine test are still cured by a sympathetic block. Thus, the predictive value of the test is low. Others have further developed the test and still use it (Raja et al. 1991).

PROGNOSIS

Children with CRPS-I seem to have milder cases compared to adults, with less atrophy and with a good short-term prognosis. Veldman and Goris (1997) found 118 cases of recurrence in 1183 consecutive patients who were mostly adults (age range 4–84 years). Recurrences especially occurred in younger patients, often in more than one limb. In a 5-year follow-up we found still higher (25%) incidence of persistent pain in children at the time of follow-up (Olsson et al. 1991). Complete resolution was seen in only half the cases in the series of 70 children with CRPS-I from Boston (Wilder et al. 1992). In a series of 1006 patients aged 10–84 years diagnosed with reflex sympathetic dystrophy, 7% developed severe complications such as infection, ulcers, chronic edema, dystonia, and myoclonus. Patients affected were younger and more often female. The skin temperature at onset was lower in these patients than in uncomplicated cases (van der Laan et al. 1998). The long-term prognosis for children must be further evaluated.

TREATMENT OF CRPS-I IN CHILDREN

Nonpharmacological approaches and sympathetic block

The following recommendations follow the guidelines for therapy of CRPS-I based on a consensus workshop in Los Angeles in November 1995 (Stanton-Hicks et al. 1998).

Reassurance. Children with CRPS-I and their parents have usually been to many different physicians and have received different explanations and suggestions for diagnosis and treatment. To gain the child's and parent's confidence that the problem is not, for example, in the foot but in the pain signal transmission takes time. We tell the child that this is not an unknown disease in the foot but a well-known and not uncommon pain syndrome that will resolve. We explain in understandable words how pain transmission works and discuss the planned diagnostic and therapeutic interventions. This conversation usually relieves a lot of stress and promotes trust. While this approach may be seen as a positive placebo effect, it still must be considered beneficial.

Sympathetic block. In Stockholm we perform an intravenous regional sympathetic block with guanethidine in an early stage (Olsson and Berde 1993). Approximately half of the children will be completely cured by one block. This result contrasts with adult studies. For example, in a double-blind, randomized multi-center study, Ramamurthy and Hoffman (1995) gave 60 patients with CRPS-I one, two, or four guanethidine blocks and found no short-term or long-term differences in pain scores. Others have confirmed these results; Kaplan et al. (1996) conclude that intravenous regional guanethidine block does not provide long-term pain relief and is associated with adverse effects in over one-third of patients. In children the block is given under general anesthesia, which may explain the good results. Majlis et al. (1997) studied the effect of intravenous sodium amytal on cutaneous limb temperatures and found that adult CRPS-I patients showed different changes in skin temperatures after sodium amytal compared to a control group. Could thiopentone, general anesthesia, or the tourniquet positively influence the outcome? Randomized double-blind studies are needed, but these must be done as multicenter studies because few centers treat sufficient numbers of patients.

In general anesthesia (we use i.v. induction with thiopentone followed by inhalation anesthesia using sevoflurane in nitrous oxide and oxygen), an i.v. cannula is inserted in the affected limb. After emptying the limb of blood, a tourniquet is applied proximal to the area of pain and a pressure of 100 mm Hg above systolic blood pressure is applied. Guanethidine 10–30 mg in 10–25 mL of saline, depending on the size of the extremity distal to the tourniquet, is injected intravenously. The tourniquet is then maintained for 20 minutes to fix the drug in the tissues. When pain is localized in a distal extremity, the tourniquet is usually applied on the lower part of the extremity to yield a high concentration of guanethidine in the affected area. Other types of sympathetic block are not used very often in children. Blocks with local anesthetics could serve as indicators of sympathetically maintained pain (SMP), but the effect is usually short. Children usually are not given regional blocks without deep sedation or general anesthesia.

Surgical and chemical destruction of sympathetic ganglia have been used, even in children. These procedures are associated with adverse effects and are traumatic and invasive. The prognosis of CRPS-I in children is believed to be better than in adults, and destructive procedures should be used very restrictively. Radiofrequency techniques have been advocated as less invasive and have also been applied in children (Wilkinsson 1996), as has thoracoscopic sympathectomy (Honjyo et al. 1997). When a sympathetic block gives pain relief, the pain is classified as SMP, and when relief is not obtained it is called sympathetically independent pain (SIP). One patient may have SMP or partial SMP while another with similar symptoms may have SIP or may manifest SMP or SIP at different times (Boas 1996).

Sympathetic block and pain alleviation can also be accomplished by continuous epidural or axillary block. It has to be performed as inpatient care, and we have used it for 3–5 days in a few therapy-resistant cases. The Boston group has used this technique more in children (Wilder et al. 1992).

Physiotherapy is advocated as a mainstay in the treatment of CRPS-I (Hood-White and Gainor 1997). Bernstein et al. (1978) hospitalized children up to 7 weeks for intense physiotherapy focused on sensory stimulation. There is no proof that physiotherapy is effective in treating CRPS-I, but its use seems plausible for several reasons. Immobilization could have negative effects. If the spinal cord corresponding to the area of pain is deprived of normal sensory input, a loss of normal segmental inhibition by LTM-fiber input may occur. Inhibitory effects of motor neuron activation could also be of value. Contracture prophylaxis is probably of less importance in most cases in children, which are usually not longstanding or therapy resistant. A physiotherapist experienced in treating children with pain syndromes is an important member of the multidisciplinary team. Early physiotherapy after trauma and avoidance of immobilization when not necessary may prevent the syndrome (Beattie 1995). After an orthopedic surgeon joined our multidisciplinary pain treatment team, the incidence of CRPS-I declined. We believe that early physiotherapy, activation, and the surgeon's simple explanation to the patient of the early signs prevented the development of severe CRPS-I in many cases. Early recognition is important, and so emergency physicians must be aware of the syndrome (Parrillo 1998).

TENS has also been advocated as effective in the treatment of CRPS-I in children (Stanton-Hicks et al. 1998). Our experience is less positive than that of the Boston group.

Psychological intervention. In Stockholm a team consisting of a pediatric psychiatrist and a psychologist is usually involved to evaluate potential stress factors and to aid in using coping strategies in therapy-resistant cases.

Dorsal column stimulation (DCS). In three girls with extremely therapy-resistant CRPS-I with high pain scores, we have used percutaneous electrodes for spinal cord stimulation. A 13-year-old girl with CRPS-I in one foot that was unresponsive to sympathetic block or any drug therapy including amitriptyline, had complete pain relief with DCS. It was recently discontinued after 3 years, and the girl seems completely cured. One 19-year-old girl has used DCS for 4 months with good to moderate effect, and one 14-year-old girl with CRPS-I in the hand after a minor trauma also had good results, but she developed an infection and the stimulator was removed. After 4 months her pain returned, and she is now scheduled for a second DCS. The patient must be conscious and cooperate during the procedure, which usually precludes the technique in younger children.

Systemic and topical pharmacological approaches

A recent review of published clinical trial data for peripheral neuropathic pain and CRPS-I (Kingery 1997) demonstrated several potential problems with current clinical practice. Studies of CRPS-I usually include few patients, often lack placebo control or double-blinding, and use inadequate statistical analyses. The author found support for the effectiveness of corticosteroids in two studies, but limited or no support for the effectiveness of other drugs. Little has been published regarding children other than case reports and clinical suggestions. It is not clear that the same treatment used in adults is appropriate for children.

Analgesics. The patient has usually tried several analgesics before admission, and we often perform analgesic tests (see above); traditional analgesics such as opioids and NSAIDs usually have no effect. Opioids in large doses have been used in the treatment of CRPS-I in adults, including opioids given intrathecally (Becker et al. 1995). We do not use large opioid doses in children, but prefer drugs that act on central transmission (Table III).

Table III
Drugs acting on central pain transmission

Tricyclic antidepressants
NMDA-blockers, ketamine
Clonidine
Local anesthetics
Antiepileptics, gabapentine
Adenosine
Capsaicin
Others

Tricyclic antidepressants. These are the most commonly administered drugs, and at our pain clinic we use amitriptyline. We start with a low dose in the evening, 10–25 mg, and over several weeks increase the dose to 2 mg/ kg depending on effectiveness and any adverse effects. If there is a positive effect we continue for 3–4 months. The drug is believed to act through enhancing serotoninergic inhibition in the dorsal horn. Modern, more selective serotonin re-uptake inhibitors have not, however, proven to be of value in the treatment of longstanding pain. Amitriptyline also has effects on the re-uptake of noradrenaline and anticholinergic effects. Amitriptyline has substantial adverse effects such as sedation, dizziness, dry mouth, and sometimes hair loss. When oral intake is not possible, amitriptyline can be administered intravenously, although experience with this approach is limited and safety and efficacy are not well established (Collins et al. 1995). Oral bioavailability of amitriptyline is 50%.

NMDA-blockers. In the acute phase we have had good effects with intravenous ketamine (see case report above). In adult neuropathic pain syndromes, ketamine has been used orally with good results (e.g., postherpetic neuralgia; Hoffman et al. 1994). We have no experience of oral ketamine in children with CRPS-I, but it should be studied. Ketamine has beneficial effects in chronic pain states with allodynia (Persson et al. 1995). Ketamine has also been infused epidurally in a 14-year-old boy with CRPS-II (causalgia) (Takahashi et al. 1998). A low dose (25 $\mu g \cdot kg^{-1} \cdot h^{-1}$) for 10 days resulted in complete pain relief when many other traditional treatment modalities had failed. After 8 months he was still pain free. However, the safe use of ketamine spinally has not been documented. On the contrary, Karpinsky et al. (1997) documented CNS toxicity.

Clonidine has, during the past decade, been increasingly used for its analgesic effects. We have used clonidine in some patients with neuropathic pain syndromes, with occasional beneficial effects. One proposed mechanism for sympathetically maintained pain is activation of peripheral adrenergic receptors. Clonidine could block the release of noradrenaline locally by activation of alpha-2 receptors on the sympathetic terminals. Topical administration of clonidine in patients with hyperalgesic skin has a beneficial effect on pain (Davis et al. 1993). Clonidine has been used epidurally with good results in refractory cases of CRPS-I. However, long-term use of epidural infusions leads to a high incidence of infections (Rauck et al. 1993).

Anticonvulsants. Gabapentine acts on voltage-sensitive sodium channels and on GABA-mediated responses. These action seems theoretically promising for the therapy of long-lasting components of neuropathic pain. In a recent study, best results were achieved in postherpetic neuralgia and diabetic neuropathy (Rosenberg et al. 1997), but gabapentine has also been proposed for adults with CRPS-I (Mellick and Mellick 1997). We have tried gabapentine in a few cases of CRPS-I in children with no positive effect on pain. Gabapentine is not especially toxic, and adverse effects are usually few and mild. Other anticonvulsants such as carbamazepine and lamotrigine have been tried in a few cases without conclusive results.

Local anesthetics such as oral mexiletine and iv. lidocaine have been advocated (Boas et al. 1982; Tanelian and Brose 1991; Wallace et al. 1997), but their use has not been documented in children with CRPS-I.

Corticosteroids are beneficial in adults with CRPS-I. Christensen et al. (1982) reported pain relief after 12 weeks of medication with prednisone compared to placebo. The benefit for children is unknown.

Adenosine is an endogenous substance that exerts an inhibitory effect on the first synapse in the dorsal horn. It has proven effective for allodynia and other types of pain. Segerdahl and colleagues (1997) demonstrated that lower concentrations of inhalation anesthetics were needed during surgery if an adenosine infusion was given. Adenosine increases the heat pain threshold in humans, which suggests a pain-reducing capacity (Ekblom et al. 1995). Belfrage et al. (1995) have shown alleviation of evoked and spontaneous peripheral neuropathic pain by an adenosine infusion. The effect of adenosine can be reversed by theophylline (Sumida et al.1998). In children with CRPS-I including allodynia, we have conducted a double-blind study of adenosine given as an infusion at 60 $\mu g \cdot kg^{-1} \cdot min^{-1}$ for 60 minutes. We found a significant reduction of the area of allodynia in most patients but no clear effect on spontaneous pain. In a 12-year-old girl who had allodynia under the heel without spontaneous pain, the allodynia disappeared and did not return. She had been using crutches for 3 months and could not bear weight on the foot before the infusion. She went out dancing the evening after adenosine administration. In the other cases, the area of allodynia returned as soon as the infusion had been completed. Adenosine can affect circulation and respiration, and the drug has been used for 20 years to promote hypotension during anesthesia. Intravenous doses for hypotension are higher, however, than those given for neuropathic pain. Doses above 50–60 µg· kg^{-1}·min^{-1} are often associated with adverse effects such as chest pain and oppression. The half-life of adenosine is 15 seconds, which makes reduction of the dose fast and effective in treating such adverse effects. Intrathecal administration of an adenosine analogue (R-PIA) was effective in treating a case of severe intractable neuropathic pain with allodynia in a 47-year-old man (Karlsten and Gordh 1995). Adenosine seems to be a promising drug in the treatment of neuropathic pain syndromes. Optimal route of administration, dosage, and duration of infusion must be further evaluated.

Topical capsaicin. Capsaicin is a selective stimulator of C-fiber nociceptors and heat receptors. It has been widely used in studies on experimental pain. Robbins et al. (1998) applied high doses of topical capsaicin under regional anesthesia in 10 patients with CRPS. Substantial analgesia lasting 1–18 weeks was reported in nine patients.

Other drugs. Beta-blockers, calcium channel blockers, topical aspirin, topical dimethylsulfoxide, intranasal calcitonin, and many other drugs seem effective in occasional cases.

CONCLUSION

The diagnosis of neuropathic pain should be made according to the symptoms the patient exhibits. The cause can be sought in history of trauma to peripheral tissue, lesions in the nervous system, or in psychological stress factors. Often no causative factors can be identified in children with CRPS-I. In addition to looking for causative factors, clinicians should focus their treatment on breaking the vicious cycle with a sympathetic block if the pain is sympathetically maintained, and otherwise by trying to strengthen inhibition of pain transmission in the CNS, which is usually not accomplished by traditional analgesics. Physiotherapy and behavioral therapy should begin soon after the diagnosis of neuropathic pain in children.

REFERENCES

Arvin AM. Varicella-zoster virus: overview and clinical manifestations. *Semin Dermatology* 1996; 15:4–7.
Bach S, Noreng MF, Tjellden NU. Phantom limb pain in amputees during the first twelve months following limb amputation after preoperative epidural blockade. *Pain* 1988; 33:297–301.
Barker FG II. Jannetta PJ, Bissonette DJ, Larkins MV, Jho HD. The long-term outcome of microvascular decompression for trigeminal neuralgia. *N Engl J Med* 1996; 334:1077–1083.

Barrera P, Van Riel PLSM, De Jong AJL, Boerbooms LBA, Van De Putte LBA. Recurrent and migratory reflex sympathetic dystrophy. *Clin Rheumatol* 1992; 11:416–421.

Beattie TF. Reflex sympathetic dystrophy in children. Active early physiotherapy is the key to prevention. *BMJ* 1995; 311:1648–1649.

Becker WJ, Ablett DP, Harris CJ, Dold ON. Long term treatment of intractable reflex sympathetic dystrophy with intrathecal morphine. *Can J Neurol Sci* 1995; 22:153–159.

Belfrage M, Sollevi A, Segerdahl M, Sjölund KF, Hansson P. Systemic adenosine infusion alleviates spontaneous and stimulus-evoked pain in patients with peripheral neuropathic pain. *Anesth Analg* 1995; 81:713–717.

Bennet GJ. Neuropathic pain. In: Wall PD, Melzack R (Eds). *Textbook of Pain.* London: Churchill Livingstone, 1994, pp 201–224.

Bernstein BH, Singsen BH, Kent JT, et al. Reflex neurovascular dystrophy in childhood. *Pediatrics* 1978; 93:211–215.

Birklein F, Riedl B, Neundorfer B, Handwerker HO. Sympathetic vasoconstrictive reflex pattern in patients with complex regional pain syndrome. *Pain* 1998; 75:93–100.

Boas RA, Covino BG, Shahnarian A. Analgesic response to i.v. lignocaine: *Br J Anaesth* 1982; 54:501–505.

Boas RA. Complex regional pain syndromes: symptoms, signs. and differential diagnosis. In: Jänig M, Stanton-Hicks M (Eds). *Reflex Sympathetic Dystrophy: a Reappraisal.* Progress in Pain Research and Management, Vol. 6. Seattle: IASP Press, 1996, p 79–92.

Chelimsky TC, Low PA, Naessens JM, et al. Value of autonomic testing in reflex sympathetic dystrophy. *Mayo Clin Proc* 1995; 70:1029–1040.

Christensen K, Jensen EM, Noer L. The reflex sympathetic dystrophy syndrome response to treatment with systemic corticosteroids. *Acta Chir Scand* 1982; 148:653–655.

Ciccone DS, Bandilla EB, Wu W. Psychological dysfunction in patients with reflex sympathetic dystrophy. *Pain* 1997; 71:323–333.

Collins JJ, Kerner J, Sentivany S, Berde CB. Intravenous amitriptyline in pediatrics. *J Pain Symptom Manage* 1995; 10:471–475.

Dangel T. Chronic pain management in children. Part I: cancer and phantom pain. *Paediatr Anaesth* 1998; 8:5–10.

Davis KD, Treede RD, Raja SN, Meyer RA, Campbell JN. Topical application of clonidine relieves hyperalgesia in patients with sympathetically maintained pain. *Pain* 1993; 54:361–362.

Egle UT, Hoffman SO. Psychosomatische Zusammenhänge bei sympatischer Reflexdystrophie (Morbus Zudeck). *Psychother Psychosom Med Psychol* 1990; 40:123–135.

Ekblom A, Segerdahl M, Sollevi A. Adenosine increase the cutaneous heat pain threshold in healthy volunteers. *Acta Anaesth Scand* 1995; 39:717–722.

Escolar DM, Jones HR Jr. Pediatric radial mononeuropathies: a clinical and electromyographic study of sixteen children with review of the literature. *Muscle Nerve* 1996; 19:876–883.

Ferrera PC, Curran CB, Swanson H. Etiology of pediatric ischemic stroke. *Am J Emerg Med* 1997; 15:671–679.

Galer BS, Butler S, Jensen MP. Case reports and hypothesis: a neglect-like syndrome may be responsible for the motor disturbance in CRPS-I. *J Pain Symptom Manage* 1995; 10:385–391.

Gallagher AC, Trounce JQ. Cerebral aqueduct stenosis presenting with limb pain. *Dev Med Child Neurology* 1998; 49:349–351.

Geertzen JHB, de Bruijn H, de Bruijn-Kofman AT, Arendzen JH. Reflex sympathetic dystrophy: early treatment and psychological aspects. *Arch Phys Med Rehabil* 1994; 75:442–445.

Gilbert A. Long term evaluation of brachial plexus surgery in obstetrical palsy. *Hand Clin* 1995; 11:583–594.

Goodman JE, McGrath PJ. The epidemiology of pain in children and adolescents: a review. *Pain* 1991; 46:247–264.

Gruener G, Dyck PJ. Quantitative sensory testing: methodology, applications and future direction. *J Clin Neurophys* 1994; 11:568–583.

Heyck H. *Headache and Facial Pain.* Chicago: Yearbook Medical Publishers, 1981, pp 125–126.

Hoffman V, Coppejans H, Vercauteren M, Adriaensen H. Successful treatment of postherpetic neuralgia with oral ketamine. *Clin J Pain* 1994; 10:240–242.

Honjyo K, Hamasaki Y, Kita M, et al. An 11-year-old girl with reflex sympathetic dystrophy successfully treated by thoracoscopic sympathectomy. *Acta Paediatr* 1997; 86:903–905.

Hood-White R, Gainor J. Reflex sympathetic dystrophy in a 8-year old: successful treatment by physical therapy. *Orthopedics* 1997; 20:73–74.

Jänig W. The puzzle of reflex sympathetic dystrophy: mechanisms, hypotheses, open questions. In: Jänig M, Stanton-Hicks M (Eds). *Reflex Sympathetic Dystrophy: a Reappraisal.* Progress in Pain Research and Management, Vol. 6. Seattle: IASP Press, 1996.

Kakourou T, Theodoridou M, Mostrou G, et al. Herpes zoster in children. *J Am Academy Derm* 1998; 39:207–210.

Kaplan R, Claudio M, Kepes E, Gu XF. Intravenous guanethidine in patients with reflex sympathetic dystrophy. *Acta Anaesthesiol Scand* 1996; 40:1216–1222.

Karlsten R, Gordh T Jr. An A1-selective adenosine agonist abolishes allodynia elicited by vibration and touch after intrathecal injection. *Anesth Analg* 1995; 80:844–847.

Karpinski N, Dunn J, Hansen L, Masliah E. Subpial vacuolar myelopathy after intrathecal ketamine: report of a case. *Pain* 1997; 73:103–105.

Kingery WS. A critical review of controlled clinical trials for peripheral neuropathic pain and complex regional pain syndromes. *Pain* 1997; 73:123–139.

Krane EJ, Heller LB. The prevalence of phantom sensation and pain in pediatric amputees. *J Pain Symptom Manage* 1995; 10:21–29.

Kurvers HA, Jacobs MJ, Beuk RJ, et al. Reflex sympathetic dystrophy: evolution of microcirculatory disturbances in time. *Pain* 1995; 60:333–340.

Lloyd-Thomas AR, Lauder G. Reflex sympathetic dystrophy in children. *BMJ* 1995; 310:1648–1649.

Lynch ME. Psychological aspects of reflex sympathetic dystrophy: a review of the adult and paediatric literature. *Pain* 1992; 49:337–347.

Majlis A, Plapler P, Ashby P, Shoichet R, Roe S. Effect of intravenous sodium amytal on cutaneous limb temperatures and sympathetic skin responses in normal subjects and pain patients with and without CRPS. *Pain* 1997; 70:59–68.

Meh D, Denislic M. Subclinical neuropathy in type I diabetic children. *Electroencephalogr Clin Neurophysiol* 1998; 109:274–280.

Mellick GA, Mellick LB. Reflex sympathetic dystrophy treated with gabapentine. *Arch Phys Med Rehabil* 1997; 78:98–105.

Melzack R, Israel R, Lacroix R, Schutz G. Phantom limbs in people with congenital limb deficiency or amputation in early childhood. *Brain* 1997; 120:1603–1620.

Merskey H, Bogduk N. *Classification of Chronic Pain: Description of Chronic Pain Syndromes and Definition of Terms,* 2nd ed. Seattle: IASP Press, 1994.

Mikkelsson M, Salminen JJ, Sourander A, Kautiainen H. Contributing factors to the persistence of musculoskeletal pain in preadolescents: a prospective 1-year follow-up study. *Pain* 1998; 77:67–72.

Ochoa JL. Guest editorial: essence, investigation, and management of "neuropathic" pains: hopes from acknowledgement of chaos. *Muscle Nerve* 1993; 16:997–1008.

Ochoa JL. Editorial: Reflex? Sympathetic? Dystrophy? Triple questioned again. *Mayo Clinic Proc* 1995; 70:1124–1126.

Olsson GL. Morphine test as a diagnostic tool in long-standing pain. *Proceedings of the 3rd International Symposium on Pediatric Pain.* Philadelphia: IASP, 1994, p 186.

Olsson GL, Berde CB. Neuropathic pain in children and adolescents. In: Schechter NL, Berde CB, Yaster M (Eds). *Pain in Infants, Children and Adolescents.* Baltimore: Williams and Wilkins, 1993, pp 473–493.

Olsson GL, Arnér S, Hirsch G. Reflex sympathetic dystrophy in children. *Adv Pain Research Therapy* 1990; 15:323–331.

Olsson GL, Lönnqvist PA, Lundeberg S. Reflex sympathetic dystrophy in children: a five year follow-up. *Proceedings of the 2nd International Symposium on Pediatric Pain.* Montreal: IASP, 1991.

Parrillo SJ. Reflex sympathetic dystrophy in children. *Pediatr Emerg Care* 1998; 14:217–220.

Persson J, Axelsson G, Hallin RG, Gustafsson LL. Beneficial effects of ketamine in a chronic pain state with allodynia, possibly due to central sensitization. *Pain* 1995; 60:217–222.

Raja SN, Treede R-D, Davis KD, Campbell JN. Systemic alpha-adrenergic blockade with phentolamine: a diagnostic test for sympathetically maintained pain. *Anesthesiology* 1991; 74:691–698.

Ramamurthy S, Hoffman J. The guanethidine study group. Intravenous regional guanethidine in the treatment of reflex sympathetic dystrophy/causalgia: a randomized, double-blind study. *Anesth Analg* 1995; 81:718–723.

Rauck RL, Eisenach JC, Jackson K, Young LD, Southern J. Epidural clonidine treatment for refractory reflex sympathetic dystrophy. *Anesthesiology* 1993; 79:1163–1169.

Robbins WR, Staats PS, Levine J, et al. Treatment of intractable pain with topical large-dose capsaicin: preliminary report. *Anesth Analg* 1998; 86:579–583.

Rosenberg JM, Harrel C, Ristic H, Werner RA, Michael de Rosayro. The effect of gabapentine on neuropathic pain. *Clin J Pain* 1997; 13:251–255.

Santinelli R, Tolone C, Toraldo R, et al. Familiar idiopathic intracranial hypertension with spinal and radicular pain. *Arch Neurol* 1998; 55:854–856.

Schondorf R. The role of the sympathetic skin response in the assessment of autonomic function. In: Low PA (Ed). *Clinical Autonomic Disorders.* New York: Little and Brown, 1993, pp 231–241.

Schiffenbauer J, Fagien M. Reflex sympathetic dystrophy involving multiple extremities. *J Rheumatol* 1993; 20:165–169.

Segerdahl M, Irestedt L, Sollevi A. Antinociceptive effect of peroperative adenosine infusion in abdominal hysterectomy. *Acta Anaesth Scand* 1997; 41:473–479

Sherry DD, Weisman R. Psychologic aspects of childhood reflex neurovascular dystrophy. *Pediatrics* 1988; 81:572–578.

Stanton-Hicks M, Jänig W, Hassenbusch S, et al. Reflex sympathetic dystrophy: changing concept and taxonomy. *Pain* 1995; 63:127–133.

Stanton-Hicks M, Baron R, Boas R, et al. Complex regional pain syndromes: guidelines for therapy. *Clin J Pain* 1998; 12:155–166.

Sumida T, Smith MA, Maehara Y, Collins JG, Kitahata. Spinal R-phenyl-isopropyl adenosine inhibits spinal dorsal horn neurons responding to noxious heat stimulation in the absence and presence of sensitization. *Pain* 1998; 74:307–313.

Takahashi H, Miyazaki M, Nambu T, Yamagida H, Morita S. The NMDA-receptor antagonist ketamine abolishes neuropathic pain after epidural administration in a clinical case. *Pain* 1998; 75:391–394.

Tanelian DL, Brose WG. Neuropathic pain can be relieved by drugs that are use-dependent sodium channel blockers: lidocaine, carbamazepine, and mexiletine. *Anesthesiology* 1991; 74:949–951.

Torebjörk HE, Lundberg LE, LaMotte RH. Central changes in processing of mechanoreceptive input in capsaicin-induced secondary hyperalgesia in humans. *J Physiol* 1992; 448:765–780.

van der Laan L, Veldman PH, Goris RJ. Severe complications of reflex sympathetic dystrophy: infections, ulcers, chronic edema, dystonia, and myoclonus. *Arch Phys Med Rehab* 1998; 79:424–429.

Veldman PH, Goris RJ. Multiple RSD. Which patients are at risk for developing a recurrence of RSD in the same or another limb. *Pain* 1997; 71:207–208.

Walker SM, Cousins MJ. Complex regional pain syndromes: including the "reflex sympathetic dystrophy" and "causalgia." *Anaesth Int Care* 1997; 25:113–125.

Wallace MS, Laitin S, Licht D, Yaksh TL. Concentration-effect relations for intravenous lidocaine infusions in human volunteers: effect on acute sensory thresholds and capsaicin-evoked hyperpathia. *Anesthesiology* 1997; 86:1262–1272.

Weintraub M, Adde MA, Venzon DJ, et al. Severe atypical neuropathy associated with administration of hematopoietic colony-stimulating factors and vincristine. *J Clin Oncol* 1996; 14:935–940.

Wilder RT, Berde CB, Wolohan M, et al. Reflex sympathetic dystrophy in children. Clinical characteristics and follow-up of seventy patients. *J Bone Joint Surg Am* 1992; 74:910–919.

Wilder RT. Reflex sympathetic dystrophy in children and adolescents: differences from adults. In: Jänig M, Stanton-Hicks M (Eds). *Reflex Sympathetic Dystrophy: a Reappraisal.* Progress in Pain Research and Management, Vol. 6. Seattle: IASP Press 1996, pp 67–77.

Wilkins KL, McGrath PJ, Finley GA, Katz J. Phantom limb sensations and phantom limb pain in child and adolescent amputees. *Pain* 1998; 78:7–12.

Wilkinsson HA. Percutaneous radiofrequency upper thoracic sympathectomy. *Neurosurgery* 1996; 38:715–725.

Yglesias A, Narbona J, Vanaclocha V, Artieda J. Chiari type I malformation, glossopharyngeal neuralgia and central sleep apnea in a child. *Dev Med Child Neurology* 1996; 38:1126–1130.

Correspondence to: Gunnar L. Olsson, MD, PhD, Pain Treatment Services, Astrid Lindgren Children's Hospital, Karolinska Hospital, S-17176 Stockholm, Sweden. Tel: 46-8-51777270; Fax: 46-8-51777265; email: gunol@ child.ks.se.

Chronic and Recurrent Pain in Children and Adolescents, Progress in Pain Research and Management, Vol. 13, edited by Patrick J. McGrath and G. Allen Finley, IASP Press, Seattle, © 1999.

6

The Management of Pain in Sickle Cell Disease

Neil L. Schechter

Department of Pediatrics, St. Francis Hospital and Medical Center, Hartford, Connecticut, USA

Sickle cell disease is the name given to a genetically inherited group of disorders characterized by large amounts of hemoglobin S in the red blood cells. Although sickle cell disease is often accompanied by various pain problems that may make it incapacitating and require hospitalization, there has been little research on the treatment of pain in this disease. This lack of research, coupled with the socioeconomic and racial disparity that frequently sets sickle cell patients apart from their providers, allows for the frequent undertreatment of pain in this population.

Sickle cell disease typically occurs in patients of African ancestry. This hemoglobin anomaly may offer some protection against malaria, as it appears that the morbidity and mortality of malaria are decreased in patients with sickle cell disease and that the frequency of cerebral malaria is dramatically reduced. This finding may account for the persistence of the gene.

Sickle cells were first described by Herrick in 1910. In 1949, Linus Pauling and colleagues threw light on sickle cell disease at the molecular level when they demonstrated that hemoglobin S had a different electrophoretic pattern than "normal" hemoglobin. It was eventually discovered that sickle cell disease results from a mutation on the sixth chromosome where valine is substituted for glutamic acid (Bunn and Forget 1986). This understanding has led to a variety of therapies for sickle cell disease, but no cure is available. Therefore, the symptoms of sickle cell disease (anemia, delayed secondary sexual characteristics, shortened lifespan, and episodes of severe pain) must be treated individually.

Sickle cell disease affects more than 50,000 Americans and approximately 1 in 375 African Americans, and is among the most prevalent genetic diseases in the United States (Sickle Cell Disease Guideline Panel 1993).

Eight percent of the African American population have sickle cell trait, essentially a benign condition without anemia or vaso-occlusive pain episodes, although some studies have reported an increased risk for hematuria and sudden death (Ballas 1998).

PAIN SYNDROMES IN SICKLE CELL DISEASE

Although the pain associated with sickle cell disease manifests itself in many different ways, the dominant pain is that associated with unpredictable and relentless vaso-occlusive episodes. The terms for sickle cell disease in a variety of African languages emphasize this point (Shapiro 1993). In Banyangi, the term for sickle cell disease is "Adep," which means "beaten up." In Ewe, sickle cell disease is known as "Nuidudui," which means "body chewing," and in Ga, it is called "chwechwechwe," which means "relentless, repetitive chewing." These terms demonstrate the unending, gnawing quality of pain associated with vaso-occlusive episodes.

Several pain syndromes are associated with sickle cell disease, as is the case with many chronic diseases. These include acute pain, chronic pain, and pain secondary to diagnosis or treatment. The predominant source of acute pain is vaso-occlusive pain. Bone infarction and bone marrow infarction are also sources of pain, as are infections such as osteomyelitis or cholecystitis. The acute chest syndrome that frequently occurs during vaso-occlusive episodes is characterized by pleuritic chest, hypoxia, and pulmonary infiltrates, and is another source of severe, acute pain. Finally, bowel infarction and priapism are also sources of acute pain in sickle cell disease.

Sickle cell disease is also associated with various chronic pains. These are more frequent in adults than in children, and may result from aseptic necrosis or bone infarction. Various arthropathies may be another source of chronic pain, as may vertebral body collapse, which may be associated with chronic back pain, and poor circulation leading to persistent leg ulcers.

Pain from diagnosis and treatment is not uncommon in sickle cell disease and other chronic diseases. Pain related to diagnosis may be caused by biopsies or multiple venipunctures and i.v. line placements. Treatment-related pain includes postoperative pain, for example from cholecystectomy or surgical removal of bowel infarction.

Pain in sickle cell disease differs in many ways from pain in cancer (Ballas 1998). Pain is frequently a hallmark of sickle cell disease, while it is not inevitable in cancer. The pain in sickle cell disease is mostly acute, with recurrent episodes of severe pain early on yielding to chronic pain later in life. In cancer, the pain is often chronic and relatively stable, except when there is disease extension. In sickle cell disease, the pain is usually generalized, while in cancer it is typically localized to the area affected. In sickle cell disease, although the lifespan can be reduced, it often extends over many decades, while cancer, if not cured, may cause death within a few months or years. In sickle cell disease, families tend to be socioeconomically disadvantaged and are often African American, whereas in cancer, socioeconomic status is variable, as are the affected ethnic and racial groups. Finally, and very significantly, in sickle cell disease, the attitude of providers has historically been somewhat negative and distrustful, while in cancer the attitude is often quite positive and supportive.

VASO-OCCLUSIVE EPISODES

By far the most common source of pain in sickle cell disease is the vaso-occlusive episode or pain crisis. Pain appears to stem from red blood cells that contain inflexible hemoglobin S becoming trapped in smaller vessels in the microcirculation. Occlusion slows capillary blood flow, which yields hypoxemia and produces further sickling, which yields further occlusion and hypoxemia. Ischemia, infarction, and tissue necrosis may result.

These episodes may be provoked by high altitude, extremes of temperature, infection, dehydration, or stress and fatigue. There may be no obvious initiating cause, however. Pain tends to be widespread during these episodes and most commonly occurs in the lumbar spine, abdomen, femoral shaft, ribs, and knees (Serjeant et al. 1994). There is some relationship of pain site to age. Very young children often suffer from dactylitis (a swelling of the hands), while long bone pain is more common among school-aged children. In adolescence, abdominal pain is more frequent, and in young and later adulthood, pain in the back predominates, particularly in the lumbar area.

Vaso-occlusive episodes do not occur in every person with sickle cell disease. Approximately 30–40% of patients rarely or never experience pain. Fifty percent have several episodes per year, and 20% have frequent episodes. In fact, 5% of sickle cell disease patients account for 30% of all vaso-occlusive episodes (Platt et al. 1991). Platt and colleagues also suggest that pain is a measure of the clinical severity of the illness and that the number of vaso-occlusive episodes correlates directly with mortality.

Although a typical vaso-occlusive episode lasts between 2 and 11 days, Ballas (1995) has defined a number of phases within each episode. These include the prodromal phase, which occurs before the episode begins and during which up to 58% of patients report unusual feelings such as tingling or parasthesias. This phase may last up to 2 days prior to the onset of the episode. Following the prodromal phase is the initial phase or evolving infarctive phase, which lasts 1–2 days. At this point the typical pain associated with the episode begins and reaches its peak. Following the initial phase is the established phase, also known as the postinfarctive or inflammatory phase, which lasts approximately 3–7 days. During this phase, the pain is persistent, severe, and steady. Finally, the resolving phase, also called the recovery or post-episode phase, brings with it a gradual decrease in pain severity over 1–2 days.

BARRIERS TO CARE

Although pain is one of the hallmarks of sickle cell disease and constitutes a huge source of suffering and disability in this population, remarkably little research has documented the pain or evaluated modalities to ameliorate it. At least in part, this has resulted from the ethnocultural disparity between the health care provider and the patient. Frequently, because of their minority status, these patients are poor and less well educated than are their providers. This yields potential distrust on the part of the providers as well as significant concerns about opioid addiction and potential opioid diversion. Undertreatment is further supported by the lack of adequate research. It is striking that the Agency for Health Care Policy and Research Guidelines on acute pain management (Acute Pain Management Guideline Panel 1992) and even the panel addressing sickle cell disease (Sickle Cell Disease Guideline Panel 1993) have little to report on the treatment of pain in sickle cell disease.

These issues have created a cycle of undertreatment (see Fig. 1) in which providers distrust their patients and typically provide inadequate analgesia (Schechter et al. 1988). Patients who remain in pain often become more manipulative and melodramatic in an attempt to obtain adequate analgesia. However, providers interpret such behavior as further support for opioid addiction, which causes them to further undertreat, and so the cycle continues.

Another barrier to adequate pain management is the lack of continuity of care within most institutions for this population. Sickle cell patients require specialized treatment, and providers often require specialized knowledge. Unfortunately, these patients are frequently treated in many different parts of the institution (the emergency room, clinics, and inpatient units), and as a result, there is often a disparity of knowledge among providers and a discontinuity in treatment among sites.

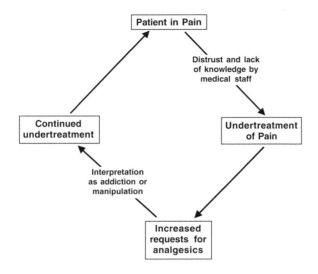

Fig. 1. Cycle of undertreatment in sickle cell disease.

PRINCIPLES OF CHRONIC PAIN MANAGEMENT

A number of general principles are important in chronic pain management and in particular in the pain associated with sickle cell disease in children. The goal of therapy should be adequate pain control as defined by the child and the family. Families should be asked about their expectations regarding treatment. Normal behavior should be encouraged as much as possible, and school attendance should be supported. In one study, children with sickle cell disease missed 21% of their school days, but only half of those days were lost to pain episodes (Shapiro et al. 1995). The other days were perhaps lost because of perceived vulnerability by parents. Missing so much school puts students at an enormous disadvantage and may further decrease self-esteem in this already compromised population. Every effort should be made to help keep children in school and to maintain academic performance at grade level. A further problem is that small strokes may be far more frequent among children with sickle cell disease than was previously surmised. Such strokes may create neuropsychological deficits and learning disabilities, which may further limit academic success unless recognized and addressed (Craft et al. 1993).

Parents need to be actively involved in treatment decisions and in treatment itself. This will require culturally sensitive education of patients and their families. The Sickle Cell Disease Association of America (SCDAA, 200 Corporate Pointe, Suite 495, Culver City, CA 90230, USA) has materials that may be helpful, and can connect families to support groups in their own areas.

It should be recognized that severe pain episodes are emergencies and must be treated expeditiously. Children should not have to wait for hours in an emergency department for decisions about analgesia to be made. Pain from diagnostic and treatment procedures should be aggressively treated, because inadequate treatment will set the stage for fear of subsequent medical procedures, which may generalize to fear and distrust of all health care providers (Weisman et al. 1997). This problem can be reduced by aggressive pharmacological and behavioral measures to relieve the pain of medical procedures.

Finally, assessment of pain should be integrated into the treatment plan. Assessment is the cornerstone of adequate treatment, and without frequent assessment and reassessment, an appropriate pain plan cannot be devised. Assessment should be developmentally appropriate and culturally sensitive. For example, the African American Oucher scale (Denyes and Villarruel 1991) should be considered for children between the ages of 3 and 8, while older children can use a visual analogue or numeric rating scale. For children younger than 3, physiological and behavioral parameters must be incorporated into assessment.

GENERAL APPROACH TO SICKLE CELL DISEASE PAIN

The pain of sickle cell disease needs to be approached at multiple levels—the treatment of the disease, the education of patients and medical staff, behavioral and physical strategies, and finally, pharmacological strategies.

SICKLE CELL TREATMENT

Obviously, reduction of sickling and concomitant decrease in vaso-occlusion can reduce pain. Blood transfusions by which the amount of sickle hemoglobin is diluted sometimes help ameliorate the pain of vaso-occlusive episodes. Chronic blood transfusion protocols are helpful for certain children, but have major long-term ramifications such as hemochromatosis.

A significant advance is the use of hydroxyurea, an agent that increases hemoglobin F. Initial reports suggest that hydroxyurea may decrease vaso-occlusive episodes by up to 44% in adults and 65% in children (Charache et al. 1995). Long-term consequences of chronic administration of this agent are unknown.

Finally, bone marrow transplantation has been advocated for significantly incapacitated persons with sickle cell disease. In the available studies, those who have survived bone marrow transplantation have often been cured of their disease. However, significant morbidity and mortality are associated with the procedure itself. The significant risks involved with this procedure, as well as the associated costs, will clearly limit its use for sickle cell disease.

EDUCATION

Helping individuals who have sickle cell disease understand the causes of their illness and its treatment may help children and families cope more effectively with this problem. A better understanding of the disease may also help families identify symptoms that are potentially life-threatening and require medical intervention, while reducing their worry about symptoms that are probably insignificant. Educational materials must be culturally sensitive and geared toward the educational level of this often socio-economically disadvantaged population.

The education of medical staff is also essential. Because sickle cell pain may have no objective markers and because of the racial and socioeconomic disparities between patient and provider, the clinical visit is often accompanied by suspicion. Providers should be aware that the pain of sickle cell vaso-occlusive episodes is significantly greater than typical postoperative pain and requires approximately twice the analgesia (Shapiro et al. 1993). They should also be aware that no laboratory markers clearly denote the beginning or end of a vaso-occlusive episode.

To address some of these issues, Johnson et al. (1995) have developed a medical "passport" that patients can carry with them. It contains information about pain management during the last hospitalization or emergency department visit, and the type and dose of analgesia that successfully alleviated their pain. Many patients have found this particularly empowering, as they have a physical document that validates their treatment in the past and may predict their present needs.

PSYCHOLOGICAL AND PHYSICAL APPROACHES TO PAIN

Several techniques are available that do not involve the use of analgesic drugs. Before undergoing painful procedures, children and their parents should receive a direct explanation of what will happen and participate in a discussion of how it will feel. Parents need to be actively involved in all phases of care, from decisions about the treatment to coaching their children through painful procedures.

Several cognitive-behavioral approaches have been identified as extremely useful (Zeltzer and LeBaron 1982; Kuttner 1989; French et al. 1994). Most of these techniques (e.g., distraction, visual imagery, and biofeedback) are useful during painful procedures, while other techniques such as meditation, self-hypnosis, and relaxation may well have more generalized value. Distraction techniques can be extremely helpful during painful procedures and include deep breathing, blowing bubbles, and the use of party blowers and pinwheels. They may involve reading a favorite story or play or looking at novel stimuli such as pop-up books. The literature on self-hypnosis and relaxation for children with sickle cell disease includes two studies of note. One study in adults with sickle cell disease (Gil et al. 1996) involves the use of a three-session intervention where the experimental group learned six different cognitive coping techniques while the control group received disease education. Individuals in the experimental group used more coping strategies, had fewer negative thoughts, and reported less pain during laboratory-induced pain. A more comprehensive and expensive weekly intervention that lasted for 6 months was studied for children with sickle cell disease, and found to decrease the number of bad "pain days" and "bad sleep" nights (Dinges et al. 1997). Other distraction techniques, such as actively involving the child in a fantasy or suggesting that the child imagine turning off a pain switch or using an imaginary glove, which the child is told has anesthetic properties, have not been formally studied in sickle cell disease.

Physical methods such as a transcutaneous electrical nerve stimulation (TENS) unit and physical therapy may also play a role in pain control. The use of the TENS unit is clearly limited, however, because vaso-occlusive episodes tend to be widespread, whereas TENS units are more successful in treating clearly localized pain. No formal studies have investigated the use of TENS units for sickle cell disease. Physical therapy approaches, such as immobilization of the limbs with splints and local application of heat and cold, may also be part of the overall treatment plan, but again, there has been no rigorous study of their effectiveness in controlling the pain of sickle cell disease.

PHARMACOLOGICAL APPROACHES TO PAIN

Several general principles apply to the use of analgesic drugs in children. As in the case of adults, these include a preventative approach, individualization of the drug dose and the route of administration, anticipation of side effects, and use of the World Health Organization (WHO) ladder. In this schema, mild pain is treated with acetaminophen or nonsteroidal anti-inflammatory drugs (NSAIDs), moderate pain with NSAIDs and a weak opioid, and severe pain with a strong opioid. For children, it is especially imperative that painful routes of administration such as intramuscular and rectal routes should be minimized.

LOCAL ANESTHETICS

Local anesthetics should be used if possible for all needle procedures, especially for children who will require frequent phlebotomy and venous cannulation. The choices include EMLA cream, injected or iontophoresed lidocaine, a vapocoolant spray, and amethocaine gel. EMLA provides 2–4 mm of anesthesia, which is usually adequate for phlebotomy or venous cannulation, but it requires approximately 60 minutes and an occlusive dressing to work (Koren 1993). The recent release of the EMLA anesthetic disk may make its application somewhat easier. Lidocaine can be injected with a narrow-gauge needle, but it often burns when placed beneath the skin. The burning sensation can be reduced by buffering 9:1 with sodium bicarbonate (Bartfield et al. 1990). Lidocaine can also be introduced with one of several commercially available devices that use battery-induced electric current. Iontophoresis provides deeper anesthesia, but some children find it uncomfortable, and burns have been associated with its use (Zempsky et al. 1998). Vapocoolant can be sprayed directly onto the skin or applied with a cotton ball. The depth of anesthesia has not been yet ascertained. In the only study to have examined its efficacy, vapocoolant provided equivalent immediate pain control to EMLA (Reis and Holubkov 1997). Amethocaine gel is not yet available in the United States. It reportedly provides more rapid onset of anesthesia than EMLA (Lawson et al. 1995), but its side effects are unclear.

ACETAMINOPHEN AND ANTI-INFLAMMATORY DRUGS

Acetaminophen and NSAIDs are appropriate for mild pain, and can be used for moderate to severe pain in conjunction with an opioid. These agents have two problems with regard to sickle cell pain—unlike the opioids, they have a ceiling effect (a dose beyond which further drug will produce no substantial effect), and they also have significant potential side effects. Acetaminophen is hepatotoxic when used at high doses; the effect on the liver of its chronic administration in moderate doses is unknown. NSAIDs can induce gastritis and ulcers, as well as renal disease. Mild bleeding associated with gastritis may be even more significant in sickle cell patients, who may already have significantly reduced levels of hemoglobin. A new modification of the NSAIDs, the COX-2 inhibitors (Bolten 1998), may reduce the burden of these side effects (see Chapter 11). These agents, not yet approved for use in children, inhibit cyclooxygenase-2, thus targeting a more specific enzyme than the other NSAIDs; they appear to have little effect on the gastrointestinal, renal, or hematologic systems. They may represent a significant advance for persons with long-term pain who require chronic analgesic administration.

Nonetheless, the NSAIDs should still be part of the treatment of vaso-occlusive pain because of their anti-inflammatory effect. They can be used without an opioid, with a weak opioid, or even as an adjunct to potent opioids. Parental administration of ketorolac has been used for vaso-occlusive pain (Perlin et al. 1994), but its efficacy remains somewhat unclear, and the degree to which it spares morphine is not known. Other anti-inflammatory agents should be considered. A study on the use of intravenous methylprednisone at a dose of 15 mg/kg suggested a shortened duration of analgesic therapy, but rebound pain was common (Griffin et al. 1994).

OPIOIDS

Several key factors govern the use of opioids in sickle cell disease. As in any other condition, the right dose is the dose that relieves the pain. With sickle cell disease, however, there is enormous interpatient variability. In one study, plasma morphine clearances ranged from 6.2 to 59.1 $mL \cdot min^{-1} \cdot kg^{-1}$ during steady-state infusion (Dampier et al. 1995). Opioid addiction is another concern. Waldrop and Mandry (1995) examined the perception of health professionals regarding opioid addiction in emergency department patients, specifically focusing on those with sickle cell disease. Emergency department staff, residents, and nurses estimated the overall percentage of addiction to be 4%, 9%, and 7%, respectively, for all patients, and 8%, 17%, and 13% for those with sickle cell disease. All groups of health professionals overestimated opioid dependence in sickle cell patients, rating it far higher than actual dependence rates reported by previous surveys and far in excess of other groups with chronic pain problems. The frequent use of agonist-antagonist compounds (e.g., nalbuphine, pentazocine, and butorphanol) in this population is a concrete example of this concern, as these agents are not indicated for chronic pain problems according to standard clinical practice guidelines.

The route of opioid administration depends on the site where the drugs are being administered (i.e., at home or in the hospital or clinic), but in all cases, emphasis should be placed on avoiding painful procedures. Typically, "weak" opioids such as codeine or oxycodone are given at home, while morphine and meperidine are given intravenously in the hospital. New studies suggest that controlled-release morphine preparations can be administered at home and may reduce the need for hospitalization. However, studies indicate that meperidine is an inappropriate drug for use in this or any other chronic pain problem because its breakdown product, normeperidine, may cause seizures and central nervous system hyperexcitability (Tang et al. 1980; Kaiko et al. 1983). Despite this fact, meperidine remains the drug of choice for many patients with sickle cell disease who have achieved relief with it in the past and are concerned that other drugs may not provide adequate relief.

In the emergency department and inpatient units, continuous infusion and patient-controlled analgesia (PCA) are the most efficacious methods for administering morphine. As noted earlier, studies indicate that doses almost twice as high as those necessary for postoperative pain relief are necessary to relieve vaso-occlusive episodes. Although PCA seems the ideal route of administration for chronic disease patients, allowing them to control their own medication and decreasing the possibility of misperceptions by hospital staff (Schechter et al. 1988), debate continues about the administration of basal infusion in conjunction with PCA. Shapiro and colleagues (1993) reported unexpected hypoxemia at night in patients receiving a basal infusion in addition to their PCA dose. Trentadue and colleagues (1998) compared subjects using high-dose PCA and low-dose basal infusion with another group using low-dose PCA and high-dose basal infusion and found that the former group used less morphine, were hospitalized for fewer days, and reported lower pain scores. PCA should be introduced when the patient is free of pain, as it is difficult to learn the appropriate techniques in the middle of a painful episode. Meanwhile, low-dose basal infusion should be used, or long-acting oral drugs can provide a background infusion equivalent.

ANESTHETIC APPROACHES

Yaster and colleagues (1994) reported on the use of epidural analgesia for patients with pain below the fourth thoracic dermatome. They used local anesthetics supplemented by fentanyl as necessary, and reported significantly decreased pain, improved oxygenation, and dramatic improvement of acute chest syndrome. At present, however, this technique is appropriate only for children for whom conventional therapy has failed.

ADJUVANT DRUGS

Several agents that were not designed to produce analgesia may be of benefit in sickle cell pain problems. These agents may be effective at decreasing opioid sedation, addressing neuropathic pain, and improving sleep. The stimulants dextroamphetamine and methylphenidate have been found to decrease sedation associated with chronic opioid administration in cancer patients (Bruera et al. 1992). They also seem to increase the "joy of life" in certain patients. There is no literature on their use in sickle cell disease. Several of the tricyclic antidepressants, such as amitryptiline or nortriptyline, and a number of anticonvulsants such as gabapentin and carbamezapine have been successful in both children and adults with neuropathic pain (pain associated with nerve injury). This is probably not a common source of discomfort for children with sickle cell disease. Such drugs may be of use, however, in children with vertebral collapse, a crushed nerve, or other nerve entrapment injuries with nerve-related pain.

TREATMENT STRATEGIES BY SITE

HOME MANAGEMENT

The importance of education in home management cannot be overemphasized. Parents need to be taught how to manage their child's pain and when to call their primary care physician or sickle cell service. Analgesic treatment at home primarily consists of "weak" opioids such as codeine or oxycodone in conjunction with NSAIDs. Use of controlled-release opioids at home has not been rigorously studied at this time but seems promising. If such measures provide inadequate control of pain, the parents are often instructed to bring their child to the emergency department.

EMERGENCY DEPARTMENT

In the emergency department, rapid pain relief is the key. Most children who arrive have found no relief from conventional oral therapies, and therefore immediate i.v. cannulation is imperative. If high doses of oral opioids have been used at home, then 1–1.5 times the traditional starting dose of 0.1 mg/kg (i.e., 0.15 mg/kg of morphine i.v.) is appropriate with rapid titration upward. If, however, administration of opioids at home was suboptimal, then a high dose may be given intravenously followed by long-acting opioids. Jacobson and co-workers (1997) compared children who received an intravenous loading dose and then were assigned either long-acting oral morphine or intravenous morphine at a continuous infusion rate They reported similar amounts of breakthrough pain and similar pain scores for both methods, suggesting that controlled-release preparations may be suitable for treating breakthrough pain at home after initial stabilization at the emergency department. If high doses of oral analgesics have been used at home without adequate analgesia, then hospitalization may be appropriate.

DAY HOSPITAL OR SICKLE CELL DISEASE UNIT

The day hospital is a special section of the emergency department or an entirely separate unit for children with sickle cell disease. This concept has been promoted by a number of major sickle cell centers. Children enter the emergency department and are immediately triaged to this unit. There is either 8- or 24-hour coverage. Children are cared for by individuals who know sickle cell disease and have easy access to their records. Intravenous medication can be administered in a comfortable, pediatric-oriented setting. Patients are spared the indignity of convincing others of their discomfort or beginning an inappropriately slow titration regimen to achicve relief. There is little information on the financial, physical, or psychological impact of day hospitals on sickle cell treatment, and it remains to be seen whether aggressive early treatment of sickle cell vaso-occlusive episodes diminishes the need for subsequent hospitalization.

INPATIENT CARE

Children are admitted to inpatient care if they have inadequately responded to medications at home or in the emergency department. A continuous infusion is often begun in children under the age of 6, and patient-controlled analgesia with a low-dose basal infusion is started in children over 6. An oral NSAID or intravenous ketorolac is often used as well. Frequent assessment is necessary, and rapid titration is essential. Depending on the severity of the episode, children remain in the hospital anywhere from 2 to 12 days. A number of weaning strategies have been devcloped, but in general the pain should be adequately controlled solely by oral medications before discharge is contemplated.

SUMMARY

The severity and unpredictability of the pain, the lack of objective markers, and the racial and socioeconomic disparity between the patients and providers make pain in sickle cell disease particularly difficult to manage. An air of distrust has permeated the clinical arena and leads to frequent undertreatment. Inadequate pain relief yields prolonged discomfort and convinces patients that they need to be more aggressive in their requests for analgesia, which confirms in the minds of clinicians that the patients are drug seeking. It is imperative that this cycle be broken.

Effective strategies for a comprehensive approach to the pain of sickle cell disease include education, cognitive-behavioral approaches, and a host of analgesic agents. New interventions to control the disease itself may also reduce the burden of pain. Available techniques clearly can reduce the pain associated with sickle cell disease if they are used expeditiously. Specific research is urgently needed to further reduce the pain associated with this problem.

REFERENCES

Acute Pain Management Guideline Panel. Acute pain management: operative or medical procedures and trauma. *Clinical Practice Guideline.* AHCPR Pub No 92-0032. Rockville, MD: Agency for Health Care Policy and Research, Public Health Service, US Department of Health and Human Services, 1992.

Ballas SK. The sickle cell painful crisis in adults: phases and objective signs. *Hemoglobin* 1995; 19:323–333.

Ballas SK. *Sickle Cell Pain.* Seattle: IASP Press, 1998, pp 14–16.

Bartfield JM, Gennis P, Barbera J, et al. Buffered versus plain lidocaine as a local anesthetic for simple laceration repair. *Ann Emerg Med* 1990; 19:1387–1389.

Bolten WW. Scientific rationale for specific inhibition of cox 2. *J Rheumatol* 1998; 51(Suppl):2–7.

Bruera E, Fainsinger R, MacEachern T, Hanson J. The use of methylphenidate in patients with incident cancer pain receiving regular opiates. A preliminary report. *Pain* 1992; 50:75–77.

Bunn HF, Forget BG (Eds). *Hemoglobin: Molecular, Clinical, and Genetic Aspects.* Philadelphia: Saunders, 1986.

Charache S. Terrin ML, Moore RD, et al. Effect of hydroxyurea on the frequency of painful crises in sickle cell anemia. *N Engl J Med* 1995; 332:1317–1322.

Craft S, Schatz J, Glauser TA, et al. Neuropsychologic effects of stroke in children with sickle cell anemia. *J Pediatr* 1993; 123:712–717.

Dampier CD, Setty BN, Logan J, et al. Intravenous morphine pharmacokinetics in pediatric patients with sickle cell disease. *J Pediatr* 1995; 126:461–467.

Denyes MJ, Villarruel AM. *The African American Version of the Oucher.* Detroit, MI: Wayne State University, 1991.

Dinges DF, Whitehouse WG, Orne EC, et al. Self-hypnosis training as an adjunctive treatment in management of pain associated with sickle cell disease. *Int J Clin Exp Hypn* 1997; 45:417–432.

French FM, Painter EC, Coury DL. Blowing away shot pain: a technique for pain management during immunization. *Pediatrics* 1994; 93:384–388.

Gil KM, Wilson JJ, Edens JJ, et al. Effects of cognitive coping skills training on coping strategies and experimental pain sensitivity in African American adults with sickle cell disease. *Health Psychol* 1996; 15:3–10.

Griffin TC, McIntire D, Buchanan G. High dose intravenous methylprednisolone therapy for pain in children and adolescents with sickle cell disease. *N Engl J Med* 1994; 330:733–737.

Herrick JB. Peculiar elongated and sickle-shaped red blood corpuscles in a case of severe anemia. *Arch Intern Med* 1910; 6:517–521.

Jacobson SJ, Kopecky EA, Joshi P, Babul N. Randomized trial of oral morphine for painful episodes of sickle cell disease in children. *Lancet* 1997; 350:1358–1361.

Johnson SS, Odesina V, Schechter NL, et al. A parent/patient held sickle cell pain relief record [Abstract]. Annual Meeting, National Sickle Cell Program, Boston, 1995.

Kaiko RF, Foley KM, Grabinski PY, et al. Central nervous system excitatory effects of meperidine in cancer patients. *Ann Neurol* 1983; 13:180–185.

Koren G. Use of eutectic mixture of local anesthetics in young children for procedure related pain. *J Pediatr* 1993; 122(5), part 2:30–35.

Kuttner L. Management of young children's acute pain and anxiety during invasive medical procedures. *Pediatrician* 1989; 16:39–44.

Lawson RA, Smart NG, Gudgeon AC, Morton NS. Evaluation of an amethocaine gel preparation for percutaneous analgesia before venous cannulation in children. *Br J Anaesth* 1995; 75:282–285.

Pauling L, Itano H, Singer SJ, Wells IC. Sickle cell anemia: a molecular disease. *Science* 1949; 110:543–548.

Perlin E, Finke H, Castro O, et al. Enhancement of pain control with ketorolac tromethamine in patients with sickle cell vaso occlusive crisis. *Am J Hematol* 1994; 46:43–47.

Platt OS, Thorington BD, Brambilla DJ, et al. Pain in sickle cell disease: rates and risk factors. *N Engl J Med* 1991; 325:11–16.

Reis EC, Holubkov R. Vapocoolant spray is equally effective as EMLA cream in reducing immunization pain in school-aged children. *Pediatrics* 1997; 100:6:e5.

Schechter NL, Berrien FB, Katz SM. The use of patient controlled analgesia in adolescents with sickle cell pain crisis: a preliminary report. *J Pain Symptom Manage* 1988; 3:109–113.

Serjeant GR, Ceulaer CD, Lethbridge et al. The painful crisis of homozygous sickle cell disease: clinical features. *Br J Haematol* 1994; 87:586–591.

Shapiro BS. Management of painful episodes in sickle cell disease. In: Schechter NL, Berde CB, Yaster M (Eds). *Pain in Infants, Children, and Adolescents.* Baltimore: Williams and Wilkins, 1993, pp 385–410.

Shapiro BS, Cohen DE, Howe CJ. Patient controlled analgesia in sickle cell related pain. *J Pain Symptom Manage* 1993; 8:22–28.

Shapiro BS, Dinges DF, Orne EC, et al. Home management of sickle cell related pain in children and adolescents: natural history and impact on school. *Pain* 1995; 61:139–144.

Sickle Cell Disease Guideline Panel. Clinical practice guideline for sickle cell disease: screening, diagnosis, management and counseling in newborns and infants. AHCPR Pub No 93-0562. Rockville, MD: Agency for Health Care Policy and Research, Public Health Service, US Department of Health and Human Services, 1993.

Tang R, Shimomura S, Rotblatt M. Meperidine induced seizures in sickle cell patients. *Hospital Formulary* 1980; 76:764–772.

Trentadue NO, Kachoyeanos MK, Lea G. A comparison of two regimens of patient controlled analgesia for children with sickle cell disease. *J Pediatric Nurs* 1998; 13:15–19.

Waldrop RD, Mandry C. Health professionals perceptions of opioid dependence among patients with pain. *Am J Emerg Med* 1995; 13:529–531.

Weisman SJ, Bernstein B, Schechter NL. The consequences of inadequate analgesia during painful procedures in children. *Arch Pediatr Adolesc Med* 1997; 152:147–149.

Yaster M, Tobin JR, Billet C, et al. Epidural analgesia in the management of severe vaso-occlusive sickle cell crisis. *Pediatrics* 1994; 93:310–315.

Zeltzer L, LeBaron S. Hypnotic and nonhypnotic techniques for reduction of pain and anxiety during painful procedures in children and adolescents with cancer. *J Pediatr* 1982; 101:1032–1035.

Zempsky WT, Anand KJ, Sullivan KM, et al. Lidocaine iontophoresis for topical anesthesia before intravenous line placement in children. *J Pediatr* 1998; 132:1061–1063.

Correspondence to: Neil L. Schechter, MD, Department of Pediatrics, St. Francis Hospital and Medical Center, 114 Woodland Street, Hartford, CT 06105, USA. Tel: 860-714-4874; Fax: 860-714-8054; email: nschecht@stfranciscare.org.

Chronic and Recurrent Pain in Children and Adolescents, Progress in Pain Research and Management, Vol. 13, edited by Patrick J. McGrath and G. Allen Finley, IASP Press, Seattle, © 1999.

7

Recurrent Headaches in Children and Adolescents

Bo Larsson

Department of Public Health and Caring Sciences, Uppsala University, Uppsala, Sweden

Epidemiological surveys conducted in various countries indicate that recurrent, nonorganic headaches are one of the most common somatic complaints in schoolchildren and adolescents (Passchier and Orlebeke 1985; Larsson 1991). Headaches are among the most common health complaints in adolescents, as reported by the adolescents themselves (Berg Kelly et al. 1991), by their mothers (Newacheck et al. 1991), and by health professionals (DiMario 1992). Headache is the most extensively investigated pain complaint in nonclinical populations of school-aged children and adolescents (Goodman and McGrath 1991). Children with recurrent headaches are more likely to have other types of pain, such as back or abdominal pain (Carlsson 1996a).

Earlier epidemiological studies relied primarily on parent reports for information on headaches in children and adolescents. However, parents and their children provide inconsistent reports of various types of internal problems (Achenbach et al. 1987). For example, Deubner (1977) found that reports from adolescents (aged 10–20 years) differed significantly from those of their parents in an epidemiological study of headache. In another study, Larsson (1995) estimated correlations between adolescent, parent, and teacher reports of headaches in typical everyday life situations. For home-based activities, the overall correlation between adolescent and parent reports was statistically significant but low ($r = 0.35$), while the relationship between adolescents' and teachers' reports of headaches at school was almost zero. In eight typical everyday activities (e.g., "leaving home for school" or "in the classroom"), the overall concordance rates between adolescent and parent reports of headaches were consistently low. These findings emphasize the importance of the source of information when evaluating estimates of headache prevalence in adolescents.

HEADACHE CLASSIFICATION

Previous research on the prevalence of headaches in children and adolescents has used various sets of diagnostic criteria. In Scandinavian countries the criteria suggested by Vahlquist (1955) and Bille (1962) have been preferred, although criticism has been raised because the criteria include family aggregation of migraine. For migraine and tension headaches, the Ad Hoc Committee definitions of headaches in adults have most often been used and extended to children and adolescents with recurrent headaches (Ad Hoc Committee 1962). Other diagnostic criteria used in research include those defined by Prensky and Sommer and Hockaday, published by Barlow (1984) and Hockaday (1988).

The International Headache Society (IHS) has developed a detailed system for the classification of headaches (Headache Classification Committee of the International Headache Society 1988), which has been widely adopted for use both in research and in clinical practice. However, in recent years it has been argued that the IHS criteria need some modification for children (e.g., Mortimer et al. 1992; Metsähonkala and Sillanpää 1994). This concern has mainly focused on the duration of migraine attacks, which tends to be shorter in children and adolescents. However, epidemiologists have noticed little difference in the sensitivity for migraine of the criteria outlined by the Ad Hoc Committee (1962), Vahlquist (1955), Bille (1962), and the IHS. The differences in prevalence rates based on the three sets of criteria were less than 1% (Mortimer et al. 1992), and they were even smaller when the two latter sets were compared (Metsähonkala and Sillanpää 1994).

Table I
The IHS criteria for diagnosis of migraine without aura

A) At least five attacks fulfilling criteria B–D

B) Headache attacks lasting 2–72 h

C) At least two of the following characteristics:
  1) Pulsating quality
  2) Moderate or severe intensity (inhibits or prohibits daily activities)
  3) Unilateral location
  4) Aggravation during routine physical activity (e.g., walking)

D) During headache at least one of the following:
  1) Nausea and/or vomiting
  2) Photophobia and phonophobia

Table II
The IHS diagnostic criteria for episodic and chronic tension-type headaches

A) At least 10 previous headache episodes fulfilling criteria B–D

B) Headache duration of 30 min–7 d

C) At least two of the following pain characteristics:
   1) Pressing or tightening quality
   2) Mild or moderate intensity (may inhibit but not prohibit everyday activities)
   3) Bilateral or variable location
   4) No aggravation during routine physical activity (e.g., walking)

D) All of the following:
   1) No vomiting; mild nausea or anorexia may occur but no moderate or severe nausea
   2) Photophobia or phonophobia of the moderate to severe form may be present, but not both

Episodic tension-type headache: headache episodes <180 days/year

Chronic tension-type headache: headache episodes >180 days/year for at least 6 mo

Both episodic and chronic TTH may be associated with a disorder of the pericranial muscles, including at least one of the following:
   1) Muscle tenderness (as measured by manual palpation or pressure algometer)
   2) Increased EMG levels at rest or during functional tests

HEADACHE TYPES

The most common types of recurrent headaches in children and adolescents are migraine and tension-type headaches (TTH). Horton's headaches are rare in childhood and adolescence (Maytal et al. 1992). The IHS criteria for diagnosis of migraine headaches without aura are presented in Table I. On the basis of frequency, TTH is classified into *episodic* and *chronic* types, and the criteria for the diagnoses are presented in Table II.

Some of the problems in the diagnostic assessment of headaches in clinical samples of children are related to descriptions of headache quality in younger children (Seshia et al. 1994; Wöber-Bingöl et al. 1995). A clinical study found that children under 10 years of age were unable to provide information about several features of their headaches more often than older children (Wöber-Bingöl et al. 1995). A study of 8–9-year-old children found that parents had problems in providing information on the quality of their children's headaches, and that they also had difficulty describing aura phenomena (Svensson et al., submitted).

HEADACHE ASSESSMENT

Headache diaries are one of the most valuable tools in the assessment of headaches in adults (Blanchard and Andrasik 1985). In studies of adolescent headaches Larsson and colleagues have used a diary format initially developed by Epstein and Abel (1977) and adapted from the Budzynski et al. (1973) headache rating scale where subjects are asked to rate degree of pain and impairment on a scale of 0–5 four times daily at breakfast, lunch, in the afternoon, and at bedtime, in addition to listing medication taken for headaches.

Several measures based on the headache diary have been used for clinical and research purposes: (1) Headache index: the total weekly headache activity score based on 28 recordings per week (0–140). (2) Headache-free days: the number of days in a week when no headache was registered (0–7). (3) Headache frequency: the number of discrete weekly headache episodes (only two episodes per day can be recorded, with the total varying from 0 to 14). (4) Average headache duration: average number of recorded time points per headache episode (0–4/day) per week. (5) Peak headache intensity: the single highest headache intensity rating per week. (6) Mean headache intensity: the average of all 28 headache recordings per week.

Adolescents can be taught how to use the diary during a 15-minute instruction period, but follow-up contacts are recommended to discuss various problems that might arise. Children need assistance and supervision from their parents to follow through in their daily recordings. For adolescents with chronic TTH (daily or almost daily), diary ratings over a 3-week period usually suffice to obtain a good picture of the severity of their headaches. Diary recordings of frequent migraine headaches (more than once a week) can also provide valuable information, in particular because migraines are often combined with TTH. However, less frequent headaches can more easily be recorded in an episode- or event-related diary.

In a recent study, Metsähonkala and her colleagues (1997) found that 11–13-year-old children with migraine or nonmigrainous headaches reported similar frequencies of headaches when interviewed, as compared to a 2–7-month period of event-based headache diary recordings. Overall, the agreement between information obtained in an interview and in a diary was 60% for migraine and 67% for nonmigrainous headaches. About half the children who received a diagnosis of migraine in the interview were found to have nonmigrainous headaches when headaches were recorded. Information obtained in the interview underestimated the duration of headache episodes as compared to the diary recordings. Somewhat surprisingly, many children reported new migraine features in the diary. About half of them reported vomiting and aura symptoms for the first time, and about one-third of the children reported nausea, unilaterality, and pulsatility. In the interview very few children stated that they had two types of headaches, but diary recordings revealed that 86% had both migraine and nonmigrainous headaches. The findings of Metsähonkala et al. contrast with the results of a clinical study of children with migraine, in which headache frequency was overestimated in an interview as compared to diary information for both children and parents (Andrasik et al. 1985). The latter study found a high level of agreement between parent and child reports.

Larsson and colleagues (1987a,b), in treatment studies on adolescents in high school, compared self-reported headache change based on diary recordings to information obtained from a significant other, parent, or friend. Only the parents of students treated with self-help relaxation regarded the students' headache activity as significantly improved, and their ratings correlated significantly with the students' self-reported change. Blanchard et al. (1981) reported similar findings for adult headache sufferers. In studies of adult headache sufferers, global self-reports have overestimated the headache change by about 35% as compared to diary recordings. Thus, the headache diary data provide conservative measures of improvement rates.

Overall, headache diaries provide the most valuable and systematic information on headache occurrence and degree of pain, and should therefore be used in clinical practice and in research as a complement to an interview. The most useful measures that can be extracted from the diary are the total headache activity (headache index), number of headache-free days, and frequency of headaches. The type of diary used should primarily depend on the frequency of headache episodes.

PREVALENCE OF HEADACHE

The prevalence of recurrent headaches has been documented in well-designed epidemiological studies conducted in several countries and cultures (see reviews by Goodman and McGrath 1991; Metsähonkala 1997). However, some of the methodological problems with those studies should be mentioned. In particular, in early prevalence studies, parents were commonly the sole informants in rating the headaches of their children. However, as previously noted, the overall agreement in epidemiological studies between child and parent reports regarding headaches in children is low to moderate (Deubner 1977). Higher rates of agreement have been found in clinical studies of school-aged children (Richardson et al. 1983; Andrasik et al. 1985). Further, most epidemiological studies have used questionnaires, and only a few have conducted direct interviews (Deubner 1977; Sparks 1978) or telephone interviews with children and their parents (Linet et al. 1989). In addition, many epidemiological investigations have been restricted to the study of headache prevalence in children and adolescents living in urban areas and big cities (McGrath and Larsson 1997). The vast majority of these studies have focused on the assessment of unspecified headaches or migraine in school-aged children. Finally, different terms have been used to assess headache prevalence, and different sets of criteria have been used in the diagnosis of migraine.

UNSPECIFIED HEADACHES

Although few studies have focused on the prevalence of headaches in 3–5-year-old preschool children, their results indicate that recurrent headaches in this age group are quite rare and occur in only 3% of individuals (Zuckerman et al. 1987); frequent headaches affect less than 1% of children of this age (Sillanpää et al. 1991; Borge et al. 1994). A recent Finnish study found that 15% of 6-year-old children had headaches that disturbed their daily activities (Aromaa et al. 1998). Overall, headache prevalences in preschool ages have varied from 5.9% to 37.7%, most likely reflecting the different definitions used in the various studies as well as true differences in prevalence rates.

In studies of headache in school-aged children in community and school settings, the prevalence rates of unspecified headaches have varied greatly, ranging from 3% to 82% (Goodman and McGrath 1991). For unspecified headaches occurring once a month or more, prevalence rates have varied from 23% to 51% (Egermark-Eriksson 1982; Sillanpää 1983a,b; Kristjansdottir and Wahlberg 1993; Carlsson 1996a). More frequent unspecified headaches occurring once a week or more have been reported by 7–22% of schoolchildren (Egermark-Eriksson 1982; Sillanpää 1983a,b; Larsson 1988; Brattberg and Wickman 1992; Kristjansdottir and Wahlberg 1993), and about 0.3–1.2% of schoolchildren experience daily headaches (Egermark-Eriksson 1982; Sillanpää 1983a,b).

Few gender differences have been reported prior to puberty, but during adolescence recurrent headaches become much more common among girls (Bille 1962; Egermark-Eriksson 1982; Sillanpää 1983a,b; Linet et al. 1989; Kristjansdottir and Wahlberg 1993). The prevalence of headaches is also higher in socially unstable residential areas and in lower socioeconomic groups (Sillanpää and Anttila 1996; Metsähonkala 1997).

MIGRAINE

The prevalence rates for migraine among preschoolers are quite consistent and vary from 3% to 7.4% (Metsähonkala 1997). Bille (1962) studied the prevalence of migraine headaches in the entire school population of Uppsala, Sweden, in 1955 (9000 pupils). Parent and child information was used in the assessment, which was carried out with a two-stage design (screening with questionnaires and a subsequent interview). The prevalence rate was 2.5% at school entry and twice as high during adolescence. Since Bille's classic study, numerous studies have examined the prevalence of migraine in children and adolescents in community and school settings. Most studies show that 2.5–10% of children experience migraines (Goodman and McGrath 1991; Metsähonkala 1997). Higher rates have been reported, but they are most likely explained by different sets of criteria and assessment methods used (e.g., Deubner 1977). Most child migraine sufferers experience migraine attacks less than once a month, although about 30% experience attacks once a month or more (Sparks 1978; Mortimer et al. 1992).

The prevalence rates of migraine obtained in more recent studies that used the IHS criteria in different countries are very similar and vary from 3% to 11% of the general population (Abu Arefeh and Russell 1994; Pothman et al. 1994; Raieli et al. 1995; Barea et al. 1996). It can therefore be concluded that the overall estimates of prevalence rates of migraine among school-aged children are reliable and show a consistent pattern.

TENSION-TYPE HEADACHES

Few well-designed investigations have examined the prevalence of TTH as defined by the IHS criteria. In an early Swedish study, Vahlquist (1955) found that infrequent nonmigrainous headaches affected 82% of 10–12-year-olds and 74% of 16–19-year-olds. Bille (1962) reported that approximately half of the 7–15-year-old schoolchildren sampled experienced such headaches. In the Vahlquist study, the corresponding figures for frequent nonmigrainous headaches in the two age groups were 13.3% and 18.6%, respectively. Bille found that 2.5% of the children in the 7–15-year-old group had such headaches, whereas they were more common (15.7%) among 15-year-old schoolchildren. In an Italian study, Saraceni and colleagues (1989) found that 25% of preadolescent schoolchildren had nonmigrainous headache.

Using IHS criteria, Pothmann and his collaborators (1994) found that about 50% of school-aged children had experienced TTH. More girls than boys had TTH, and prevalence rates increased during adolescence. It is

likely that most schoolchildren with nonmigrainous headaches in early studies experienced headaches that we now would label as TTH of the episodic
and chronic types with the IHS criteria. Abu-Arefeh and Russell (1994)
reported that about 1% of school-aged children had chronic TTH.

Researchers and clinicians have speculated that the prevalence of headaches has increased during previous decades. In a recent study of children
starting school conducted in two Finnish cities, Sillanpää and Anttila (1996)
found a striking increase in the prevalence of migraine and unspecified
headaches over a 20-year period. They studied the same age group of children from the same urban area and used identical assessment methods. The
authors suggest that changes in the psychosocial environment might explain
the observed increase in headache prevalence. Similar results were obtained
in a recent Swedish study where the prevalence rates of frequent headaches
among schoolchildren had increased over a decade, in particular among
adolescent girls (Marklund 1997). Thus, there is some evidence for an increase in headache prevalence among school-aged children in Scandinavian
countries.

Although the IHS criteria (Headache Classification Committee 1988)
were originally proposed for diagnosing migraine and TTH in adults, they
may also help to standardize the assessment of headaches in pediatric populations and reduce the variation in prevalence rates due to different sets of
diagnostic criteria.

PROGNOSIS

In a recent study of prepubertal children with migraine, Metsähonkala
and her colleagues (1997) found that 8–9-year-old boys had a worse prognosis than girls when reassessed after about 2–3 years. Overall, boys had
more frequent attacks than girls. On reassessment about 80% of all children
still had migraine attacks, 10% no longer had migraines but had developed
TTH or other headaches, and only 5% had become headache free.

Over the course of a 6-year follow-up period, Bille (1962) found that
approximately 15% of schoolchildren with migraine or pronounced migraine
were unimproved, and found similar rates for children with nonmigrainous
headaches. However, two-thirds of the children in the latter group were
headache-free, in contrast to about a third in the group with pronounced
migraine. The annual recovery rate for children with migraine aged 7–20
years was estimated to be 10%. In a similar follow-up study over 7 years,
Sillanpää (1983b) found that 22% of schoolchildren with migraine had become migraine free, whereas 41% were unimproved.

The long-term prognosis for childhood migraine has been examined in clinical follow-up studies of adults. Overall, the prognosis is good for at least half of the cases (Hockaday 1988), and attacks cease for about one-third of children. The prognosis appears to be better for boys than girls. In Bille's long-term follow-up of his original sample of 73 children (7–15 years old) with pronounced migraine (more than once a month), he found that 50% continued to have migraine attacks over a 40-year period. About one-third of the adults had suffered annual attacks since childhood. Although the attacks had been less frequent in adulthood, the intensity was often reported to be similar to that experienced in childhood (Bille 1997). The long-term prognosis was better for men, who became migraine free more often than women. Although most subjects (both men and women) had been migraine free during puberty and as young adults, many of them relapsed in adulthood.

Surprisingly, our knowledge about the prognosis for TTH in children and adolescents is much more limited. In a Swedish study, Wänman (1987) found that about 50% of the adolescents suffering from unspecified recurrent headaches (once a week or more often, mostly consisting of TTH) had improved over a 1-year period. In another Swedish study (Brattberg and Wickman 1993) about 30% of schoolchildren reported recurrent headaches (in answer to the question, "Do you usually have headaches"?) at both assessments over a 2-year period. Such headaches were about twice as common among girls than boys. In the study by Metsähonkala (1997) more than half of the 8–9-year-old children continued to experience nonmigrainous headache when they were 11–13 years of age, one-third had developed migraine instead, and about 10% had become headache free.

In conclusion, the short-term prognosis for children and adolescents with pronounced migraine (more than once a month) or frequent TTH (more than once a week) is poor without intervention (Larsson and Melin 1988c).

INCIDENCE

Bille's (1962) study of children with migraine reported an annual incidence (percentage of new cases per year) of about 0.6%. However, this figure is based on cases with frequent migraine headache. The cumulative annual incidence rate for recurrent headaches among 10–17-year-old Swedish schoolchildren is estimated at 11–26% (Brattberg and Wickman 1993).

PATHOPHYSIOLOGY

MIGRAINE

During recent years our knowledge about pathophysiology of migraine has advanced considerably, but almost all research has been carried out on adults. Although vascular and neurogenic theories have dominated our hypotheses about the mechanisms involved in migraine, biochemical mechanisms also play an important role. Various types of neuropeptides cause vasodilatation and inflammation peripherally, and centrally they convey nociceptive information to neurons in the trigeminal nerves. New knowledge about the pharmacokinetics of the triptans has also helped us to understand the mechanisms involved in migraine headaches. The pain of migraine arises from the distension of the pial arteries and the sensitization of periarterial nociceptors (Olesen et al. 1993).

TENSION-TYPE HEADACHES

Our understanding of the pathophysiology of TTH has lagged behind that of migraine. Researchers have long assumed that muscular tension plays a role in TTH, previously called "muscle-contraction headache," for example in the Ad Hoc Committee definitions of headaches (1962). However, extensive studies of adults with TTH have shown inconsistent results concerning, for example, increased electromyogram (EMG) levels during headaches. Evidence suggests that headache sufferers respond to stress with more muscle tension than do headache-free individuals (Martin 1993). Recently, adults with chronic TTH with a muscular disorder have shown lower pressure detection thresholds and tolerances than those without a disorder in various pericranial locations (Jensen et al. 1998). Jensen also suggested that prolonged nociceptive stimuli from the pericranial muscles might sensitize the central nervous system and thereby lead to an increased general sensitivity of pain. The relative importance of central and peripheral mechanisms may change in episodic versus chronic tension headache (Olesen et al. 1993).

Although most research on the mechanisms involved in TTH has been conducted on adults, schoolchildren with frequent headaches have also shown an increased sensitivity to pressure stimuli in the pericranial muscles (Carlsson 1996b). Children with nonorganic recurrent abdominal pain (RAP) have shown lower pain pressure thresholds, not only in the umbilical area but also in some of the pericranial muscles (Alfvén 1993). Similar findings have been reported for adolescents with chronic arthritis (Hogeweg et al. 1995). Thus, reduced pain tolerance thresholds in various muscles of the body seem to be related to the experience of a longstanding pain disorder in children and adolescents, and such a disorder might have similar consequences on the central nervous system.

ETIOLOGY

FAMILY AGGREGATION AND HEREDITY

Community and clinical studies have found a strong familial occurrence of migraine; more than 50% of other members of a migraine sufferer's immediate family also suffer from headaches (Ziegler et al. 1988). However, for nonmigrainous headaches familial aggregation is lower (Larsson 1988; Metsähonkala 1997). Genetic epidemiological investigations of large-scale, nonselected twin samples or adoption studies are needed to estimate the relative importance of environmental and genetic contributions to the occurrence of various types of headaches.

Recent large-scale twin studies have shown that about 40–60% of the liability to migraine in adults was explained by genetic factors (Honkasalo et al. 1995; Larsson et al. 1995). Concordance rates for migraine were consistently higher among monozygotic than dizygotic same-sexed twins (48% and 31%, respectively). A weaker genetic contribution was found for a mixed group of headaches, possibly including TTH (Larsson et al. 1995). In this group, environmental factors played a more important role. Environmental factors, which may be unique to each twin in the pair, might consist of exposure to illness or stressful events. The influence of genetic factors was somewhat stronger for females than males. A study that compared sets of adult twins who had grown up together with others who were raised separately found that 50% of the susceptibility for migraine was genetically determined (Ziegler et al. 1998). A study of 8–9-year-old twins found a higher correlation for recurrent headache susceptibility in same-sexed monozygotic twins (about 70% of boys and girls) than in same-sexed dizygotic twins (23% of boys and 33% of girls), but in different-sexed dizygotic twins the correlation was zero (Svensson et al., submitted). However, only small differences in concordance rates between migraine and nonmigrainous headaches were found.

STRESS

The role of stress has long been considered an important etiological factor for migraine and TTH in children (Bille 1962; Passchier and Orlebeke 1985). Both mental and physical stress are significant (Bille 1962; Leviton et al. 1984). However, in a recent study, adolescents with nonmigrainous headaches reported a trigger more often than those with migraine (Osterhaus 1998). In controlled studies, adolescents reported more stress symptoms than did headache-free subjects, and they were more likely to live in divorced families (Larsson 1988). Their daily stress often consists of feeling pressured and frustrated. Studies of young adults have found that headache sufferers are not exposed to higher levels of external stressors but that their subjective experience of such stressors is more negative than that of non-headache subjects (Holm et al. 1986). Schoolchildren with headaches experience more stress, fear of failure, and problems than others (Passchier and Orlebeke 1985), in addition to being bullied more often (Metsähonkala 1997).

Many headaches in schoolchildren occur during school hours (Bille 1962). Data are surprisingly scarce on environmental factors such as classroom temperature, levels of carbon dioxide, and noise, which might influence the occurrence of headaches in children. However, larger school classes are related to a higher incidence of headaches in children (Carlsson 1996a). In studies of adults, elevated levels of subjective stress seem to occur about 2 days prior to a migraine attack (Sorbi et al. 1994). It is also well known that migraine headaches tend to occur when slowing down at the end of the week or after a stressful event such as a school test.

OTHER ETIOLOGICAL FACTORS

Irregular, poor, or extended sleep over the weekend may also elicit migraine attacks in children (Bille 1962). Dietary factors have also been studied. Irregular meals may be linked to headaches (Dalton and Dalton 1979). A small subgroup of migraine sufferers appear to be sensitive to tyramine (Hanington 1967) and react to various foods, such as cheese, but other foods such as chocolate or fruits may also elicit attacks in certain children with migraine. Although some evidence supports a radical (oligoantigenic) elimination diet in the treatment of frequent migraine in children, such an intervention cannot be generally recommended because of its high cost and heavy pressure on the child and parents (e.g., Egger et al. 1983).

PSYCHOSOCIAL FUNCTIONING

PSYCHOLOGICAL SYMPTOMS

It is unclear whether various types of psychological symptoms often found in adults as well as children and adolescents with recurrent headaches are causes or consequences of longstanding headaches. Studies of adults with recurrent headaches have found anxiety, depression, and somatic complaints other than headaches to be more common in those with chronic TTH than in migraine sufferers (Blanchard and Andrasik 1985). Such findings suggest that "headache density" plays an important role in the development of psychological symptoms. That is, the more frequent or intense the headaches, the greater the number of psychological symptoms reported. Studies of adults treated with psychological methods show that anxiety and depression decrease with treatment regardless of change in headache frequency, whereas somatic complaints were related to headache change (Blanchard et al. 1991). Our own studies of adolescents treated with relaxation training approaches have found inconsistent results regarding relationships between degree of headache change and accompanying psychological symptoms.

Several clinical studies have shown that anxiety, depression, and somatic complaints are more common in children with migraine than in those free of headaches (e.g., Bille 1962; Cunningham et al. 1987; Andrasik et al. 1988). However, a study of children and adolescents with headaches, using other types of pain as controls, found that anxiety and depression may be due to the pain itself (Cunningham et al. 1987). The results of similar studies of nonmigrainous headaches (mostly TTH) have shown that adolescents with headaches report more somatic complaints and anxiety than do headache-free subjects (Larsson 1988). In addition, parents and teachers also found anxiety and depression to be more common in adolescent headache sufferers. In line with findings for adult chronic headache sufferers (Blanchard and Andrasik 1985), schoolchildren with chronic TTH as well as migraine have reported more psychological problems than those with migraine alone (Carlsson et al. 1996), thus supporting the headache density hypothesis. However, it should be noted that several correlation studies report inconsistent results regarding the role of headache severity or chronicity for psychological symptoms in children and adolescents.

Until recently, little information has existed on recurrent headaches in children and adolescents diagnosed with various types of psychiatric disorders through standardized interviews using criteria from the *Diagnostic and Statistical Manual of Mental Disorders* (DSM-IV) (American Psychiatric Association 1994). However, Egger et al. (1998) found that girls with depression or anxiety disorder had a greater prevalence of recurrent headaches than did girls without such disorders. Only depressed girls with recurrent headaches missed school because of headaches, and they took medication more often than did nondepressed girls with headaches. Girls with depression reported more frequent headaches and said that headaches affected their lives more severely than did girls with anxiety disorders. In boys, recurrent headaches were significantly associated with disruptive behavior in school (conduct disorder). The authors suggest that a dysfunction in central pain regulation could explain the gender difference in psychopathology associated with recurrent headaches and might be an underlying cause common to both depression and recurrent headaches.

Recently, Langeveldt and colleagues (1996) developed a more comprehensive approach to measure quality of life in adolescents with recurrent headaches. They developed a questionnaire to assess psychological functioning, functional status, physical status, and social functioning that has shown good psychometric properties. Changes in headache activity were related to changes in the areas of psychological functioning, functional status, and the subscales "satisfaction with life in general" and "health" (Langeveldt et al. 1997). The effects of headache on quality of life seem to be greater in adolescents who experience higher levels of stress in their lives.

A note of caution applies to the assessment of psychosocial functioning in young adults. Holroyd and his collaborators (1993) found that various psychological symptoms were elevated only in subjects who had a headache at the time of assessment. However, locus of control was not affected by the subjects' pain state. One conclusion of these findings is that elevated psychological symptoms reflect a transient negative bias caused by the headache episode. Subjects who experienced headaches at assessment also reported higher levels of headache activity during the previous month than did headache-free subjects. It is very likely that such biased ratings in the assessment of headache activity and psychosocial functioning also influence the reports of children and adolescents.

SCHOOL ABSENCE, HELP-SEEKING, AND MEDICATION

Children who seek help for headaches at a pediatric clinic are not typical of headache sufferers in the population. They are more likely to have severe headaches, to have unusual headaches such as those accompanied by neurological symptoms, or to be handicapped by headaches and unable to participate in normal activities. Pediatric clinics more commonly treat migraine headaches than either frequent TTH or TTH combined with migraine (Wöber-Bingöl et al. 1995). Metsähonkala and her colleagues (1996) found that children with migraine who consulted a doctor (usually a specialist) had more symptoms such as aura and nausea, a higher frequency of attacks, and more absences from school than did nonconsulters.

Intensity of headaches has been closely related to disability in clinic samples of children and adolescents (Hämäläinen 1997). Almost all children with migraine were bedridden during migraine attacks, whereas only two-thirds of children with other headaches stayed in bed. In studies of adolescents with frequent headaches (more than once a week for more than a year), 90% of those with migraine reported that their headaches were "severe enough to disturb their school work" or "unbearable." About 30% of those with chronic TTH reported such disability levels, but most of them stated that their headaches were "mild" or "difficult but not interrupting their work." Although these figures are based on children and adolescents seeking help because of their recurrent headaches, in an unselected school sample about one-quarter of schoolchildren were able to continue their activities, whereas about a third needed to "stop or rest" or "go to bed" (Pothmann et al. 1994). In a Swedish study, about 25% of schoolchildren reported that their headache did not disturb their daily life, and somewhat fewer stated that the pain made it "difficult to concentrate" (Brattberg and Wickman 1991).

Most children with headache do not miss school and function well in spite of their pain, and among those who do miss school, almost all are absent from school 1 day or less (Collin et al. 1985). In a Swedish study, about 5% reported that they sometimes missed school due to headaches (Brattberg and Wickman 1991). However, school absence seems to be greater in children and adolescents with migraine than among those with infrequent nonmigrainous headaches (Bille 1962; Larsson 1988).

About 30–60% of children with migraine headaches have consulted a physician because of their headaches (Bille 1962; Sparks 1978; Metsähonkala et al. 1996). In studies of adolescents with primarily nonmigrainous headaches, about 25% had consulted a physician (Larsson 1988). As expected, in unselected school populations the consultation rates were much lower and varied from 2% to 10% in a Swedish study (Egermark-Eriksson 1982). In another Swedish study, about 25% of schoolchildren had sought help for headaches, and were equally likely to consult the school nurse as the school physician (Brattberg and Wickman 1991). However, schoolchildren with headaches at least once a week consulted the school nurse (but not the school physician) more often than those with less frequent headaches (Kristjansdottir and Wahlberg 1993).

In a Scandinavian survey of schoolchildren, about one-third of 15-year-olds surveyed reported that they used medication regularly to treat their headaches (Due et al. 1991). In a similar study, about 50% of schoolchildren with weekly headaches reported that they had used medication the previous month; the figure for those with more frequent headaches was even higher (70%) (Kristjansdottir and Wahlberg 1993). Studies of adolescents with headaches more than once a week who sought care found that 14% of those with TTH and 25% of those with migraine used analgesic drugs "daily or almost daily."

Changes in medication and school absence have commonly been used to assess the social consequences of recurrent headaches in children and adolescents. However, research has not found them to be useful measures of treatment outcome due to the low frequency of medication usage school absence recorded in headache diaries in spite of a high frequency of headaches (Larsson and Melin 1988b; McGrath et al. 1992). Future research must evaluate other aspects of social functioning such as peer relations, school work, and leisure time activities.

COPING WITH HEADACHE

In the past decade, researchers have shown increased interest in different aspects of coping with various health problems in children and adolescents. In our studies on adolescents with frequent headaches, we found that about 50% of the subjects went to bed (if possible), 40% used medication, 34% "tried to relax," and 25% used relaxation techniques of some kind (Larsson and Melin 1988a). The first two strategies were rated as most effective in dealing with recurrent headaches. An Australian study of 10–18-year-old schoolchildren (King and Sharpley 1990) and a German study of schoolchildren (Pothmann et al. 1994) found similar results. The Australian children used the following statements during headache episodes: "It will pass ... I will get over it" (41%), "Don't think about anything" (27%), and "This is terrible ... I wish I'd die" (18%).

Recently, Reid and colleagues (1998) developed the Pain Coping Questionnaire (PCQ), a comprehensive assessment tool for various types of pain. The PCQ has been tested on healthy children and children with headaches or arthritis. Higher levels of avoidance behavior were related to higher levels of anxiety, depression, and pain distress in the headache sample. However, none of the coping scales were related to the intensity or duration of headaches or to functional disability related to headaches.

Mothers of noncoping children with various types of pain may discourage coping behavior in their children, who display more negative behavior, express more pain, and are on-task less often than copers (Dunn-Geier et al. 1986).

TREATMENT

The first step in clinical assessment is to establish a headache diagnosis and rule out any significant organic pathology. The second task is to develop a treatment plan and assess the degree of motivation of the child as well as the parents, who need to support the child during treatment. Adolescents can be treated individually and in groups after attending information meetings along with their parents.

The treatment plan depends on the frequency of the headaches and the degree of disability. For example, if migraine attacks are mild and infrequent, then providing information about the diagnosis and prognosis, together with reassurance and appropriate analgesic drugs, will often be sufficient (Forsythe and Hockaday 1988). However, systematic headache recordings in a diary may reveal that headache activity is higher than reported in an interview. Health care providers should delay starting treatments such as psychological interventions until they obtain a definitive picture of the headache activity.

It is also important to identify and avoid specific environmental triggers of migraine and TTH. The first line of defense may include wearing sunglasses to limit exposure to glaring light (Good et al. 1991), ensuring that meals are not skipped, or reducing certain stressors, such as physical exertion. Surprisingly little research has focused on improvement of the child's school environment, for example, in attempts to change the temperature, the air, or the noise level. More attention needs to be directed to this neglected area in future research.

PHARMACOLOGICAL TREATMENT

Pharmacological treatment of headaches can be palliative, abortive, or prophylactic. *Palliative* relief of the symptom is most often directed at the pain, but nausea might also be the target. In clinical practice acetaminophen is often the *abortive* treatment of choice for both migraine and TTH because it is often effective and has few side effects. Other alternatives are nonsteroidal anti-inflammatory drugs (NSAIDs) or aspirin. However, aspirin must be used with care due to the slight risk of Reye's syndrome.

In adults, numerous controlled outcome studies have evaluated the effects of acetaminophen, NSAIDs, ergotamine, and various triptans on recurrent headaches. In contrast, only a few controlled studies have considered their effects in children and adolescents. Recent research by Hämäläinen (1997) has shown that more than 50% of children with migraine improved within 2 hours of treatment with a single dose of acetaminophen (15 mg/kg) or ibuprofen (10 mg/kg). Although the effects of acetaminophen were more rapid, ibuprofen gave better overall relief. More than half of those who did not respond to these drugs improved after a single dose of dihydroergotamine (20–40 μg/kg). A poor response to sumatriptan was found among those who did not respond to any of the previous treatments. Similar findings have been reported after oral administration of sumatriptan to adolescents, which was found to be ineffective in a large-scale controlled multinational trial (Korsgaard 1995). However, subcutaneous administration of sumatriptan to children and adolescents with migraine seems to be as effective as in adults (Linder 1995).

Adolescents often wait about 1 hour from the onset of a headache before taking analgesics (Forward et al. 1996; Chambers et al. 1997). Children and adolescents and their parents must be carefully instructed to take acetaminophen or NSAIDs at the very onset of a headache for optimum performance.

Prophylactic drugs such as clonidine, pizotifen, beta-blockers, and calcium channel blockers are often prescribed to children and adolescents with disabling migraines that occur at least twice a month or more often (Barlow 1984; Forsythe and Hockaday 1988). However, controlled empirical studies have not yet shown that prophylactic medications are effective in the prevention of migraine in children and adolescents (Symon 1995). The results of a meta-analysis suggest that beta-blockers may be valuable (Hermann et al. 1995).

PSYCHOLOGICAL TREATMENT

Extensive research on adults has found relaxation training or EMG biofeedback to be effective alone or in combination in the treatment of chronic TTH (Blanchard and Andrasik 1985). Relaxation training was somewhat less effective in the treatment of migraine, but when combined with thermal (finger temperature) biofeedback showed an improved outcome. A recent review showed that minimal therapist contact and the use of home-based interventions for both migraine and TTH were shown to be much more cost-effective in both adult and pediatric populations (Rowan and Andrasik 1996).

If recurrent headaches in school-aged children are moderate or severe and occur more than once a week, extended and intense treatments such as stress management are likely to be useful and can be recommended to motivated headache sufferers and their parents. However, children under 8 years of age are unlikely to be able to follow simple treatment protocols, even with support from their parents (Blanchard and Andrasik 1985). Stress management, cognitive behavioral therapy, and relaxation training are the treatments of choice for tension or migraine headaches that interfere with activities and occur often enough to be perceived as a problem.

Psychological treatment approaches that are valuable for adults with various types of recurrent headaches have been examined in controlled outcome studies on children and adolescents. The first comparative group study was published in 1984 by Labbé and Williamson. Since then several studies have been conducted, but most have focused on migraine in clinical samples of children and adolescents, while only a few have evaluated TTH, primarily in school adolescents. The results show that relaxation, biofeedback training procedures, and cognitive approaches are valuable in the treatment of children 8 years of age or older (Hermann et al. 1995; Osterhaus et al. 1997). Most studies have used at least eight sessions administered once or twice a week. In a recent study a brief cognitive-behavioral group treatment (two 90-minute sessions) for prepubertal children was ineffective, probably due to the brevity of treatment (Barry and von Baeyer 1997). However, with one exception (McGrath et al. 1988), all controlled group studies had a positive outcome when active treatments were compared to placebo or waiting-list control conditions. Because various psychological approaches were used, either alone or combined, it is not possible to conclude that any one of the procedures is more efficacious than the others. More comprehensive treatment packages (Osterhaus et al. 1993, 1997) have achieved improvements equal to the outcome of single treatment procedures administered to children and adolescents (Fentress et al. 1986; Richter et al. 1986).

Usually, psychological therapy has involved one-on-one sessions with trained therapists. However, cognitive behavior therapy and relaxation training can be delivered in a group format or with reduced therapist contact. Therapist-reduced formats involve a few sessions with a therapist followed by use of tapes, telephone calls, and self-help books (for example, *Help Yourself: A Treatment for Migraine Headaches* by McGrath et al. 1990). A largely self-administered, home-based treatment approach can be just as effective as clinical treatment for adolescents with migraine (McGrath et al. 1992). Moreover, the self-administered treatment was about three times more cost-effective than the therapist-administered treatment.

Studies of adolescents with TTH (headaches at least once a week for more than a year, mostly consisting of almost daily or daily headaches) have used a standardized relaxation training program (Larsson 1995). The program includes discrimination training administered over two or three sessions (mostly with three or four subjects in a group). Participants then learn a rapid relaxation technique (two or three sessions), with training on how to apply the techniques to everyday life situations during the final session. The program has been administered at school, often in the school nurse's office, twice a week in 20–30 minute sessions over a 6–8-week period.

Therapist-assisted relaxation training reduced the adolescents' headache activity by 59%, whereas home-based training was less effective and reduced headaches by 25%. Adolescents who monitored their headaches did not improve, and those who were treated with attention-control procedures improved only slightly (5%) (Larsson and Melin 1988a). The improvements were well maintained at 6-month follow-up evaluations (Larsson and Melin 1988b). More than 50% of the adolescents treated with therapist-based relaxation achieved a 50% improvement or more, a clinically significant change in headache research (Blanchard and Andrasik 1985). These adolescents rated the relaxation training as highly credible at the beginning of treatment and still found it valuable at the end of treatment. Total headache activity and frequency showed the greatest improvement among adolescents (Osterhaus et al. 1997). Long-term improvement has been maintained among children and adolescents with various types of headaches 3–4 years after relaxation training (Larsson and Melin 1989; Engel et al. 1992).

PREDICTORS OF TREATMENT OUTCOME

Studies that analyzed predictors of headache change found that treatment type was important (relaxation training fared better than alternative treatment or no treatment), that more severe headaches responded better to relaxation training, and that adolescents who were unhappy at school or at home also showed more improvement from psychological treatment (Larsson and Melin 1988b). In direct comparisons, adolescents with TTH responded better than those with migraine (25%). Osterhaus and her collaborators (1997) have reported similar results and have noted that youngsters with a longer headache history profited less than those with a shorter history. Interestingly, the child's report of maternal rewarding of illness behavior predicted a worse outcome. In line with our own findings for the treatment of TTH in adolescents, Richter and colleagues (1986) reported a better improvement for more severe migraine headaches. In home-based biofeedback training of children with migraine, Hermann et al. (1997) found that younger children responded better to the treatment, and that psychosomatic distress and externalizing behaviors were also related to outcome. However, contradictory results have been reported on the importance of compliance with home practices (Allen and McKeen 1991; Hermann et al. 1997).

TREATMENT RECOMMENDATIONS

Children and adolescents with moderate or severe migraine or tension-type headaches should be advised to take a single dose of acetaminophen (paracetamol) (15 mg/kg) or ibuprofen (10 mg/kg) at the first sign of a headache. If symptoms recur, another dose can be taken. For those with migraine who do not respond to such mild analgesics, dihydroergotamine can be given. The benefits of sumatriptan in childhood migraine sufferers are still unclear, so this drug is not recommended.

Psychological treatment can be recommended to school-aged children with moderate or severe nonorganic migraine or tension-type headaches occurring more than once a week and for at least 6 months.

DIRECTIONS FOR FUTURE RESEARCH

Our knowledge of various aspects of recurrent headaches in children and adolescents has increased considerably during the past decade, but several important issues need to be addressed in future research. First, in contrast to our extensive information on the prevalence, incidence, and short- and long-term stability of migraine in children and adolescents, our knowledge about TTH is much more limited. More research must be directed to the treatment of TTH in children and should focus on developing cost-effective approaches for migraine and TTH and examining the characteristics of individuals who respond to such treatment approaches. Can more cost-effective treatments be administered to larger groups, for example by the school nurse? Are single treatment methods better for some individuals than treatment packages that include cognitive training, relaxation, and biofeedback? What treatments work best for those with chronic daily headaches, and which individuals with frequent migraine or TTH will benefit from combined psychological and pharmacological treatment?

Future research should focus on some of these issues so that children and adolescents with recurrent headaches, a neglected area in research and often an undertreated problem in practice, will receive better management that may prevent them from becoming adult headache sufferers.

REFERENCES

Abu-Arefeh I, Russell G. Prevalence of headache and migraine in school children. *BMJ* 1994; 309:765–769.

Achenbach TM, McConaughy SH, Howell CT. Child/adolescent behavioral and emotional problems: implications of cross-informant correlations for situational specificity. *Psychol Bull* 1987; 101:213–232.

Ad Hoc Committee on the Classification of Headaches. Classification of headaches. *JAMA* 1962; 179:717–718.

Alfvén G. The pressure pain threshold (PPT) of certain muscles in children suffering from recurrent abdominal pain of non-organic origin. An algometric study. *Acta Paediatr Scand* 1993; 82:481–483.

Allen KD, McKeen LR. Home-based multicomponent treatment of pediatric migraine. *Headache* 1991; 31:467–472.

American Psychiatric Association. *Diagnostic and Statistical Manual of Mental Disorders*, 4th ed. Washington, DC: American Psychiatric Association, 1994.

Andrasik F, Burke EJ, Attanasio V, Rosenblum EL. Child, parent, and physician reports of a child's headache pain: relationships prior to and following treatment. *Headache* 1985; 25:421–425.

Andrasik F, Kabela E, Quinn S, et al. Psychological functioning of children with recurrent migraine. *Pain* 1988; 34:43–52.

Aromaa M, Rautava P, Helenius H, Sillanpää M. Factors of early life as predictors of headache in children as school entry. *Headache* 1998; 38:23–30.

Barea LM, Tannhauser M, Rotta NT. An epidemiological study of headache among children and adolescents of southern Brazil. *Cephalalgia* 1996; 16:545–549.

Barlow CF. *Headaches and Migraine in Childhood*. London: Spastics International Medical Publications, 1984.

Barry J, von Baeyer CL. Brief cognitive-behavioral group treatment for children's headache. *Clin J Pain* 1997; 13:215–220,

Berg Kelly K, Erhvér M, Erneholm T, et al. Self-reported health status and use of medical care by 3500 adolescents in Western Sweden. I. *Acta Paediatr Scand* 1991; 80:837–843.

Bille B. Migraine in schoolchildren. *Acta Paediatr Scand* 1962; 51(Suppl 136):1–151.

Bille B. A 40-year follow-up of school children with migraine. *Cephalalgia* 1997; 17:488–491.

Blanchard EB, Andrasik F. *Management of Chronic Headaches. A Psychological Approach.* New York: Pergamon Press, 1985.

Blanchard EB, Andrasik F, Neff DF, Jurish S, O'Keefe DM. Social validation of the headache diary. *Behav Ther* 1981; 12:711–715.

Blanchard EB, Steffek BD, Jaccard J, Nicholson NL. Psychological changes accompanying non-pharmacological treatment of chronic headache: the effects of outcome. *Headache* 1991; 31:249–253.

Borge AIH, Nordhagen R, Moe B, Bakketeig LS. Prevalence and persistence of stomach ache and headache among children. Follow-up of a cohort of Norwegian children. *Acta Paediatr Scand* 1994; 83:433–437.

Brattberg G, Wickman V. Ryggont och huvudvärk vanligtbland skolelever. [Back pain and headaches are common in schoolchildren.] *Läkartidningen* 1991; 88:2155–2157.

Brattberg G, Wickman V. Prevalence of back pain and headache in Swedish school children: a questionnaire. *The Pain Clinic* 1992; 5:211–220.

Brattberg G, Wickman V. Longitudinell studie av skolelever.Rehabilitera tidigt vid ryggont och huvudvärk. [A longitudinal study of schoolchildren.] *Läkartidningen* 1993; 90:1452–1460.

Budzynski TH, Stoyva JM, Adler CS, Mullaney DJ. EMG biofeedback and tension headache: a controlled outcome study. *Psychosom Med* 1973; 6:509–514.

Carlsson J. Prevalence of headache in schoolchildren: relation to family and school factors. *Acta Paediatr Scand* 1996a; 85:692–696.

Carlsson J. Tenderness in pericranial muscles in school children with headache. *Pain Clinic* 1996b; 9:49–56.

Carlsson J, Larsson B, Mark A. Psychosocial functioning in schoolchildren with recurrent headaches. *Headache* 1996; 36:77–82.

Chambers CT, Reid GJ, McGrath PJ, et al. Self-administration of over-the-counter medication for pain among adolescents. *Arch Pediatr Adolesc Med* 1997; 151:449–451.

Collin C, Hockaday JM, Waters WE. Headache and school absence. *Arch Dis Child* 1985; 60:245–247.

Cunningham SJ, McGrath PJ, Ferguson HB et al. Personality and behavioural characteristics in pediatric migraine. *Headache* 1987; 27:16–20.

Dalton K, Dalton ME. Food intake before migraine attacks in children. *J Royal Coll Gen Pract* 1979; 29:662–665.

Deubner DC. An epidemiologic study of migraine and headache in 10–20 year olds. *Headache* 1977; 17:173–180.

DiMario FJ. Childhood headaches. A school nurse perspective. *Clin Pediatr* 1992; 31:279–282.

Due P, Holstein BE, Marklund U. Selvrapporteret helbred blandt skolelever i Norden. [Self-reported health among schoolchildren in the Nordic countries.] *Nord Med* 1991; 106:71–74.

Dunn-Geier BJ, McGrath PJ, Rourke BP, Latter J, D'Astous JD. Adolescent chronic pain: the ability to cope. *Pain* 1986; 26:23–32.

Egermark-Eriksson I. Prevalence of headache in Swedish schoolchildren. A questionnaire survey. *Acta Paediatr Scand* 1982; 71:135–140.

Egger J, Carter CM, Soothill JF, Turner MW, Wilson J. Controlled trial of diet in migraine. *Arch Dis Child* 1983; 58:648.

Egger HL, Angold A, Costello EJ. Headaches and psychopathology in children and adolescents. *J Am Acad Child Adolesc Psychiatry* 1998; 37:951–958.

Engel JM, Rapoff MA, Pressman AR. Long-term follow-up of relaxation training for pediatric headache disorders. *Headache* 1992; 32:152–156.

Epstein LH, Abel GG. An analysis of biofeedback training effects for tension headache patients. *Behav Ther* 1977; 8:37–47.

Fentress DW, Masek BJ, Mehegan JE, Bensen H. Biofeedback and relaxation-response training in the treatment of pediatric migraine. *Dev Med Child Neurol* 1986; 28:139–146.

Forsythe I, Hockaday JM. Management of childhood migraine. In: Hockaday JM (Ed). *Migraine in Childhood.* London: Butterworths, 1988.

Forward SP, Brown TL, McGrath PJ. Mothers' attitudes and behaviour toward medicating children's pain. *Pain* 1996; 67:469–475.

Good PA, Taylor RH, Mortimer MJ. The use of tinted glasses in childhood migraine. *Headache* 1991; 31:533–536.

Goodman JE, McGrath PJ. The epidemiology of pain in children and adolescents: a review. *Pain* 1991; 46:247–264.

Hämäläinen ML. Optimal drug treatment of recurrent headaches and migraine in children. Thesis. Helsinki: Helsinki University, 1997.

Hanington E. Preliminary report on tyramine headache. *BMJ* 1967; 1:550–551.

Headache Classification Committee of the International Headache Society. Classification and diagnostic criteria for headache disorders, cranial neuralgias and facial pain. *Cephalalgia* 1988; 8(Suppl 17):1–96.

Hermann C, Kim M, Blanchard EB. Behavioral and prophylactic intervention studies of pediatric migraine: an exploratory meta-analysis. *Pain* 1995; 60:239–256.

Hermann C, Blanchard EB, Flor H. Biofeedback treatment for pediatric migraine: prediction of treatment outcome. *J Consult Clin Psychol* 1997; 55:611–616.

Hockaday JM. Definitions, clinical features, and diagnosis of childhood migraine. In: Hockaday J (Ed). *Migraine in Childhood.* Butterworths: London, 1988, p 16.

Hogeweg JA, Kuis W, Huygen ACJ, et al. The pain threshold in juvenile chronic arthritis. *Br J Rheumatol* 1995; 34:61–67.

Holm JE, Holroyd KA, Hursey KG, Penzien DB. The role of stress in recurrent tension headache. *Headache* 1986; 26:160–167.

Holroyd KA, France JL, Nash J.M, Hursey KG. Pain state as artifact in the psychological assessment of recurrent headache sufferers. *Pain* 1993; 53:229–235.

Honkasalo M-L, Kaprio J, Winter MA, et al. Migraine and concomitant symptoms among 8167 adult twin pairs. *Headache* 1995; 35:70–78.

Jensen R, Berndtsen L, Olesen J. Muscular factors are of importance in tension-type headache. *Headache* 1998; 38:10–17.

King NJ, Sharpley CF. Headache activity in children and adolescents. *J Paediatr Child Health* 1990; 26:50–54.

Korsgaard AG. The tolerability, safety and efficacy of oral sumatriptan 50 mg and 100 mg for the acute treatment of migraine in adolescents. Poster presented at the 3rd International Congress on headache in childhood and adolescents. Budapest, 1995.

Kristjansdottir G, Wahlberg V. Sociodemographic differences in the prevalence of self-reported headaches in Icelandic school-children. *Headache* 1993; 33:376–380.

Labbé EE, Williamson DA. Treatment of childhood migraine using autogenic feedback training. *J Consult Clin Psychol* 1984; 52:968–976.

Langeveldt JH, Koot HM, Loonen MCB, et al. A quality of life instrument for adolescents with chronic headache. *Cephalalgia* 1996; 16:183–196.

Langeveldt JH, Koot HM, Passchier J. How are changes in headache intensity in adolescents related to changes in experienced quality of life? *Headache* 1997; 37:37–42.

Larsson BS. The role of psychological, health behaviour and medical factors in adolescent headache. *Dev Med Child Neurol* 1988; 30:616–625.

Larsson BS. Somatic complaints and their relationship to depressive symptoms in Swedish adolescents. *J Child Psychol Psychiatry* 1991; 32:821–832.

Larsson B. School-based treatment of recurrent headaches in adolescents. In: Wallander JL, Sigel LJ (Eds). *Behavioral Perspective on Adolescent Health*. New York: Guilford Publications, 1995, pp 248–264.

Larsson B, Melin L. Relaxation training in the treatment of recurrent pediatric headache: the Uppsala studies. *Scand Behav Ther* 1988a; 17:125–137.

Larsson B, Melin L. The psychological treatment of recurrent headache in adolescents— short-term outcome and its prediction. *Headache* 1988b; 28:187–195.

Larsson B, Melin L. Follow-up on behavioral treatment of recurrent headache in adolescents. *Headache* 1989; 29:249–253.

Larsson B, Daleflod B, Håkansson L, Melin L. Therapist-assisted versus self-help relaxation of chronic headaches in adolescents: a school-based intervention. *J Child Psychol Psychiatry* 1987a; 28:127–136.

Larsson B, Melin L, Lamminen ML, Ullstedt E. A school-based treatment of chronic headaches in adolescents. *J Pediatr Psychol* 1987b; 12:553–566.

Larsson B, Bille B, Pedersen N. Genetic influence in headaches: A Swedish twin study. *Headache* 1995; 35:513–519.

Leviton A, Slack WV, Masek B, Bana D, Graham JR. A computerized behavioral assessment for children with headaches. *Headache* 1984; 24:182–185.

Linder SL. Subcutaneous sumatriptan in the clinical setting: the first fifty consecutive patients with acute migraine in a pediatric neurology office practice. Poster presented at the 3rd International Congress on headache in childhood and adolescents. Budapest, 1995.

Linet MS, Stewart W F, Celentano DD, Ziegler DK, Sprecher M. An epidemiologic study of headache among adolescents and young adults. *JAMA* 1989; 261:2211–2216.

Marklund U. *Skolbarns hälsovanor under ett decennium. Tabellrapport. Health Behaviour in School-aged Children. A WHO Collaborative Study*. Stockholm: Folkhälsoinstitutet, Garnisonstryckeriet AB, 1997.

Martin PR. *Psychological Management of Chronic Headaches*. New York: Guilford Press, 1993.

Maytal J, Lipton RB, Solomon S, Shinnar S. Childhood onset cluster headaches. *Headache* 1992; 32:275–279.

McGrath PJ, Larsson B. Headache in children and adolescents. *Child Adolesc Psychiatr Clin N Am* 1997; 6(4):843–861.

McGrath PJ, Humphreys P, Goodman JT, Keene D. Relaxation prophylaxis for childhood migraine: a randomized placebo-controlled trial. *Dev Med Child Neurol* 1988; 30:626–631.

McGrath PJ, Cunningham SJ, Lascelles MA, Humphreys P. *Help Yourself: A Treatment for Migraine Headaches: Patient Manual*. Ottawa: University of Ottawa Press, 1990.

McGrath PJ, Humphreys P, Keene D, et al. The efficacy and efficiency of a self-administered treatment for adolescent migraine. *Pain* 1992; 49:321–324.

Metsähonkala L. Migraine in childhood. Thesis, Turku University, Medica-odontologica 266, 1997.

Metsähonkala L, Sillanpää M. Migraine in children—an evaluation of the IHS criteria. *Cephalalgia* 1994; 14:285–290.

Metsähonkala L. Sillanpää M, Tuominen J. Use of health care services in childhood migraine. *Headache* 1996; 36:423–428.

Metsähonkala L, Sillanpää M, Tuominen J. Outcome of early school-age migraine. *Cephalalgia* 1997; 17:662–665.

Mortimer MJ, Kay J, Jaron A. Epidemiology of headache and childhood migraine in an urban general practice using Ad Hoc, Vahlquist and IHS criteria. *Dev Med Child Neurol* 1992; 34:1095–1101.

Newachek PW, McManus MA, Harriette BF. Prevalence and impact of chronic illness among adolescents. *Amer J Dis Child* 1991; 145:1367–1373.

Olesen J, Tfelt-Hansen P, Welch KMA (Eds). *The Headaches.* New York: Raven Press, 1993.

Osterhaus SOL. Recurrent headaches in youngsters. Measurement, behavioral treatment, stress and family factors. Thesis, University of Amsterdam, 1998.

Osterhaus SOL, Passchier J, van der Helm Hylkema H, et al. Effects of behavioral psychophysiological treatment on schoolchildren with migraine in a nonclinical setting: predictors and process variables. *J Pediatr Psychol* 1993; 18:697–711.

Osterhaus SOL, Lange A, Linssen WHJP, Passchier J. A behavioral treatment of young migrainous and nonmigrainous headache patients: prediction of treatment success. *Int J Behav Med* 1997; 4:378–396.

Passchier J, Orlebeke JF. Headaches and stress in schoolchildren: an epidemiological study. *Cephalalgia* 1985; 5:167–176.

Pothmann R, Frankenberg SV, Muller B, Sartory G, Hellmeier W. Epidemiology of headache in children and adolescents: evidence of high prevalence of migraine among girls under 10. *Int J Behav Med* 1994; 1:76–89.

Raieli V, Raimondo R, Camarda R. Migraine headaches in adolescents: a student population-based study in Montreal. *Cephalalgia* 1995; 15:5–12.

Reid GJ, Gilbert CA, McGrath PJ. The Pain Coping Questionnaire: preliminary validation. *Pain* 1998; 76:83–96.

Richardson GM, McGrath PJ, Cunningham SJ, Humphreys P. Validity of the headache diary for children. *Headache* 1983; 23:184–187.

Richter IL, McGrath PJ, Humphreys PJ, Goodman JT. Cognitive and relaxation treatment of paediatric migraine. *Pain* 1986; 25:195–203.

Rowan AB, Andrasik F. Efficacy and cost-effectiveness of minimal therapist contact treatments of chronic headaches: a review. *Behav Ther* 1996; 27:207–234.

Saraceni G, Armani S, Bottazzo S, Gesmundo E. Prevalence of migraine in 901 Venetian school children between 6 and 13 years. In: Lanzi G, Balotin U, Cernibori (Eds). *Headache in Children and Adolescents.* Amsterdam: Elsevier Science, 1989, pp 181–184.

Seshia SS, Wolstein JR, Adams C, Booth FA, Reggin JD. International Headache Society criteria and childhood headache. *Dev Med Child Neurol* 1994; 36:419–428.

Sillanpää M. Prevalence of headache in prepuberty. *Headache* 1983a; 23:10–14.

Sillanpää M. Changes in the prevalence of migraine and other headaches during the first seven school years. *Headache* 1983b; 23:15–19.

Sillanpää M, Anttila P. Increasing prevalence of headache in 7-year-old school-children. *Headache* 1996; 36:446–470.

Sillanpää M, Piekkala P, Kero P. Prevalence of headache at preschool age in an unselected child population. *Cephalalgia* 1991; 11:239–242.

Sorbi MJ, Haimowitz BR, Spierings ELH, Tellegen B. Daily hassles and mood changes preceding the migraine attack. In: Hogenhuis LAH, Steiner TJ (Eds). *Headache and Migraine 3.* Wetenschappelijke Uitgeverij Bunge, 1994, pp 29–41.

Sparks JP. The incidence of migraine in schoolchildren. A survey by the Medical Officers of Schools Association. *Practitioner* 1978; 221:407–411.

Svensson DA, Larsson B, Bille B, Lichtenstein P. Genetic and environmental influences of recurrent headaches in childhood. Submitted.

Symon D. Paediatric migraine—a literature review of placebo controlled clinical trials. Poster presented at the 3rd International Congress on headache in childhood and adolescents. Budapest, 1995.

Vahlquist B. Migraine in children. *Int Arch Allergy* 1955; 7:348–355.

Wänman A. Recurrent headaches and craniomandibular disorders in adolescents: a longitudinal study. *J Craniomandib Dis* 1987; 1:227–236.

Wöber-Bingöl C, Wöber C, Karwautz A, et al. Diagnosis of headache in childhood and adolescence: a study in 437 patients. *Cephalalgia* 1995; 15:13–21.

Ziegler DK, Hur Y-Mi, Bouchard TJ, Hassanein RS, Barter R. Migraine in twins raised together and apart. *Headache* 1998; 38:417–422.

Zuckerman B, Stevenson J, Bailey V. Stomachaches and headaches in a community sample of preschool children. *Pediatrics* 1987; 79:677–682.

Correspondence to: Bo Larsson, Department of Public Health and Caring Sciences, Uppsala University, 75183 Uppsala, Sweden. Tel: +46-18-4713483; Fax: +46-18-4713490; email: bo.larsson@ccs.uu.se.

Chronic and Recurrent Pain in Children and Adolescents, Progress in Pain Research and Management, Vol. 13, edited by Patrick J. McGrath and G. Allen Finley, IASP Press, Seattle, © 1999.

8

The Evolution of Research on Recurrent Abdominal Pain: History, Assumptions, and a Conceptual Model

Lynn S. Walker

Division of Adolescent Medicine, Department of Pediatrics, Vanderbilt University School of Medicine, Nashville, Tennessee, USA

In the four decades since Apley published his observations of English schoolchildren with recurrent episodes of abdominal pain, what have we learned? This chapter describes the evolution of research on recurrent abdominal pain (RAP). It organizes the literature into three historical periods and focuses on the conceptual models, methodological approaches, and major findings associated with each. Assumptions that limit our current knowledge are discussed. Finally, a conceptual model is proposed that draws on theories of child development to identify psychosocial mechanisms that lead some children with RAP to develop chronic sick role behavior, that is, frequent somatic complaints, activity restriction, and dependence on caretakers (Mechanic 1986).

HISTORY OF RESEARCH ON RECURRENT ABDOMINAL PAIN

EARLY INVESTIGATIONS: DEFINING RAP AND RULING OUT ORGANIC DISEASE

In 1958, Apley and Naish published the results of a field survey of 1000 schoolchildren who received routine school medical examinations in Bristol, England. During the course of this survey, they conducted detailed clinical evaluations of a subgroup of children with RAP, defined as "at least three bouts of pain, severe enough to affect [their] activities, over a period of not less than three months, with attacks continuing in the year preceding the examination" (Apley and Naish 1958, p. 165). Although RAP had previously received some attention in the pediatric literature (e.g., Conway 1951; MacKeith and O'Neill 1951), the work by Apley and Naish established RAP as a common pediatric problem and was the impetus for research by other investigators. Indeed, the criteria for sample selection used by Apley and Naish were subsequently adopted as the defining characteristics of RAP.

Apley's study of unselected schoolchildren (Apley and Naish 1958) and his later investigation of hospitalized children (Apley 1975) identified important characteristics of RAP. Specifically, these studies documented that RAP occurred in about 10% of the population of school-aged children, was more common in girls than in boys, and was most prevalent during middle childhood. Apley also reported that RAP is frequently associated with other somatic symptoms such as vomiting and headaches. In addition, his studies found that family members of children with RAP had a higher incidence of abdominal and other pain complaints compared to family members of control children. Most important, although incidental anomalies were found in a few patients in the hospital study, results of medical evaluations generally failed to uncover organic disease that could account for the children's abdominal pain. Apley observed that patients with RAP tended to be "anxious, timid, fussy, and over-conscientious, taking the ordinary difficulties of life (especially of school life) too much to heart" (Apley and Naish 1958, p.170). He concluded that emotional disturbance is more common in children with RAP than in other children.

Other investigations built on Apley's work, replicating and extending his findings during the 1960s and 1970s. These studies aimed to describe the course and symptoms of RAP. They replicated Apley's findings that children with RAP reported multiple somatic complaints (Stone and Barbero 1970; Liebman 1978) and that their abdominal pain rarely had an identifiable organic etiology (Stickler and Murphy 1979; Christensen and Mortensen 1975). Moreover, long-term follow-up studies demonstrated that a third to half of patients with RAP continued to complain of abdominal pain and other nonspecific somatic symptoms years or even decades after their initial medical evaluation (Apley and Hale 1973; Christensen and Mortensen 1975; Stickler and Murphy 1979). Like Apley, other investigators speculated that psychological factors are likely to play a significant role in RAP.

Contributions of early investigations

These early investigations were based on clinical interviews and results of medical diagnostic procedures. The investigators were physicians whose subjects generally were their own patients. Their observations provided a rich description of children with RAP. Many of their clinical findings were later replicated with more sophisticated research methods.

A clinical problem provided the impetus for these initial investigations— the need for pediatricians to differentiate children whose abdominal pain was associated with serious organic disease from those whose pain, while disabling, rarely reflected disease. As Apley put it, "the differentiation between primarily organic and primarily non-organic disorder remains one of the basic tenets of medical practice" (Apley 1975, p. 68). Apley warned that positive evidence of emotional factors should be identified rather than assumed. Nonetheless, the literature generally reflected a dualistic view of pain in the widespread tendency to speculate that abdominal pain must be psychogenic when no organic etiology is identified. Although several investigators considered physiological factors that might contribute to RAP, including lactose or sucrose intolerance (Barr et al. 1979; Liebman 1979), gut transit time (Dimson 1971), and autonomic dysfunction (Kopel et al. 1967; Rubin et al. 1967; Apley et al. 1971), these tended to be isolated studies that did not generate conclusive findings. Thus, the bottom line for the body of research on RAP conducted before 1980 seems to be: "It's not organic; it's probably psychogenic."

THE 1980s: SEARCHING FOR OTHER CAUSES OF RAP

The consistent finding that RAP was not associated with apparent organic disease led to a search for other causes in the 1980s. This decade marked the entry of psychiatry and psychology into the study of RAP. Numerous studies described psychosocial correlates of RAP with the implicit notion that they might provide clues to the etiology of RAP. Three major sets of psychosocial variables were examined: (1) psychiatric disorder and emotional/behavioral problems, (2) stressful life events, and (3) family environment. Major findings in each of these areas are reviewed below.

Psychiatric disorders and emotional/behavioral problems

Several studies during the 1980s found evidence of higher levels of internalizing emotional symptoms in children with RAP compared to well children. For example, RAP patients tended to score higher than control children on standardized measures of anxiety and depression (Raymer et al. 1984; Hodges et al. 1985a,b; Wasserman et al. 1988; Walker and Greene 1989). Similarly, reports of clinical observations by psychiatric consultation and liaison services suggested that most children hospitalized for RAP met the criteria for a psychiatric disorder, particularly anxiety or depression

(Astrada et al. 1981; Hughes 1984). Other investigators pursued the hypothesis that RAP might be a precursor of somatization disorder and reported that pediatric patients with RAP scored higher on measures of nonspecific somatic symptoms and had more relatives with somatization disorder compared to patients with an identified organic etiology for abdominal pain (Ernst et al. 1984; Routh and Ernst 1984; Routh et al. 1988; Walker et al. 1991).

However, not all investigators found evidence linking RAP to internalizing symptoms: McGrath and colleagues (1983) reported that measures of emotional and behavioral problems did not differentiate patients with RAP from well children. Furthermore, the finding that emotional distress was elevated both in children with RAP and in those with an organic etiology for abdominal pain (Sawyer et al. 1987; Walker and Greene 1989) raised the possibility that distress associated with RAP could be a result rather than a cause of pain.

Stressful life events

Based on his clinical observations, Apley had concluded that "in a large proportion of children with recurrent abdominal pain the criteria of a stress disorder are fulfilled" (Apley 1975, p. 93). In the 1980s, this notion was examined empirically using measures of stressful life events. The results suggested that, in comparison to well children, patients with RAP had experienced more events related to family illness and death (Wasserman et al. 1988; Hodges et al. 1984) but had not experienced more total life events (McGrath et al. 1983; Wasserman et al. 1988). Thus, it appeared that illness-related events might be more common in patients with RAP; however, these studies assessed life events occurring during a broad time period prior to clinic referral and did not establish the relation of these events to the onset or exacerbation of pain episodes.

Family environment

During the 1980s, studies of family functioning (Wasserman et al. 1988) and marital adjustment (McGrath et al. 1983) demonstrated that families of children with RAP were no different from families of well children on global measures of family functioning. With respect to parent functioning, however, Walker and Greene (1989) reported that mothers (but not fathers) of children with RAP had higher levels of anxiety, depression, and somatization symptoms than did mothers of well children. Studies of family medical history yielded mixed results: one study found a higher incidence of current and prior painful gastrointestinal disorders among family members of children with RAP compared to family members of well children (Wasserman et al. 1988), but another found no difference (McGrath et al. 1983).

Conceptual models of RAP

Two important conceptual models of RAP were published during this decade, although neither was adopted as a framework to guide research. First, Barr and colleagues proposed a "tripartite" model of RAP (Barr 1983; Barr and Feuerstein 1983; Hunziker and Barr 1984). They argued that in a large percentage of children with RAP, pain is neither organic nor psychogenic but rather is "dysfunctional." They defined dysfunctional abdominal pain as associated with a nonpathological biological mechanism, such as lactose intolerance, that is indicative neither of organic disease nor psychopathology. This model classifies children into groups based on the etiology of their pain. A single cause is assumed to predominate for each child. For example, there is no category for a case in which organic and psychological causes both contribute to a child's pain.

Levine and Rappaport (1984) proposed a multivariate model of RAP, the "primary forces model," which held that RAP was a function of four forces: (1) somatic predisposition, dysfunction, or disorder; (2) lifestyle and habit; (3) milieu and critical events; and (4) temperament and learned response patterns. The primary forces model is similar to the tripartite model in suggesting that the absence of organic disease does not necessarily reflect a psychogenic etiology but in some cases can be explained by relatively common, benign physiological dysfunctions. In addition, the primary forces model allows for multiple causes, although it does not specify how these might interact to produce pain.

These were the first explicit conceptual models of RAP. They are especially important contributions to the literature because each model recognizes that the cause of RAP is not *either* organic *or* psychogenic, but also may be a function of normal biological mechanisms. A few investigators continued the effort to identify those mechanisms. For example, a study of gastroduodenal motility in eight adolescents with RAP concluded that altered intestinal motility might be the underlying mechanism in some children (Pineiro-Carrero et al. 1988). Another study exposed children with RAP to a cold pressor stimulus and found no evidence of a deficit in autonomic nervous system recovery to this stressor (Feuerstein et al. 1982).

Contributions of the 1980s

During the 1980s, studies of the psychosocial characteristics of RAP introduced several methodological features not present in prior literature. Assessment procedures were strengthened by the use of standardized psychiatric diagnostic interviews (e.g., Astrada et al. 1981; Wasserman et al. 1988) and validated measures of emotional symptoms, stressful life events, and family functioning (e.g., McGrath et al. 1983). Comparison groups were used more frequently than in earlier years, and included well children (e.g., Wasserman et al. 1988), children with organic etiologies for abdominal pain (e.g., Routh and Ernst 1984; Walker and Greene 1989), and children with emotional/behavioral disorders referred to a child psychiatry clinic (e.g., Hodges et al. 1985a). Finally, statistical tests were routinely applied to evaluate the significance of differences between groups.

Despite the introduction of nondualistic models of RAP early in the decade, the fact that the empirical literature focused on identification of psychosocial etiologies for this syndrome gives the impression that it was still viewed in dualistic terms as organic or psychogenic. The most reliable findings of the decade were that patients with RAP tended to be characterized by high levels of internalizing symptoms, including anxiety, depression, and nonspecific somatic symptoms, and that their family members tended to report frequent health problems and pain complaints. These findings were consistent with clinical observations of earlier decades and were based on more rigorous methodologies. An important new finding was that standardized measures of emotional distress were not useful in differentiating abdominal pain patients with and without organic disease.

THE 1990s: IDENTIFYING INDIVIDUAL DIFFERENCES AND INTERACTIVE EFFECTS

During the 1990s, several investigators have continued to replicate earlier findings linking RAP to internalizing emotional symptoms (Garber et al. 1990; Walker et al. 1993; Woodbury 1993) and to a high incidence of pain complaints by family members (Robinson et al. 1990; Walker et al. 1993). In addition, findings of important similarities between families of patients with RAP and families of well children have been replicated: family functioning, marital adjustment, and exposure to non-illness-related stressful life events appear to be within normal limits in families of patients with RAP (Walker et al. 1993). These studies have used the categorical approach that characterized prior research on RAP, i.e., children with RAP are compared as a group to well children and to other patient groups. This approach is useful to identify features that are characteristic of most children with RAP, but it neglects individual differences among RAP patients.

In recent years, attention has shifted to identifying individual differences that are predictive of differences in health outcomes among RAP patients. This shift is consistent with a move away from a disease model in which the expression of disease is expected to be the same for all patients. Several innovations in research have accompanied the focus on individual differences including assessment of the severity of abdominal symptoms and disability, testing of conceptual models with multivariate statistical approaches, and identification of subgroups of children with RAP. Progress in these areas is laying the groundwork for the development of treatment programs that take into account such individual differences.

Measures of severity

Variation in symptom severity is an important individual difference variable. When RAP is described only by Apley's criteria (three or more episodes of abdominal pain that occur over at least 3 months and are severe enough to interfere with activities), it is unclear how to track the course of illness or to assess treatment response. How does a clinician describe exacerbations or improvements in the condition or determine when the child has recovered? Early outcome studies reported whether children with RAP continued to experience abdominal pain at follow-up, but did not systematically assess the frequency and severity of their pain (e.g., Apley and Hale 1973; Christensen and Mortensen 1975; Stickler and Murphy 1979). The mere presence versus absence of pain is unsatisfactory as an outcome measure for RAP, given the importance of related symptoms and disability as additional outcome measures, as well as the high frequency of abdominal pain in otherwise healthy schoolchildren (Garber et al. 1991; Hyams et al. 1996).

Recently, standardized measures of children's symptom severity and disability have been developed and validated specifically for use with RAP patients. The development of multiple outcome measures means that patients with RAP not only can be classified by Apley's criteria, but also can be described and compared in the frequency, duration, and intensity of their abdominal pain (e.g., Abdominal Pain Index; Walker et al. 1997), the level of other nonspecific somatic symptoms (e.g., Children's Somatization Inventory; Walker and Greene 1989; Garber et al. 1991), and the degree to which they are disabled by their pain (e.g., Functional Disability Inventory, Walker and Zeman 1992). The availability of both parent-report and child-report versions of these measures means that we no longer have to rely solely on parent reports, which may be biased by parent characteristics (Garber et al. 1998). These measures of outcomes specific to RAP, as well as standardized measures of other relevant outcomes such as depression, have been used in prospective studies to describe changes in the severity of abdominal pain, emotional and somatic symptoms, and functional disability across time (Walker et al. 1991, 1993, 1995b; Walker and Greene 1991).

Acknowledgment of individual differences in the severity of RAP reflects an important change in thinking: it now can be viewed not only as a diagnostic entity, but also as a set of symptoms and disability that range on a continuum from mild to severe. This dimensional approach also implies that symptoms of RAP may be found at lower levels in healthy children, and that at higher levels these symptoms may reflect an exaggeration of normal biopsychosocial processes (cf. Costa and McCrae 1985).

Empirical tests of multivariate models

Although Levine and Rappaport introduced a multivariate model of the etiology of RAP in 1984, it was not until the 1990s that multivariate models were tested empirically. For example, Walker and colleagues have examined the interaction of stressful life events with various risk and protective factors in predicting the course of RAP. In a prospective study of pediatric patients evaluated for RAP, they found that the combination of high levels of negative family life events and low social competence predicted high symptom levels 1 year following the initial clinic evaluation (Walker et al. 1994). This finding suggests that the ability to obtain social support from peers may buffer children from the effect of family stressors on their health. Furthermore, results of a 5-year follow-up study of these pain patients indicated that a passive style of coping with pain is a risk factor for continued somatic symptoms (Walker et al. 1997).

Another study using a multivariate model found that abdominal pain and related bowel symptoms were more likely to be associated with functional disability in adolescents with low perceived academic competence than in adolescents with high perceived competence (Lewis et al., in press). Specifically, among teens who perceived themselves as doing poorly at school, higher symptom levels were associated with greater disability. Among teens who viewed themselves as doing well in school, disability was low, even for those with high levels of bowel symptoms. Thus, there may be a vicious cycle in which (1) pain-related disability is reinforced in adolescents with lower academic competence because it allows them to avoid a threatening situation, and (2) adolescents with more severe symptoms and disability suffer decrements in actual or perceived academic competence due to restricted participation at school. In this sense, low academic competence may be a risk factor for increased disability in teens with abdominal pain and related somatic symptoms.

Multivariate conceptual models and statistics have allowed us to examine the interaction between health status and psychosocial variables in prospective studies predicting patient outcomes. For example, after controlling for initial symptom severity and pain duration in pediatric patients with abdominal pain, Walker and Heflinger (1998) found that measures of functional disability, depression, and academic competence obtained at the clinic visit significantly predicted later recovery. Another study examined the relative utility of biomedical findings and psychosocial variables in predicting abdominal pain. Results suggested that psychosocial variables, such as use of passive coping strategies, are better predictors of child pain reports than are biomedical findings regarding the severity of tissue damage (Stutts et al. 1998). Considered together, the findings of these multivariate studies indicate that assessment of psychosocial factors is important in identifying abdominal pain patients at risk for poor recovery.

Identification of subgroups

Recent clinical and theoretical literatures have emphasized the heterogeneity of biological processes that may underlie symptoms of RAP (Boyle 1991, 1997). Organic disease is found in only a small percentage of cases (Stickler and Murphy 1979; Walker et al. 1995b); the remainder are considered "functional" in nature. Although the term "functional" refers only to the absence of organic disease, it often is inferred to mean that biological processes are irrelevant and that a psychogenic etiology must account for the symptoms. However, even in the absence of organic disease, physiologic abnormalities may underlie symptoms of functional gastrointestinal disorders (Drossman 1994). Over the years, investigators have attempted to identify some of these physiological abnormalities with studies of lactose intolerance (Barr et al. 1979), gastrointestinal motility (e.g., Pineiro-Carrero et al. 1988), and autonomic dysfunction (e.g., Feuerstein et al. 1982). Recent research has focused on visceral hyperalgesia (Hyams and Hyman 1998) and hormone levels (Alfvén and Uvnas-Moberg 1993; Alfvén et al. 1994) as potential contributors to abdominal distress. Thus, some functional gastrointestinal symptoms may be explained by physiological abnormalities that do not constitute disease but rather represent a benign physiological deviation.

Considerable additional research is needed before it will be possible to develop laboratory tests that reliably identify physiological abnormalities associated with various functional gastrointestinal disorders. However, clusters of functional gastrointestinal symptoms tend to aggregate together, making it possible to generate symptom-based diagnostic criteria that identify sub-groups of these disorders (Drossman 1994). International working teams of experts in gastroenterology have established symptom-based diagnostic criteria for functional gastrointestinal disorders in adults (Drossman 1994). A similar symptom-based classification system for pediatric functional gastrointestinal disorders is under development (Hyman et al., in press).

Once such a classification system is validated, it will be possible to differentiate children who meet Apley's broad criteria for RAP into sub-groups characterized by symptom clusters that may reflect different under-lying physiological processes. For example, in the absence of identifiable organic disease, a child with abdominal pain of several months' duration might be classified into one of several groups: (1) functional dyspepsia, characterized by pain centered in the upper abdomen; (2) irritable bowel syndrome, characterized by pain that is relieved with defecation and associated with changes in stool frequency or consistency; (3) functional constipation, characterized by fecal retention; and (4) functional abdominal pain, characterized by periumbilical abdominal pain that is unrelated to food intake or bowel habits.

Thus, a two-stage classification system may be applied to RAP: children first may be identified as meeting Apley's broad criteria for RAP and then further classified into subgroups according to more specific symptom descriptions (von Baeyer and Walker, in press). This approach should facilitate research investigating differences among subgroups with respect to etiology, course, and treatment needs.

Matching patients to treatment

Treatment of RAP has been limited by our inability to reliably identify subgroups of children who may differ in their treatment needs. In some instances, a single treatment may be offered to all children, with inconsistent results. For example, mixed results from studies of the efficacy of fiber treatments for RAP (Feldman et al. 1985; Christensen 1986) may be due to heterogeneity among the patients, some of whom may not have had constipation and therefore would not be expected to benefit from fiber treatment.

Another approach has been to design treatment programs with multiple components that address a variety of patient needs. For example, Sanders and his colleagues in Australia included relaxation training, cognitive self-control strategies, parent reinforcement of appropriate coping behaviors, and differential reinforcement of competing activities in a cognitive-behav-ioral treatment program for children who met Apley's broad criteria for RAP (Sanders et al. 1989, 1994). Although this program demonstrated some success, considerable savings in time and resources could be gained if it were possible to identify children who needed particular treatment components but not others. In this vein, Finney has argued for multicomponent targeted therapy that matches patients to treatment components according to their presenting symptoms (Finney et al. 1989; Edwards et al. 1991).

Ongoing research investigating individual differences among RAP patients should provide a knowledge base for better matching of patients with specific treatments. It will be important to identify both psychosocial and biological factors that influence outcomes and to integrate both types of factors into treatment programs. For example, fiber treatment might be offered to a patient with functional constipation and not to a patient with functional dyspepsia, but both might benefit from a stress management intervention.

Contributions of the 1990s

During this decade, children with RAP came to be viewed as a heterogeneous group. It now appears that identification of differences among individuals within the group, rather than differences between RAP and other groups, may hold the key to understanding the etiology and course of RAP. This change in thinking is reflected in other changes in the literature, summarized in Table I. Specifically, Apley's original criteria are being supplemented with symptom-based diagnostic criteria that promise to identify distinct subgroups within the broad category of RAP. New diagnostic procedures for the medical evaluation of abdominal pain (e.g., endoscopy, ultrasound) are enhancing our ability to identify biological contributions to RAP. Research

Table I
Changes in the literature on recurrent abdominal pain (RAP)

Characteristic	Early Literature	Current Literature
View of RAP	Homogeneous	Heterogeneous
Classification system	Apley's criteria (1958)	Symptom-based diagnostic criteria
Medical evaluation	Limited medical evaluation	New diagnostic procedures; measures of symptom severity
Psychosocial evaluation	Clinical observation	Standard instrumentation
Conceptual models	Main effects	Interactive effects
Statistics	Univariate	Multivariate
Outcomes	Presence/absence of pain	Changes in severity on multiple dimensions

methods have moved beyond clinical observation to include standardized measures of symptoms and disability that allow assessment of individual differences in the severity and course of RAP. Conceptual models have been elaborated to include the interactive effects of several factors on the severity and course of RAP. Univariate statistical approaches have been supplemented with multivariate approaches. Finally, the assessment of outcomes has moved beyond a focus on the presence or absence of pain to address changes in the severity of multiple outcomes.

ASSUMPTIONS IN THE LITERATURE

Despite these advances in our methods and in our understanding of RAP, significant gaps remain. Three characteristics of the current literature maintain implicit assumptions that limit our progress.

ASSUMPTION 1: RAP IS A PROBLEM

Research to date has focused primarily on a restricted group of children with RAP, which puts us in danger of concluding that this group represents the whole. The course of RAP is depicted in Fig. 1. Like any other condition, it has antecedents, an onset, and a course. Some time after the onset of the illness, some children become patients while others do not. Later, some of these general practice patients become referral patients at specialty clinics.

Most of the research on RAP is based on referral patients seen in tertiary care settings. There are a few exceptions: Apley's 1958 survey was conducted in a community field setting, and a later study by Faull and Nicol (1986) investigated the incidence of abdominal pain in a community sample of 5- to 6-year-olds. Two recent studies have used samples of unselected schoolchildren (Sharrer and Ryan-Wenger 1991; Hyams et al. 1996). With these exceptions, our empirical knowledge of RAP is a knowledge of tertiary care referral patients. No studies to date have assessed differences between patients and nonpatients (i.e., those who do not seek medical help), or between primary care and tertiary care patients. Thus, it is impossible to

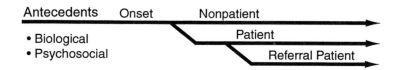

Fig. 1. The course of recurrent abdominal pain.

know the degree to which our findings represent characteristics of tertiary care patients versus characteristics of the general population of children with RAP. The adult literature on patients and nonpatients with irritable bowel syndrome (e.g, Drossman et al. 1988) suggests that such comparisons might substantially change our thinking about RAP. Specifically, we might find that features assumed to characterize RAP, such as internalizing emotional symptoms, in fact characterize pediatric tertiary care patients in general.

Tertiary care patients, by definition, have progressed some distance in the course of their illness. Research relying on these patients is similar to that using pain clinic samples to study chronic pain in adults (cf. Dworkin et al. 1992)—both have limited generalizability. Patients referred to pediatric gastroenterology clinics are those whose symptoms did not respond to the standard treatment available in primary care settings. They may be particularly complex or resistant to treatment. Furthermore, whatever the initial cause of their pain, these patients and their families have suffered the consequences of living with pain for some time. Thus, our research samples to date tend to represent children with the most severe psychosocial and biological sequelae of pain.

This reliance on samples of patients with the most extreme symptoms and disability has led to an implicit assumption that RAP is always a problem. We know little about the early course of RAP or about those children and families who manage pain without seeking medical consultation. A focus on the early course and on the entire continuum of symptom severity would help us understand the potential range of adaptation to RAP. In addition, this broader focus may teach us to what extent similar mechanisms explain RAP that occurs in the context of normal development as well as that associated with extensive disability and internalizing emotional symptoms.

ASSUMPTION 2: RAP IS IN THE CHILD

Our research questions have generally focused on the child as the unit of analysis and have considered RAP as a characteristic of the child in much the way that a disease entity is viewed as residing within an individual. In contrast, Bronfenbrenner (1977) argued that to understand the child's behavior we must consider the multiple contexts in which a child functions. Fig. 2 applies this ecological perspective and depicts the child with RAP within the larger social context. The most proximal interdependent contexts include the family, school, and health care system—all situated within the community, which is situated within a culture.

The bulk of clinical and empirical literature on RAP has focused on the

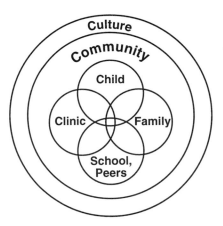

Fig. 2. The social context of recurrent abdominal pain.

child and, to a lesser extent, the family. Children's academic performance is sometimes assessed, but the classroom setting has not been examined. For example, no one has addressed the potential effects of teaching style and classroom environments on the development of RAP. The role of the health care setting has been addressed at the level of recommendations for clinical assessment and treatment, but no studies have examined how variables such as the extent and outcome of the medical evaluation, the relationship with the provider, or the way in which results of the medical evaluation are presented may affect the course of the syndrome.

Similarly, nothing is known about the relation of the broader community and culture to RAP. Research in Western nations has not explored potential differences among ethnic subgroups in the presentation and course of RAP, and non-Western studies are rare. Indeed, the existence and incidence of this problem in non-Western cultures are unknown. Given the important role of culture in the socialization of sick role behavior and attitudes (e.g., Mechanic 1986; Landrine and Klonoff 1992), a cross-cultural approach might be helpful in identifying processes that we may not see from the vantage point of our own culture.

The lack of attention in the literature to the multiple contexts of RAP reflects an implicit assumption that the problem is within the child. An alternative perspective is to move beyond the individual as the unit of analysis and to conceptualize RAP as a system of multiple units including the family, school and peers, and health care providers, all interdependent and embedded within a particular community and culture.

ASSUMPTION 3: RAP IS DISCONTINUOUS WITH NORMAL DEVELOPMENT

Finally, in neglecting the role of child development in RAP, the research reflects an implicit assumption that RAP is discontinuous with normal development. Apley and others have reported that the incidence of RAP is greatest during middle childhood, at approximately 7–11 years of age (Apley and Naish 1958; Bury 1987; Sharrer and Ryan-Wenger 1991). This observation suggests the possibility that something about the typical environment and developmental processes during middle childhood may increase children's vulnerability to RAP.

In his theory of personality development, Erikson (1964) describes middle childhood as the period of "industry versus inferiority." During middle childhood, ability becomes a major concern. Children are in grade school and must develop a wide array of new skills. According to Erikson, successful application of these skills builds a sense of industry, whereas failure produces a sense of inferiority. Earlier developmental tasks (learning to trust, to be autonomous, and to take initiative) were tackled within the context of the family, but many tasks of middle childhood involve activities outside the home, comparison with peers, and evaluative feedback from people other than family members. In our efforts to understand problems of middle childhood, it is important that we view the child within this social and developmental context.

Rothbaum and Weisz (1989), like Erikson, identify perceived inferiority as a major risk in middle childhood, noting that "inferiority results from increased awareness of relative failure and relative ability," which develops during this stage (p. 69). They argue that children are predisposed to certain kinds of problems at each stage of intellectual development. During middle childhood, children develop an understanding of stable dispositional constructs (e.g., ability to perform tasks) and how to compare them. Children become aware of ability as an explanation for their performance, and they evaluate their ability in comparison to others. However, children at this stage tend to overuse dispositional constructs in explaining behavior. They have difficulty coordinating dispositional and situational cues and, as a consequence, are vulnerable to self-attributions for failure, even in situations where chance or task difficulty are obvious alternative explanations. According to Rothbaum and Weisz (1989), some children deal with dispositional self-attributions for failure by engaging in externalizing behavior; for example, they may engage in hostile aggression aimed at increasing their relative standing in comparison to peers. Other children, in contrast, react with internalizing behavior in the form of perceived inferiority; these children

may exhibit negative self-evaluations, symptoms of anxiety, and self-de-
feating behaviors such as extreme passivity and withdrawal.

This description of grade-schoolers who react to perceived inadequacy
with internalizing behavior bears much in common with descriptions of patients with RAP, who are characterized by internalizing emotional symptoms. They exhibit passivity and withdrawal in the form of pain-related
disability. Their frequent absence from school and other peer activities may
help them to avoid potentially negative evaluation. Perhaps RAP, when it is
associated with high levels of sick role behavior, is a manifestation of the
struggle with inferiority that is common in middle childhood. The way in
which a child is meeting normative developmental tasks may predict how
the child deals with RAP, and furthermore, the way in which a child deals
with RAP may affect his or her ability, for better or worse, to confront future
developmental tasks. Thus, attention to theories of child development might
provide clues regarding normative issues that make children particularly
vulnerable to RAP during middle childhood and lead some children to develop chronic sick role behavior while others continue their activities despite pain.

NEW DIRECTIONS: A MODEL OF THE ROLE OF PSYCHOSOCIAL FACTORS

A proposed conceptual model of the role of psychosocial factors in the
course of RAP in middle childhood acknowledges the importance of both
biological and psychosocial factors, but focuses on the course of illness
rather than its etiology. This model addresses three features that have received little attention in prior literature: (1) some children with RAP do not
become patients, (2) the social context of pain, and (3) the contribution of
developmental issues. The model draws on the current literature and the
author's clinical experience; hypotheses suggested by the model must be
examined carefully in empirical research.

The model begins with the occurrence of abdominal pain and proposes
multiple "forks in the road." Some children and their families take forks
leading to increasing levels of child disability and family caretaking; this
path exacerbates children's skill deficits and perceived inferiority relative
to peers. Other children and their families take forks leading to resumption
of normal activities; this path increases children's mastery of skills and
development of competence. Thus, the model encompasses a continuum of
health that ranges from dysfunction to positive health (cf. Seeman 1989).

As illustrated in Fig. 3a, the first fork in the road occurs soon after the onset of episodes of abdominal pain. Surveys of schoolchildren suggest that as many as 15–20% report weekly episodes of abdominal pain (Aro et al. 1987; Garber et al. 1991). Following one or more of these episodes, some children restrict their activities. It is likely that other children continue their normal activities despite pain, although data are not available regarding these children. The literature on the sick role suggests that the child and family's appraisal of the meaning of the pain along several dimensions (e.g., severity, course) is critical in determining whether the child is defined as ill and the extent to which the child's normal activities are maintained or restricted (Myfanwy et al. 1985; Leventhal 1986; Walker et al. 1995a).

For children who restrict their activities, a second fork in the road emerges: some children will find the sick role rewarding and others (after the initial novelty wears off) will find it aversive (Fig. 3b). Characteristics of both the child and the environment determine the extent to which the sick role will be experienced as rewarding or aversive. First, the degree to which the child has been successful in accomplishing normative developmental tasks is likely to influence his or her experience of the sick role. Drawing on the observation that development of competence in new domains is an important task of middle childhood, we might expect that children who have recently experienced (or who anticipate) personally significant failures and who attribute these failures to inadequate ability would find it a welcome relief to be excused from activities that carry the threat of failure. Rothbaum and Weisz (1989) noted that perceived inferiority may cause grade-schoolers to avoid public evaluation and to take on the role of victim as a way to gain control. The sick role may provide a legitimate means of doing this and thereby protect children from the threat of evaluation that might reveal relative inability in comparison to peers. Of course, the sick role may serve this protective function without children's conscious intention.

In addition to the child's perceived inferiority, characteristics of the activity settings of middle childhood may increase the degree to which the sick role is experienced as a safe haven. Many activities of middle childhood (school, sports, and so on) carry opportunities for social comparison. If these activities are organized to be highly competitive, if the adults in charge tend to be demanding or critical, or if some children are dealing with their own perceived inferiority by attacking others, the sick role is likely to be a welcome respite. Any privileges or special attention associated with the sick role also would increase its attractiveness. It is critical to note that these factors may influence children's experience of the sick role regardless of whether organic disease is present or absent.

Children with few real or imagined personal failures and those who participate in activity settings that are low in competitiveness, in contrast,

(a)

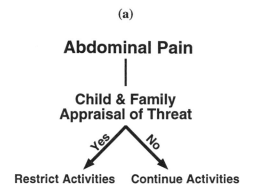

(c)

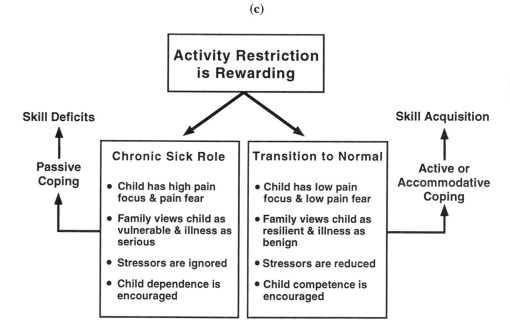

Fig. 3 **(a)** Child and family appraisal of pain. **(b)** Consequences of the sick role. **(c)** Pathways to a chronic sick role versus transition to normal role. **(d)** The course of pain: cycles of dysfunction versus positive growth.

(b)

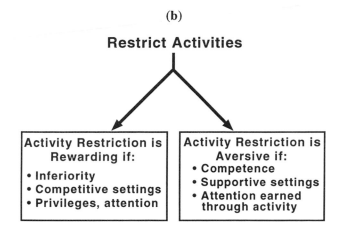

(d)

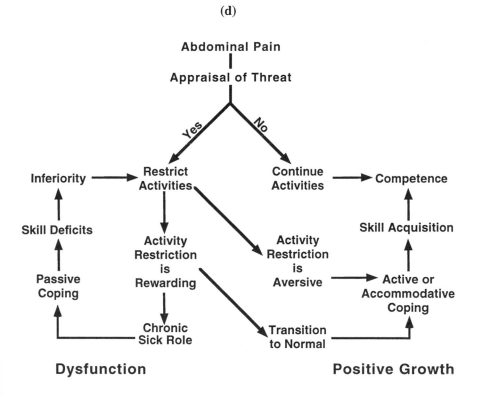

Fig. 3. Continued.

may find it aversive to be removed from the activities of their daily lives even for short periods. To the extent that these children obtain satisfaction in their roles outside the family, they are unlikely to find the privileges and extra attention of the sick role sufficiently rewarding to substitute for the attention they earn in the course of their usual activities. Thus, they are likely to engage in efforts to actively manage or accommodate to the pain and resume their activities. It is not that their coping efforts necessarily reduce or eliminate their pain; rather, their efforts may reduce the impact of the pain on their lives and allow them to continue the pursuit of new skills and competence. Again, this may occur regardless of whether organic disease is present or absent.

Among those children who find withdrawal from activities rewarding, a third fork in the road (see Fig. 3c) presents itself: will they continue in an extended sick role or return to their usual roles? This fork marks the transition from short-term acute episodes of pain (Fig. 3b) to recurrent pain that takes on a life of its own, characteristic of chronic pain syndrome (for a discussion of chronic pain syndrome in children, see McGrath [1990]). Factors that initially made the sick role rewarding (perceived inferiority in normal roles, competitive settings, attention for symptom complaints) may continue. In addition, characteristics of the child, family, school, peers, clinic, and broader social environment interact to determine whether the child will continue in an extended sick role or transition back into normal roles. The contribution of each of these factors is discussed below.

CHILD FACTORS

Children with particular characteristics may be especially vulnerable to adopting a chronic sick role. In adults, trait anxiety is related to increased vigilance and attentiveness to somatic sensations (Cameron et al. 1998). Similarly, Barr and colleagues (1994) have suggested that some children may have a "psychobiological reactivity" that makes them particularly vulnerable not only to pain but also to the effects of other stressors. In an excellent presentation of a psychobiological approach to pediatric pain, Zeltzer and colleagues argue that pain perception is a function of the child's ability to regulate focus of attention, the rapidity with which the child becomes aroused in the face of perceived threat, and the memory of past noxious events (Zeltzer et al. 1997). Children with poor ability to regulate the focus of their attention may focus on pain sensations, becoming anxious and fearful of the pain. Fear, in turn, magnifies the noxious sensory experience. Thus, some children may be predisposed to a self-perpetuating cycle of focus on pain, fear of pain, and heightened pain perception. As more is learned about the psychobiology of pain perception, it may be possible to identify child characteristics that increase the likelihood that acute pain episodes will become chronic or recurrent pain associated with high levels of disability.

FAMILY FACTORS

Just as the family and others are important in defining the child as ill, they are important in defining when the child is well. Parents who view their child as vulnerable and see the abdominal pain as particularly serious may be extremely cautious in letting their child leave the sick role. These appraisals of vulnerability and threat may be long-standing, based on prior family events. For example, Parmelee (1989) has noted that when children have frequent illnesses as infants, some parents come to lack confidence in their children's physical stamina. Parents' appraisals of such vulnerability may be communicated to the children. For example, recent evidence shows that mothers' appraisals of greater severity of their children's abdominal pain predicts children's appraisals of greater pain severity, which in turn predict children's use of more passive pain coping strategies and reports of higher symptom levels (Van Slyke 1998). Thus, parent appraisals may contribute indirectly to children's pain focus, pain fear, and heightened pain perception.

Modeling and reinforcement of symptoms and disability by family members also may influence children's illness behavior (Craig 1978), and have been cited as a factor in the development of RAP (Osborne et al. 1989; Walker and Zeman 1992; Walker et al. 1993). By observing how parents define and respond to their own episodes of pain, children may learn how to interpret symptoms and what type of behavior is appropriate. Children whose parents routinely excuse themselves from daily activities and responsibilities when ill may learn to adopt similar behavior when they are not feeling well (cf. Turkat 1982; Turkat and Guise 1983). Children whose parents are particularly solicitous in providing special attention and privileges during illness episodes may learn that illness behavior carries rewards. Indeed, some parents may themselves find their child's illness behavior rewarding if it distracts them from other problems or provides them an opportunity for greater closeness with their child (cf. Minuchin et al. 1978).

In addition, a child is more likely to develop chronic sick role behavior if the family views the illness itself as the principal threat to the child's well-being and ignores other stressors that may contribute to the illness or to the child's withdrawal from activities. These other stressors may involve the world outside the family (e.g., a competitive classroom or athletic activity), as well as stressors within the family (e.g., unresolved marital conflict, death of a grandparent). Health care providers, teachers, and other individuals can play an important role in helping the family identify potential stressors. Failure to address these stressors means that they continue to pose a threat and, as a result, the sick role may continue to represent an improved quality of life for the child (cf. Lethem et al. 1983).

Finally, families who substantially redefine their roles and their relationships to accommodate the child as patient are likely to extend the child's length of stay in the sick role. Some families make considerable accommodations. For example, arrangements may be made for a grandparent to care for the child or for a parent to take time off from work to allow the child to stay home from school. The child may be allowed to sleep with a parent. The school may be asked to excuse the child's assignments or to allow these to be completed at home and returned at a later date. The effect of these accommodations is to foster the child's dependency and passive coping with pain. Passive coping strategies are associated with maintenance of symptoms and disability (Walker et al. 1997). As disability continues, the child is likely to fall behind peers in a number of areas, with consequent increases in perceived inability. What may have begun as a fear of inability becomes a reality to the extent that the child's withdrawal interferes with new skill acquisition. In this way, an escalating cycle of activity restriction, skill deficits, and perceived inferiority may be set in motion. This deviation-amplifying cycle is illustrated in Fig. 3d.

In contrast, some children transition out of the sick role rather quickly. The families of these children are likely to view the child as resilient and the illness as benign. They do not view pain and activity as incompatible. They may recognize stressors preceding or resulting from the illness and take steps to reduce these to a manageable level. For example, they may recognize that the child feels pressured by a particular activity and may discontinue the child's participation in that activity or help the child develop more effective ways to cope with it. The stressor may not have played a causal role in the child's illness; it also is possible that the illness created the stressor (e.g., illness may lead to school absence that results in falling behind in schoolwork) or that the illness may have overtaxed the child's resources for dealing with a previously manageable stressor. Finally, rather than organizing themselves around the child as patient, these families attempt to maintain their usual roles and relationships. They provide extra support and care for the child, make some allowances in their expectations, and at the same time encourage the child's own coping efforts and competence (cf. Walker et al. 1995b). Thus, the sick role may provide a period of respite in which the bond between parents and children is strengthened as children gain confidence in their ability to cope with illness (cf. Parmelee 1986, 1989). These children renew their interest and engagement in the activities of their age group and are able to return to confront the middle childhood challenge of developing new skills and a sense of competence (Fig. 3d).

SCHOOL AND PEER FACTORS

The nature of the school environment and the child's relationship with the teacher and classmates may foster an extended sick role or a speedy recovery. It is well known that many patients with RAP have frequent school absences associated with pain episodes (Bury 1987; Wasserman et al. 1988; Walker et al. 1995b). Furthermore, approximately 20% of mothers of patients cite difficulty with the teacher or classmates as a factor contributing to their children's pain (Lewis et al., in press). For example, the child's classroom may be more competitive or the teacher more demanding than in earlier grades, resulting in greater child anxiety regarding evaluation. This increased anxiety may contribute to abdominal pain complaints through both physiological and psychosocial mechanisms (cf. Cohen and Rodriguez 1995).

In some instances, the child may be caught in the middle of conflict between parents and teacher. The teacher believes that the parents should make the child go to school; the parents believe that the child is in too much pain and that the teacher is being unreasonable. From the teacher's point of view, the parents are neglecting the child's need for education. From the parents' point of view, the teacher is neglecting the child's need for special protection. As a result, the teacher may apply increased pressure for attendance, the parents may increase their protectiveness of the child, and the child's anxiety, fear, and dependency may further increase.

In contrast, the teacher and school officials may take actions that facilitate the child's return to school. For example, they may initially allow the child to return to school for half-days and provide special assistance in catching up with classmates. In cases of bowel dysfunction, the child may be allowed to go to the restroom without requesting permission to leave the classroom. Rather than admonishing the child about his or her school absence, the teacher may welcome and support the child and encourage classmates to do the same.

HEALTH CARE SYSTEM

The interactions of the health care system with the child and family also can facilitate or impede recovery from RAP. Unnecessarily extensive medical evaluations carry the risk of prolonging and exacerbating child and family concern about the child's condition, promoting the belief that the child is vulnerable. Extensive medical evaluations also may uncover minor findings, such as "microscopic inflammation," that do not necessarily account for the child's pain (Boyle 1997) but provide a diagnostic label that maintains the family's belief that their child's activity restriction is necessary and reasonable. A reasonably limited evaluation also carries risks of an adversarial relationship between the family and the physician if the family has not been helped to understand how pain can occur without underlying disease and therefore believes that an organic etiology has been missed. It is not sufficient to rule out organic disease; the physician also must explain how normal biological and psychosocial processes contribute to functional gastrointestinal pain (for a case example, see Zeltzer 1995).

COMMUNITY FACTORS

The child, family, school, and health care system are part of a larger social system that also may affect the course of RAP. For example, in some states allocation of funds to public schools is dependent on the maintenance of high average daily attendance rates. As a result, teachers may feel considerable pressure to ensure student attendance. This demand on the teacher may conflict with interventions for RAP that use a gradual reintegration into school activities to allow time to enhance the child's confidence and skills.

The public schools in the United States provide another example of a societal influence on RAP. It is not uncommon for the restrooms in public schools to lack privacy. In some schools, the doors leading to the toilet stalls inside the restrooms have been removed, perhaps because they were broken and lack of funds prevents their replacement, or because the school administration hopes that the absence of privacy will reduce the likelihood of children engaging in illicit activities in the restrooms. Anecdotal reports from clinical interviews in our pediatric gastroenterology clinic indicate that refusal to use the toilet at school due to privacy concerns is common in children whose abdominal pain is associated with constipation. This environmental condition may contribute to the cause and maintenance of constipation with associated abdominal pain. Similarly, among children with irritable bowel syndrome, reluctance to use the school restroom may increase school absence.

CULTURAL FACTORS

Finally, the broader context of culture also may play a role in RAP. Culturally mediated values and socialization practices may suppress the development of some emotional and behavioral problems and foster the development of others (Weisz et al. 1987). Some cultures may have low tolerance for extensive disability related to RAP. For example, in societies that focus more on collective efforts than on individual accomplishments, children may be less vulnerable to a sense of inferiority that fosters withdrawal from activities. Similarly, in agricultural societies where the active participation of all family members is required for planting and harvesting, children may not receive the level of caretaking and relief from responsibility that is necessary for an extended course of RAP.

LONG-TERM OUTCOMES

We have seen how recurrent episodes of abdominal pain may develop into chronic sick role behavior for some children. What long-term trajectories are associated with RAP as children move into adolescence and adulthood? Existing studies indicate that symptoms and disability are likely to continue into adulthood for more than a third of pediatric patients (Stickler and Murphy 1979; Walker et al. 1998). However, these studies are based on tertiary care referral patients who have a less favorable prognosis compared to other children with RAP. Furthermore, even among these patients, approximately half do not exhibit negative outcomes. Thus, the incidence of negative long-term outcomes in the total population of children with RAP may not be as extensive as that documented in patient samples in the published literature.

Rutter (1989) has argued that childhood experiences that seem negative at the time may nevertheless be protective in that successful coping may foster later resistance to adversity. Similarly, according to the model proposed here, some children should experience positive outcomes from RAP. The experience of RAP may have beneficial outcomes for children who develop a sense of mastery from learning that they can recover from illness or carry on despite physical discomfort. Successful resolution of RAP also may increase parents' confidence in their children's resilience and in their own competence as parents (cf. Parmelee 1989).

Of course, the experience of RAP does have lasting negative impacts for some children, although not necessarily because of an inherent stable characteristic that must run its course. Rutter (1989) has identified various mediating factors that can account for the persistence of childhood disorders. Among these are several that may help to explain the long-term persistence of symptoms and disability observed in many patients with RAP. First, children's behavior may shape their later environment. For example, a child who misses a lot of school due to illness may be held back in school; the resulting placement in a class of younger children for the remaining years of schooling may constitute a stressful environment that contributes to the persistence of symptoms and disability. Children's behavior also may shape others' responses to them. For example, compared to other children, those with frequent somatic complaints may elicit different responses from peers (Guite et al., in press). As children develop, they also play a greater role in determining parental behavior toward them (Scarr and Deater-Deckard 1997). Children with extensive pain-related disability may elicit parental caretaking responses that maintain their dependency. Furthermore, to the extent that others view them as vulnerable, children with RAP may not be offered challenging opportunities that would help them develop their potential and prepare for adolescence.

In addition to influencing the environment and others' responses, the experience of RAP may have lasting effects on the development of children's personal resources. These resources, in turn, may influence later adaptation. For example, children with RAP who withdraw from peer activities may develop deficits in social skills that affect their later ability to obtain social support. Children who cope with pain by withdrawing from activities may come to doubt their ability to succeed at these activities. Moreover, activity restriction associated with RAP may negatively affect children's actual competence by limiting opportunities to develop skills in peer relationships, academics, sports, and so on. Thus, several mechanisms may link RAP to later emotional and behavioral dysfunction, but RAP itself does not *necessarily* lead to dysfunction.

FUTURE RESEARCH

One of the goals of future research should be to describe the mechanisms that lead some children to adapt well to recurrent episodes of abdominal pain and others to become seriously disabled. It is neither practical nor necessary to aim to prevent RAP altogether. Instead, our goal should be to maximize positive outcomes and prevent or reduce chronic sick role behavior.

In order to do so, we need to understand child sick role behavior and parent caretaker behavior in normal families. We know little about the typical patterns of interaction in families when children are ill. We tend to assume abnormal or dysfunctional interactions in families of children with exaggerated symptoms and disability, but we have no reference point that defines normal interactions. For example, how does supportive caretaking differ from overprotection and encouragement of pain behavior? Do the latter simply reflect unusually high levels of support, or is this support qualitatively different? How do teachers, health care providers, and various social structures contribute to pediatric sick role behavior that is considered adaptive? Socialization practices that enhance adaptive sick role behavior may vary according to the age of the child, the nature of the illness, and the cultural context. Increased understanding of adaptive child sick role behavior and appropriate parent caretaking behavior will provide a reference point for identification of children at risk for chronic sick role behavior and may offer clues for the design of treatment interventions that enhance adaptive functioning.

The generalizability of psychosocial processes across pain conditions is another important area for further research. Do the same psychosocial mechanisms influence the course of symptoms and disability in children with various subtypes of RAP? For that matter, are the psychosocial mechanisms that influence the course of RAP similar to those that influence the course of symptoms and disability for children with headaches, juvenile rheumatoid arthritis, and sickle cell disease? The model proposed here refers specifically to the course of RAP, but may apply in some degree to other pediatric pain processes.

Finally, our research findings must be applied in the design and evaluation of interventions for children with recurrent pain. These interventions should focus not only on ameliorating any biological disease or dysfunction, but also on enhancing positive aspects of children's growth and development (cf. Seeman 1989). This will require identifying and nurturing children's emerging competencies. In doing so, such treatments will foster a state of health that is not just the absence of pain but also the development of personal strengths that can be used in confronting future threats to health.

ACKNOWLEDGMENTS

This work was supported by a grant from the National Institute of Child Health and Human Development (HD23264).

REFERENCES

Alfvén G, Uvnas-Moberg K. Elevated cholecystokinin concentrations in plasma in children with recurrent abdominal pain. *Acta Paediatr* 1993; 82:967–970.

Alfvén G, de la Torre B, Uvnas-Moberg K. Depressed concentrations of oxytocin and cortisol in children with recurrent abdominal pain of non-organic origin. *Acta Paediatr* 1994; 83:1076–1080.

Apley J. *The Child with Abdominal Pains*. London: Blackwell, 1975.

Apley J, Hale B. Children with recurrent abdominal pain: how do they grow up? *BMJ* 1973; 7:7–9.

Apley J, Naish N. Recurrent abdominal pain: a field survey of 1,000 school children. *Arch Dis Child* 1958; 33:165–170.

Apley J, Haslam DR, Tulloh CG. Pupillary reaction in children with recurrent abdominal pain. *Arch Dis Child* 1971; 46:337–340.

Aro H, Paronen O, Aro S. Psychosomatic symptoms among 14–16 year old Finnish adolescents. *Soc Psychiatry* 1987; 22:171–176.

Astrada CA, Licamele WL, Walsh TL, Kessler ES. Recurrent abdominal pain in children and associated DSM-III diagnoses. *Am J Psychiatry* 1981; 138:687–688.

Barr RG. Recurrent abdominal pain. In: Levine MD, Corey WB, Gross RT (Eds). *Developmental Behavioral Pediatrics*. Philadelphia: Saunders, 1983.

Barr RG, Feuerstein M. Recurrent abdominal pain syndrome: how appropriate are our basic clinical assumptions? In: McGrath PJ, Firestone P (Eds). *Pediatric and Adolescent Behavioral Medicine*. New York: Springer, 1983, pp 13–27.

Barr R, Levine M, Watkins J. Recurrent abdominal pain due to lactose intolerance. *N Engl J Med* 1979; 300:1449–1452.

Barr RG, Boyce WT, Zeltzer L. The stress–illness association in children: a perspective from the biobehavioral interface. In: Haggerty RJ, Sherrod LR, Garmezy B, Rutter M (Eds). *Stress, Risk and Resilience in Children and Adolescents: Processes, Mechanisms, and Interventions*. Cambridge: Cambridge University Press, 1994, pp 182–224.

Boyle J. Recurrent abdominal pain: an update. *Pediatr Rev* 1997; 18:310–320.

Boyle JT. Chronic abdominal pain. In: Walker WA, Durie PR, Hamilton JR, Walker-Smith JA, Watkins JB (Eds). *Pediatric Gastroenterology: Pathophysiology, Diagnosis, and Management*, Vol. 1. Philadelphia: B.C. Decker, 1991, pp. 45–54.

Bronfenbrenner U. Toward an experimental ecology of human development. *Am Psychol* 1977; 32:513–531.

Bury RG. A study of 111 children with recurrent abdominal pain. *Aust Paediatr J* 1987; 23:117–119.

Cameron LD, Leventhal H, Love RR. Trait anxiety, symptom perceptions, and illness-related responses among women with breast cancer in remission during a tamoxifen clinical trial. *Health Psychol* 1998; 17:459–469.

Christensen MF. Recurrent abdominal pain and dietary fiber. *Am J Dis Child* 1986; 140:738–739.

Christensen MF, Mortensen O. Long-term prognosis in children with recurrent abdominal pain. *Arch Dis Child* 1975; 50:110–114.

Conway DJ. A study of abdominal pain in childhood. *G Ormand St J* 1951; 2:99–109.

Cohen S, Rodriguez MS. Pathways linking affective disturbances and physical disorders. *Health Psychol* 1995; 14:372–380.

Costa PT, McCrae RR. Hypochondriasis, neuroticism, and aging: when are somatic complaints unfounded? *Am Psychol* 1985; 40:19–28.

Craig KD. Modeling and social learning factors in chronic pain. In: Bonica J (Ed). *Advances in Pain Research*, Vol. 5. New York: Raven, 1978, pp 813–827.

Dimson SB. Transit time related to clinical findings in children with recurrent abdominal pain.

Pediatrics 1971; 47:666–674.

Drossman DA, McKee DC, Sandler RS, et al. Psychosocial factors in the irritable bowel syndrome: a multivariate study of patients and nonpatients with irritable bowel syndrome. *Gastroenterology* 1988; 95:701–708.

Drossman DA (Ed). *The Functional Gastrointestinal Disorders. Diagnosis, Pathophysiology, and Treatment: A Multinational Consensus.* Boston: Little, Brown, 1994, pp 1–23.

Dworkin SF, Von Korff MR, LeResche L. Epidemiologic studies of chronic pain: A dynamic-ecologic perspective. *Ann Behav Med* 1992; 14:3–11.

Edwards MC, Finney JW, Bonner M. Matching treatment with recurrent abdominal pain symptoms: an evaluation of dietary fiber and relaxation treatments. *Behav Ther* 1991; 22:257–267.

Erikson E. *Childhood and Society*, 2nd ed. New York: Norton, 1964.

Ernst AR, Routh DK, Harper DC. Abdominal pain in children and symptoms of somatization disorder. *J Ped Psychol* 1984; 9:77–85.

Faull C, Nicol AR. Abdominal pain in six-year-olds: an epidemiological study in a new town. *J Child Psychol Psychiatry* 1986; 27:251–260.

Feldman W, McGrath P, Hodgson C, Ritter H, Shipman RT. The use of dietary fiber in the management of simple, childhood, idiopathic recurrent abdominal pain. *Am J Dis Child* 1985; 139:1216–1218.

Feuerstein M, Barr RG, Francoeur TE, Houle M, Rafman S. Potential biobehavioral mechanisms of recurrent abdominal pain in children. *Pain* 1982; 13:287–298.

Finney JW, Lemanek KL, Cataldo MF, Katz HP, Fuqua RW. Pediatric psychology in primary health care: brief targeted therapy for recurrent abdominal pain. *Behav Ther* 1989; 20:283–291.

Garber J, Zeman J, Walker LS. Recurrent abdominal pain in children: psychiatric diagnoses and parental psychopathology. *J Am Acad Child Adolesc Psychiatry* 1990; 29:648–656.

Garber J, Walker LS, Zeman J. Somatization symptoms in a community sample of children and adolescents: further validation of the Children's Somatization Inventory. *Psychol Assess* 1991; 3:588–595.

Garber J, Van Slyke DA, Walker LS. Concordance between mothers' and children's reports of somatic and emotional symptoms in patients with recurrent abdominal pain or emotional disorders. *J Abnorm Child Psychol* 1998; 26:381–391.

Guite J, Walker LS, Smith C, Garber J. Children's perceptions of peers with somatic symptoms: The impact of gender, stress, and illness. *J Ped Psychol,* in press.

Hodges K, Kline JJ, Barbero G, Flanery R. Life events occurring in families of children with recurrent abdominal pain. *J Psychosom Res* 1984; 28:185–184.

Hodges K, Kline JJ, Barbero G, Flanery R. Depressive symptoms in children with recurrent abdominal pain and their families. *J Pediatr* 1985a; 107:622–626.

Hodges K, Kline J, Barbero G, Woodruff C. Anxiety in children with recurrent abdominal pain and their parents. *Psychosomatics* 1985b; 26:859–866.

Hughes MC. Recurrent abdominal pain and childhood depression: clinical observations of 23 children and their families. *Am J Orthopsychiatry* 1984; 54:146–155.

Hunziker RA, Barr RG. Recurrent abdominal pain in childhood and adolescence: Part 1. Classification and clinical strategy. *Practical Gastroenterol* 1984; 8:3–10.

Hyams JS, Hyman PE. Recurrent abdominal pain and the biopsychosocial model of medical practice. *J Pediatr* 1998; 133:473–478.

Hyams JS, Burke G, Davis PM, Rzepski B, Andrulonis PA. Abdominal pain and irritable bowel syndrome in adolescents: a community-based study. *J Pediatr* 1996; 129:220–226.

Hyman PE, Rasquin-Weber A, Cucchiara S, et al. Childhood functional gastrointestinal disorders. *Gut,* in press.

Kopel FB, Kim IC, Barbero GJ. Comparison of rectosigmoid motility in normal children, children with recurrent abdominal pain, and children with ulcerative colitis. *Pediatrics* 1967; 39:539–545.

Landrine H, Klonoff EA. Culture and health-related schemas: a review and proposal for interdisciplinary integration. *Health Psychol* 1992; 11:267–276.

Lethem J, Slade PD, Troup JDG, Bentley G. Outline of a fear-avoidance model of exaggerated pain perception, I. *Behav Res Ther* 1983; 21:401–418.

Leventhal H. Symptom reporting: a focus on process. In: McHugh S, Vallis M (Eds). *Illness Behavior: A Multidisciplinary Model*. New York: Plenum, 1986, pp 219–237.

Levine MD, Rappaport LA. Recurrent abdominal pain in school children: the loneliness of the long-distance physician. *Pediatr Clin North Amer* 1984; 31:969–991.

Lewis RE, Walker LS, Smith CS. Functional disability in adolescents and young adults with symptoms of irritable bowel syndrome: the role of academic, social, and athletic competence. *J Pediatr Psychol,* in press.

Liebman WM. Recurrent abdominal pain in children: a retrospective survey of 119 patients. *Clin Pediatr* 1978; 17:149–153.

Liebman WM. Recurrent abdominal pain: lactose and sucrose intolerance. *Pediatrics* 1979; 64:43–45.

MacKeith R, O'Neill D. Recurrent abdominal pain in children. *Lancet* 1951; 278–282.

McGrath PA. *Pain in Children: Nature, Assessment, Treatment*. New York: Guilford, 1990.

McGrath PJ, Goodman JT, Firestone P, Shipman R, Peters S. Recurrent abdominal pain: a psychogenic disorder? *Arch Dis Child* 1983; 58:888–890.

Mechanic D. The concept of illness behavior: culture, situation, and personal predisposition. *Psychol Med* 1986; 16:1–7.

Minuchin S, Rosman BL, Baker L. *Psychosomatic Families*. Cambridge, MA: Harvard University Press, 1978.

MyFanwy M, Calnan M, Manning N. *Sociological Approaches to Health and Medicine*. London: Croom Helm, 1985.

Osborne RB, Hatcher JW, Richtsmeier AJ. The role of social modeling in unexplained pediatric pain. *J Pediatr Psychol* 1989; 14:43–61.

Parmelee AH. Children's illnesses: their beneficial effects on behavioral development. *Child Dev* 1986; 57:1–10.

Parmelee AH. The child's physical health and the development of relationships. In: Sameroff AJ, Emde RN (Eds). *Relationship Disturbances in Early Childhood*. New York: Basic Press, 1989, pp 145–162.

Pineiro-Carrero VM, Andres JM, Davis RH, Mathias JR. Abnormal gastroduodenal motility in children and adolescents with recurrent functional abdominal pain. *J Pediatr* 1988; 113:820–825.

Raymer D, Weininger O, Hamilton JR. Psychological problems in children with abdominal pain. *Lancet* 1984; 1:438–439.

Robinson JO, Alverez JH, Dodge JA. Life events and family history in children with recurrent abdominal pain. *J Psychosom Res* 1990; 34:171–181.

Rothbaum F, Weisz JR. In: Kazdin AE (Ed). *Child Psychopathology and the Quest for Control*. Developmental Clinical Psychology and Psychiatry Series, Vol. 17. Newbery Park: Sage Publications, 1989.

Routh DK, Ernst AR. Somatization disorder in relatives of children and adolescents with functional abdominal pain. *J Pediatr Psychol* 1984; 9:427–437.

Routh DK, Ernst AR, Harper DC. Recurrent abdominal pain in children and somatization disorder. In: Routh DK (Ed). *Handbook of Pediatric Psychology*. New York: Guilford Press, 1988, pp 492–504.

Rubin LS, Barbero GJ, Sibinga MS. Pupillary reactivity in children with recurrent abdominal pain. *Psychosom Med* 1967; 29:119–120.

Rutter M. Pathways from childhood to adult life. *J Child Psychol Psychiatry* 1989; 30:23–51.

Sanders MR, Rebgetz M, Morrison M, et al. Cognitive-behavioral treatment of recurrent nonspecific abdominal pain in children: An analysis of generalization, maintenance, and side effects. *J Consult Clin Psychol* 1989; 57:294–300.

Sanders MR, Shepherd RW, Cleghorn G, Woolford H. The treatment of recurrent abdominal pain in children: a controlled comparison of cognitive-behavioral family intervention and standard pediatric care. *J Consult Clin Psychol* 1994; 62:306–314.

Sawyer MG, Davidson GP, Goodwin D, Crettenden AD. Recurrent abdominal pain in childhood. Relationship to psychological adjustment of children and families: a preliminary study. *Aust Paediatr J* 1987; 23:121–124.

Scarr S, Deater-Deckard K. Family effects on individual differences in development. In: Luthar S, Burack JA, Cicchetti D, Weisz JR (Eds). *Developmental Psychopathology: Perspectives on Adjustment, Risk, and Disorder*. Cambridge: Cambridge University Press, 1997, pp 115–136.

Seeman J. Toward a model of positive health. *Am Psychol* 1989; 44:1099–1109.

Sharrer VW, Ryan-Wenger NM. Measurements of stress and coping among school-aged children with and without recurrent abdominal pain. *J Sch Health* 1991; 61:86–91.

Stickler GB, Murphy DB. Recurrent abdominal pain. *Am J Dis Child* 1979; 133:486–489.

Stone RT, Barbero GJ. Recurrent abdominal pain in childhood. *Pediatrics* 1970; 45:732–738.

Stutts JT, Walker LS, Greene JW, et al. Relation of pain intensity ratings to endoscopic findings and use of passive pain coping strategies in children with recurrent abdominal pain. Presented at the Annual Meeting of the North American Society of Pediatric Gastroenterology and Nutrition, 1998.

Turkat ID. An investigation of parental modeling in the etiology of diabetic illness behavior. *Behav Res Ther* 1982; 20:547–552.

Turkat ID, Guise BJ. The effects of vicarious experience and stimulus intensity of pain termination and work avoidance. *Behav Res Ther* 1983; 21:241–245.

Van Slyke DA. Maternal influences on children's pain behavior. Dissertation, Department of Psychology and Human Development, Vanderbilt University, Nashville, 1998.

von Baeyer CL, Walker LS. Children with recurrent abdominal pain: issues in the selection and description of research participants. *J Dev Behav Pediatr,* in press.

Walker LS, Greene JW. Children with recurrent abdominal pain and their parents: more somatic complaints, anxiety, and depression than other patient families? *J Pediatr Psychol* 1989; 14:231–243.

Walker LS, Greene JW. Negative life events and symptom resolution in pediatric abdominal pain patients. *J Pediatr Psychol* 1991; 16:341–360.

Walker LS, Heflinger CA. Quality of life predictors of outcome in pediatric abdominal pain patients: Findings at initial assessment and 5-year follow-up. In: Drotar DD (Ed). *Measuring Health-Related Quality of Life in Children and Adolescents: Implications for Research and Practice*. Malwah, NJ: Lawrence Erlbaum, 1998, pp 237–252.

Walker LS, Zeman JL. Parental response to child illness behavior. *J Pediatr Psychol* 1993; 17:49–71.

Walker LS, Garber J, Greene JW. Somatization symptoms in pediatric abdominal pain patients: relation to chronicity of abdominal pain and parent somatization. *J Abnorm Child Psychol* 1991; 19:379–394.

Walker LS, Garber J, Greene JW. Psychosocial correlates of recurrent childhood pain: a comparison of pediatric patients with recurrent abdominal pain, organic illness, and psychiatric disorders. *J Abnorm Psychol* 1993; 102:248–258.

Walker LS, Garber J, Greene JW. Somatic complaints in pediatric patients: a prospective study of the role of negative life events, child social and academic competence, and parental somatic symptoms. *J Consult Clin Psychol* 1994; 62:1213–1221.

Walker LS, Garber J, Van Slyke DA. Do parents excuse the misbehavior of children with physical or emotional symptoms? An investigation of the pediatric sick role. *J Pediatr Psychol* 1995a; 20:329–345.

Walker LS, Garber J, Van Slyke DA, Greene JW. Long-term health outcomes in patients with recurrent abdominal pain. *J Pediatr Psychol* 1995b; 20:233–245.

Walker LS, Smith CA, Garber J, Van Slyke DA. Development and validation of the Pain

Response Inventory for Children. *Psychol Assess* 1997; 9:392–405.

Walker LS, Guite JW, Duke M, Barnard JA, Greene JW. Recurrent abdominal pain: a potential precursor of irritable bowel syndrome in adolescents and young adults. *J Pediatr* 1998; 132:1010–1015.

Wasserman AL, Whitington PF, Rivara FP. Psychogenic basis for abdominal pain in children and adolescents. *J Am Acad Child Adolesc Psychiatry* 1988; 27:179–184.

Weisz JR, Suwanlert S, Chaiyasit W, Walter B. Over- and undercontrolled referral problems among children and adolescents from Thailand and the United States: The "wat" and "wai" of cultural differences. *J Consult Clin Psychol* 1987; 55:719–726.

Woodbury MM. Recurrent abdominal pain in child patients seen at a pediatric gastroenterology clinic. *Psychosomatics* 1993; 6:485–493.

Zeltzer LK. Challenging case: recurrent abdominal pain. *J Dev Behav Pediatr* 1995; 16:277–281.

Zeltzer LK, Bush JP, Chen E, Riveral A. A psychobiologic approach to pediatric pain: part I. History, physiology, and assessment strategies. *Curr Probl Pediatr* 1997; 27:255–258.

Correspondence to: Lynn S. Walker, PhD, Division of Adolescent Medicine, Department of Pediatrics, Vanderbilt University School of Medicine, 436 Medical Center South, Nashville, TN 37232-3571, USA. Tel: 615-936-0252; Fax: 615-936-0202; email: walkerls@ctrvax.vanderbilt.edu.

Chronic and Recurrent Pain in Children and Adolescents, Progress in Pain Research and Management, Vol. 13, edited by Patrick J. McGrath and G. Allen Finley, IASP Press, Seattle, © 1999.

9

Musculoskeletal Pain

Patrick J. McGrath and Lynn Breau

Department of Psychology and Pain Service, Dalhousie University, and IWK Grace Health Centre, Halifax, Nova Scotia, Canada

Although common, musculoskeletal pains have received less attention than most other types of chronic and recurrent pediatric pain. Most epidemiological surveys of chronic and recurrent musculoskeletal pain have examined specific pains, usually limb pain. For example, Oster (1972b), in an early study of 2178 schoolchildren aged 6–19 years, found that approximately 15% had recurrent limb pains and 4.5% had pain sufficiently severe to interfere with activities for more than 3 months. Similarly, Larsson (1991) found that 27% of 539 children in grades 7–11 had limb pain.

However, some studies have looked at the overall prevalence of all musculoskeletal pain. For example, Mikkelsson et al. (1997a) examined musculoskeletal pain using a structured pain questionnaire in a 1-year follow-up study of 1756 third- and fifth-grade children. At follow-up, pain at least once a week persisted in 52% of the 564 children who originally reported weekly musculoskeletal pain in at least one body part, and 50% who reported pain at the time of the initial survey still had pain at the 1-year follow-up. Girls had more persistent pain than boys, and the risk for persistent pain increased 1.2 times per year of age. Neck pain was the most persistent type of pain. A child's perception that he or she was disabled (OR = 3.2; 95% CI = 1.5–6.6) and daytime tiredness (OR = 1.9; 95% CI = 1.2–3.0) were the most significant predictors of pain persistence.

This chapter will review common diffuse pain such as that secondary to arthritis and associated with fibromyalgia, and more localized pain such as back or knee pain, growing pains, and pain associated with overuse syndromes. Research, especially on treatment, is limited, and accepted "facts" are based on few or no data.

173

CHRONIC ARTHRITIS IN CHILDREN

The first English-language description of chronic arthritis in childhood was a brief description by Wells in 1810 (Still 1931). He also noted that arthritis in children was probably not one uniform syndrome. We now know that the condition called juvenile chronic arthritis or juvenile rheumatoid arthritis (JRA) represents a set of disorders.

Three types of JRA are commonly distinguished. In systemic JRA, characterized by high intermittent fever and a rash for several weeks at onset, children frequently have rather severe pain in numerous joints during the initial period of the disease and during remissions. Polyarticular JRA involves more than five joints. Children commonly have symmetrical arthritis in the small joints of the hands and involvement of the knees, ankles, elbows, and feet. Finally, pauciarticular JRA (also known as oligoarticular JRA) involves four or fewer joints.

The prevalence of arthritis in childhood has been estimated to be between 0.5 (Lovell and Walco 1989) and 1.1 per 1000 (Schaller 1984). Several recent studies have used disease registries to report the number of cases of JRA seen at pediatric rheumatology clinics (Table I). Moe and Rygg (1998) retrospectively reviewed all the cases seen at the only pediatric department treating JRA in northern Norway. They estimated a point prevalence for 1994 of 1.48 per 1000 (girls: 2.02; boys: 0.97) and an annual incidence rate over the 9 years of 2.26 per 1000 (girls: 2.94; boys: 0.16). The greatest incidence was for pauciarticular (1.18), followed by polyarticular (0.089) and systemic (0.008) arthritis.

The characteristics of pain experienced in JRA have also been investi-

Table I
Prevalence of juvenile rheumatoid arthritis (JRA) and subtypes of JRA based on Pediatric Rheumatology Disease Registries

Reference	Population	Information Source	Type	Prevalence
Bowyer and Roettcher 1996	25 centers in the United States	Pediatric Rheumatology Disease Registry, 1992–1995 ($N = 12{,}939$)	Total Pauciarticular Polyarticular Systemic	2071 1070 686 315
Symmons et al. 1996	23 centers in the United Kingdom	Pediatric Rheumatology Group National Diagnostic Register, 1990–1994 ($N = 4948$)	Total Pauciarticular Polyarticular Systemic	1831 916 311 201
Malleson et al. 1996	13 centers in Canada	Canadian Pediatric Rheumatology Association Disease Registration, 1991–1993 ($N = 3362$)	Total Pauciarticular Polyarticular Systemic	521 305 154 62

gated. For example, Beales et al. (1983) interviewed 39 children aged 6–17 years attending an outpatient clinic. Children picked words from a list of descriptors of joint sensations to rate unpleasantness and severity on a 10-cm visual analogue scale (VAS). All the children said their joints ached. Of the 24 children aged 6–11, 50% indicated some type of sharp pain (pain that cut, pricked, smacked, or pinched) and 37% indicated a burning sensation. Of the 15 children aged 12–17, 53% indicated sharp and burning pain. Older children interpreted their sensations as more unpleasant and more painful than did younger children, and the pain was more likely to suggest to older children that they were disabled. Beales concluded that the meaning the children attributed to their sensations contributed to whether their experience was interpreted as unpleasant and painful. However, other studies (e.g., Ross et al. 1989; Vandvik and Eckblad 1990; Benestad et al. 1996) have not reported increases in pain with age, leading Jaworski (1993) to suggest that Beales' findings might be spurious.

Studies asking children to report on their pain have found that current pain ratings tend to average about 3 on a 10-cm VAS (Table II). Children rated their "worst" pain much higher. Most of the children in these studies were taking medication to control their disease and their pain.

The amount of pain children experience appears to differ with the subtype of JRA. Several studies have found that children with systemic JRA experience the most severe pain and those with pauciarticular JRA experience the least (Table III). The systemic group also includes the fewest pain-free children. In a study of 293 children, 26% of those with pauciarticular JRA were pain free, compared to only 3% of those with polyarticular JRA and 4% of those with systemic JRA (Sherry et al. 1990).

Some researchers have attempted to explain arthritis pain in children by investigating physical factors such as disease severity and pain thresholds,

Table II
Pain severity reported by children with juvenile rheumatoid arthritis

Reference	Sample	Age Range	Pain Measure*	Pain Rated	Pain Rating (Mean ± 1 SD)
Varni et al. 1987	19 girls, 6 boys	4–16	10-cm VAS	Present Worst	1.63 ± 2.12 4.74 ± 3.91
Benestad et al. 1996	37 girls, 20 boys	6–18	10-cm VAS	Present Worst	1.5 ± 2.3 3.80 ± 3.3
Gragg et al. 1996	68 girls, 32 boys	8–16	100-mm VAS	Present Worst in past week	30.17 ± 31.43 53.36 ± 36.21
Schanberg et al. 1997	36 girls, 20 boys	6–20	100-mm VAS	Present	29.7 (3.5) ± 3.5

Table III
Pain severity by subtype of JRA (pauciarticular, polyarticular, systemic)

Reference	Sample	Age Range	Pain Measure	Subtype	Pain Rating*
Thompson et al. 1987	19 girls, 6 boys	4–16	Child-completed 10-cm VAS of present pain	Pauciarticular Polyarticular Systemic	0.5 1.45 1.83
Ross et al. 1989	77 girls, 24 boys	1–12 6–16	Parent-completed 10-cm VAS ($N =$ 58) of general pain severity and frequency	Pauciarticular Polyarticular	4.2 ± 2.9 4.7 ± 2.9
			Child-completed 10-cm VAS ($N =$ 43) of general pain severity and frequency	Pauciarticular Polyarticular	2.4 ± 3.3 4.9 ± 3.6
Truckenbrodt 1993	11 children	1–8	Parent report	Pauciarticular Polyarticular Systemic	<45% <30% 100%

* Data are means, means ± 1 SE, or percentage who rated their pain as severe.

while others have investigated psychosocial characteristics. Studies on the relationship between pain intensity and disease activity have produced mixed results. In a sample of 101 children, Ross et al. (1989) found that parental pain reports and a clinical variable (joint inflammation, disease activity, or morning stiffness) had a correlation of 0.40 for pauciarticular and 0.56 for polyarticular JRA. Similarly, Ilowite et al. (1992) found that parents' and doctors' ratings of pain in 18 children were correlated with joint inflammation (0.58 and 0.50, respectively), as measured by surface temperature. However, a significant correlation with joint inflammation was observed only for self-reported pain in children under 7.8 years of age. Thus, although sometimes related, measures of pain and disease severity should be considered separate variables.

In a series of studies, Hogeweg's group has found that patients with JRA have lower pressure pain thresholds at inflamed joints and at noninflamed paraspinal areas, especially those areas associated with inflammation (Hogeweg et al. 1995a,b, in press). They also reported that children with disease, but no active inflammation, had lower pain thresholds than did healthy children, that children with disease and active inflammation had the lowest pain threshold, and that pain was correlated with lower thresholds for pain. These results suggest both a central and a peripheral sensitization in children with JRA that appears to outlast active disease states.

Several studies have examined family and individual factors that influence pain in JRA. Ross et al. (1993) randomly selected 78 children from clinic attendees and instructed them to use a prospective pain diary. They found that psychological variables accounted for more variance in pain (31%) than did disease variables (12%). The psychological variables related to pain were child anxiety, child depression, mother distress, and lack of family harmony. However, behavior problems did not predict pain.

Schanberg and her colleagues (1997) studied coping and pain in 56 children with JRA. Age and disease duration accounted for a very small amount of variance, but disease activity, the ability to control and decrease pain, and the ability to avoid catastrophizing made substantial contributions. Prospective or experimental studies have not yet confirmed that psychosocial factors directly influence pain in JRA.

Treatment of pain in JRA generally occurs as an adjunct to the treatment of inflammation. Both disease treatments and a variety of NSAIDs are commonly used. Two studies have described psychological treatment for the pain of JRA. Lavigne and his colleagues (1992) used individually administered progressive relaxation, electromyelogram (EMG) biofeedback, thermal biofeedback, and autogenic training with seven girls and one boy with JRA. Using a multiple baseline to evaluate the program of six sessions, one every two weeks, they found modest reductions in pain as measured by child and maternal diaries. The authors suggest that the study provides preliminary but not conclusive support of the intervention's effectiveness. Walco et al. (1992) treated 13 children (8 girls, 5 boys) with JRA. In eight individually administered sessions, progressive relaxation, guided imagery, and meditative breathing were taught to the children. In two additional sessions, parents were taught behavioral pain management. The authors report a substantial reduction in pain and improved adaptive functioning that was maintained at the 6- and 12-month follow-ups. These results suggest that a broad-based cognitive behavioral treatment may be effective, although randomized trials are required to confirm the efficacy of this approach.

In summary, JRA is a relatively common musculoskeletal pain, and some physiological and psychological factors may relate to the severity of pain that children experience. Because studies of treatments are so few, and none have compared treatments, there is little information regarding the "best" way of managing the pain of JRA beyond efforts to manage the disease.

JUVENILE PRIMARY FIBROMYALGIA SYNDROME

Juvenile primary fibromyalgia syndrome (JPFS) is seen in children as young as 5 years of age (Yunus and Masi 1985). It is characterized by widespread chronic pain accompanied by fatigue, poor sleep, and other nonmusculoskeletal symptoms. Buskila's group (1993, 1995b) found that 6% of 338 students aged 9–15 years had JPFS, while Mikkellson's group, using a two-stage epidemiological study (1997b), found that 22 of 1756 (1.25%) third- and fifth-grade children met the criteria for JPFS. One factor that makes interpretation of these and most studies of fibromyalgia in children difficult to interpret is that two sets of criteria are used. Both these studies followed adult criteria devised by the American College of Rheumatology (Wolfe et al. 1990). However, many others used a set of revised criteria designed by Yunus and Masi (1985) to capture the pediatric manifestation of this condition (Table IV). Many researchers have noted the symptom overlap between fibromyalgia and chronic fatigue syndrome (see review by Breau et al., in press).

JPFS appears to be more common in girls. Although no large-scale epidemiological studies have been conducted, the proportion of girls has ranged from approximately 38% (Buskila et al. 1995b) to almost 94% (Yunus and Masi 1985). Data on age are also limited. Although Buskila's group found JPFS to be equally prevalent among 9–15-year-olds (Buskila et al. 1993), Yunus and Masi found that 58% of the 33 children in their study reported an age of onset between 13 and 15 years.

The prognosis for children with JPFS is unclear. In their epidemiological study, Buskila et al. (1995b) reported that, of 15 children initially meet-

Table IV
Criteria for juvenile primary fibromyalgia syndrome (patients must satisfy all three
major criteria and 3 out of 10 minor criteria)

Major Criteria	Minor Criteria
1) General musculoskeletal aching at 3 or more sites for 3 or more months in the absence of any underlying condition	1) Subjective soft tissue swelling 2) Pain modulated by physical activities 3) Pain modulated by weather factors
2) Laboratory tests normal	4) Pain modulated by anxiety/stress 5) Irritable bowel syndrome
3) Severe pain in 5 of 18 bilateral tender point sites with palpation of less than 4 kg force:* occiput; low cervical area; trapezius; supraspinatus; second rib; lateral epicondyle; gluteal, upper outer quadrant of buttock; greater trochanter; knee	6) Chronic anxiety or tension 7) Fatigue 8) Poor sleep 9) Numbness 10) Chronic headaches

Source: Yunus and Masi (1985).
* Criteria are also satisfied by 4 of 18 tender points and 5 of 10 minor criteria.

ing ACR criteria, 11 no longer met the criteria at a 30-month follow-up. However, using the criteria of Yunus and Masi, Malleson et al. (1992) followed a group of clinically referred children and found that 61% had not improved over an average of 27 months.

Little is known about the etiology of JPFS. Children with this syndrome appear not to have thyroid dysfunction (Buskila et al. 1993; Wolfe et al. 1995), serologic abnormalities (Buskila et al. 1993; Vandvik and Forseth 1994; Wolfe et al. 1995), synovitis or muscle weakness (Buskila et al. 1993), or abnormalities at tender points (Buskila et al. 1993; Wolfe et al. 1995).

Gedalia and his colleagues (1993) have proposed that joint hypermobility may be a factor in JPFS. They conducted a study in which 338 children (aged 9–15 years) from a public school were given two independent, blind assessments for hypermobility and JPFS. Their results indicated that 40% of the 43 children with hypermobility had JPFS and 81% of the 21 children with JPFS had hypermobility. In contrast, only 1% of the 295 children without JPFS were hypermobile. A recent chart review by Siegel and colleagues (1998) supports this proposal. They found that 18 of 45 children with JPFS had been diagnosed with hypermobility. However, Reid et al. (1996) reported that none of the 15 children with JPFS (aged 11–17 years) in their study were hypermobile.

Sleep disturbances or genetics could be factors in JPFS. Roizenblatt and his co-authors (1997) administered a sleep questionnaire and used nocturnal polysomnography (sleep laboratory recordings) with 34 children with JPFS (aged 9–12 years), 10 children with diffuse pain, and 17 age- and sex-matched controls. In addition to finding that their JPFS group showed more decreased sleep efficiency, arousals, intrusions on slow-wave sleep, and morning fatigue than both other groups, they also found that alpha and theta intrusions on slow-wave sleep were related to the number of tender points and to the mean tenderness threshold at tender points in the children with JPFS. Buskila's group (1996) investigated genetic factors by evaluating the 58 children of 20 mothers meeting ACR criteria for fibromyalgia. Twenty-eight percent met ACR criteria, much more than the estimated prevalence of 2% in the general population (Wolfe et al. 1995). Roizenblatt also found that 71% of the children in their study had mothers with fibromyalgia. These studies suggest that sleep anomalies may be related to JPFS and that familial aggregation occurs, but it is unclear whether either is causal.

Although psychological factors have been theorized to play a role in JPFS, results of investigations have indicated that children with JPFS are no more depressed than those with JRA (Vandvik and Forseth 1994; Reid et al. 1996). Similarly, past sexual or physical abuse has been proposed to contribute to fibromyalgia, but retrospective studies of adults have reported differing results (e.g., Boisset-Pioro et al. 1995; Taylor et al. 1995). Women with fibromyalgia who seek medical care may be more likely to have been abused than those who do not seek medical care. Studies of children do not report increased rates of abuse in those with JPFS. For example, in a retrospective chart review (Malleson et al. 1992), 9% of 40 children with diffuse idiopathic pain (35 of whom had JPFS) and 7% of 41 children with localized idiopathic pain were suspected to have experienced abuse. Comparisons with population prevalence data are difficult, but the rates are not significantly above what might be expected in the general population. Psychological factors or childhood abuse probably do not play an etiologic role in most cases of JPFS.

Many children with JPFS do not receive treatment. For example, a small 1-year follow-up study of 11 children and adolescents found that 92% had pain but only 54% were receiving treatment at the time of follow-up (Rabinovich et al. 1990). Only two studies have reported the results of pharmacological treatments for children with JPFS. Romano (1991) reported that 73% of his patients showed improvement of symptoms with cyclobenzaprine over a 2-year period. Siegel et al. (1998) also reported that improved symptoms were reported by most of the children in their study taking cyclobenzaprine.

Walco and Ilowite (1992), in the only study on the efficacy of cognitive-behavioral treatment for JPFS, reported a case series of five girls aged 8–17 years. Over 4–24 months, four of the children in their study had no pain and one reported intermittent, low-level pain that could be managed.

Much of our knowledge of JPFS is from studies using inadequate designs and small samples. Because many still question the validity of fibromyalgia as a physical disorder, and because even the diagnosis is not standardized, a great deal more research is needed before these children will experience substantial improvement in care.

BACK PAIN

Not long ago, clinicians thought that back pain was rare in children and that it was an indicator of significant pathology (King 1986). However, studies in Switzerland (Balagué et al. 1988), Australia (Erball 1994a), Iceland (Kristjánsdóttir 1996), and Finland (Taimela et al. 1997) show that back pain is common in children and adolescents (Table V). In a study of 29,424 Danes aged 12–41, the lifetime prevalence of 50% was surpassed by 18-year-old girls and 20-year-old boys, and the steepest increase in 1-year prevalence occurred between ages 13 and 14, regardless of gender (Leboeuf-

Table V
Prevalence of back pain (BP) and low back pain (LBP) in children

Reference	Age Range	Sample Size	Prevalence
Balagué et al. 1988	7–17	1715	BP ever: 42%; girls 38%, boys 32% LBP ever: 34.5% BP in past week: 16%
Erball 1994	12–19	610 boys	LBP ever: 57% LBP now: 16.7%
Balagué et al. 1995	12–17	615	BP ever: 26%
Kristjánsdóttir 1996	11–12	1005	BP once a month: 16.9% BP once a week: 7.6%
	15–16	1113	BP once a month: 29.5% BP once a week: 11.9%
Taimela et al. 1997	7–16	1171	LBP in past 12 months: boys 10.1%, girls 9.4%

Yde and Kyvik 1998). All the studies in Table V reported an increase in current and past back pain by age. Similarly, many children presenting with back pain in medical clinics have no trauma or pathology to explain their pain (Turner et al. 1989; Coombs and Caskey 1997).

Balagué and his colleagues (1988) found that only 14% of their sample with back pain, and 27% of those with low back pain, had sought medical advice. Their results also show that 27% of those who sought medical advice experienced frequent or continual pain compared to only 8% of those who had not consulted a doctor. In a study of 96 children, Newcomer and Sinaki (1996) also reported that 51% of the 96 children in their sample had experienced back pain, yet only 7% had ever sought medical attention. Thus, it appears that only those children experiencing more severe pain seek medical assistance.

It could be argued that children are unlikely to seek treatment for back pain because it is a transient problem, but this does not appear to be the case. The results of the Finnish study (Taimela et al. 1997) indicate that 26% of the boys and 30% of the girls with low back pain reported that it was recurrent, and 3% of the girls reported it to be continual. In Erball's study of adolescent boys (1994), 348 reported current or past pain. Of these, 14% said they had low back pain every day, 3% said their pain never goes away, and 46% said that they had suffered pain for over a year. Finally, Balagué et al. (1995) found that 4% of the total sample said they had back pain almost continually. Thus, many children with back pain experience frequent pain for a long time.

The low rate of help sought also does not indicate decreasing frequency of back pain. In a prospective 4-year study that began with a cohort of 216 11-year-old schoolchildren, the frequency of back pain did not decrease (Burton et al. 1996). The authors found that of the 96 children with pain, 44% reported it as recurrent at age 11, while 59% reported it as recurrent at age 15. In addition, most of those with recurrent pain at 15 had some back pain at age 11. Back pain thus appears to occur more frequently with increasing age.

Back pain may result from numerous conditions. For example, it can be related to trauma, infection, or vertebral tumors (Afshani and Kuhn 1991). However, in many children no pathophysiology is found, even in children referred to a tertiary care center. Over a 3-year period, King (1986) saw 54 patients under age 19 who complained of back pain. No diagnosis was possible in 37% of the cases. Similarly, of 61 children under 15 who visited an orthopedic department, nearly 48% were given no diagnosis (Turner et al. 1989).

Many investigators have examined the possible contributors to non-pathologic back pain. Anthropometric dimensions, spinal mobility, trunk muscle strength, and sociodemographic, familial, psychological, and lifestyle factors are among them. Studies of anthropometric differences between children with and without back pain have had mixed results. Fairbank and his colleagues (1984a) reported that 115 adolescents with pain had greater trunk length and weight relative to the 331 without pain. Similarly, Erball (1994b) found that upper body segment, sitting height, pelvic height, and suprapelvic height were greater in 38 male adolescents with idiopathic low back pain than in controls. However, weight was not a distinguishing feature. In a well-designed prospective study, Nissinen and his co-authors (1994) followed 451 boys and 408 girls, 11 years of age, for 2 years. Those reporting pain were taller at baseline, and boys with back pain also had greater sitting height and weight, although this was not the case for girls. A univariate logistic regression showed that at the 1-year follow-up, back pain in boys was predicted by height and increase of sitting height, while in girls it was predicted by trunk asymmetry. Mierau and his colleagues (1989) measured straight leg raising, an indication of sagittal mobility and hamstring flexibility, in a group of children and adolescents. They found that the 61 male adolescents (aged 14–18) with a history of low back pain had decreased flexibility in straight leg raising. However, this was not the case for the 74 female adolescents or for the 267 children aged 6–13, regardless of gender. Salminen's group examined 38 15-year-olds with low back pain and 38 controls matched for age, gender, and school class (Salminen et al. 1992).

Decreased flexibility of the hamstrings in straight leg raising was found for both boys and girls with pain, and trunk muscle strength (endurance strength of the abdominal and back muscles) was also decreased in the group with pain. However, when this same group was retested 3 years later, mobility and trunk strength still differed between the groups with and without pain, but neither mobility nor trunk muscle strength at baseline predicted future low back pain (Salminen et al. 1995). These factors are more likely to be consequences rather than causes of back pain since they show no predictive value.

Newcomer and Sinaki (1996) explored the role of back strength in a detailed prospective study of 96 children aged 10–19. They found that an increase in back flexor strength was related to low back pain 4 years later, while back extensor strength was not related to subsequent pain. However, they found that the ratio of back extensor strength to flexor strength was decreased in their pain group, although not significantly. They hypothesized that children with low back pain may be participating in activities that selectively strengthen back flexors and that the imbalance between back flexors and extensors may contribute to the occurrence of sprains and strains.

Overall, it appears that children with back pain differ on some physical measures from children without such pain. Unfortunately, because most studies have not been prospective, it is impossible to conclude whether these factors are causal. Back pain may result in behavioral changes that lead to the physical differences found between children with and without pain.

The only sociodemographic factor found to differentiate between children with and without back pain has been residential location. Kristjánsdóttir (1996) found that adolescents aged 15–16 from rural areas of Iceland had more back pain than did those from urban areas. She hypothesized that this difference may reflect a greater participation in manual labor. Lifestyle variables associated with the presence of back pain have included watching television more than 2 hours per day (Balagué et al. 1988), low physical activity (Salminen et al. 1995), increased activity (Newcomer and Sinaki 1996), and sports (Burton et al. 1996). However, only the latter two, reflecting increased physical activity, predicted low back pain. Finally, although associations between familial and psychological factors and low back pain have been reported (Balagué et al. 1995), prospective studies are needed before we can conclude that these factors are causes rather than consequences of the pain.

Treatment of back pain in children and adolescents has not been well studied; typically it involves the use of acetaminophen or NSAIDs and rest. For example, Milling et al. (1989), in a case study of behavioral treatment of chronic back pain in a 15-year-old boy, reported that a combination of biofeedback, progressive muscle relaxation, imagery, and family therapy assisted parents in shaping healthy behaviors and reducing pain behaviors. Burton (1996) recommends following adult treatment guidelines, including discouraging extended rest and encouraging children to resume activities and take analgesics for pain relief. She suggests that physical therapy may be helpful for pain lasting more than a few days, but questions the usefulness of back exercises.

To recap, most back pain in children does not have a clear underlying pathology. However, the effect of the pain on functioning can be significant. The most under-researched area is treatment. Empirically validated treatments for back pain would have a great impact on many children's lives.

KNEE PAIN

Pain in the knee that is not the result of an acute trauma can be related to a number of conditions. Patellofemoral or anterior knee pain are terms used to describe general knee pain located between the knee cap (patella) and the thigh bone (femur). Chondromalacia patellae refers to a condition in which there is pathological change in the cartilage of the patella. Patellar pain is relatively common in children and adolescents.

In one study, Fairbank and his colleagues (1984b) attempted to assess the prevalence and correlates of knee pain by measuring joint mobility and lower limb morphology in 446 schoolchildren (227 boys, 219 girls) aged 13–17 years. Measures of activity level and knee pain experienced in the past year were also taken. The overall prevalence of knee pain was 31%, and children were more likely to experience pain if they regularly participated in sporting activities. Boys and girls were equally represented in the pain group. Of this group, 25 adolescents (18%) had stopped sports because of the pain, and 40 adolescents (29%) reported visiting a doctor.

A recent study of 569 children from the fourth, seventh, and ninth grades in Norway (mean ages 10.5, 13.5, and 15.5 years, respectively) asked children to identify the location of their pain (Smedbråten et al. 1998). The most common site was the knee, reported by 29% of girls and 32% of boys.

In a group of younger urban minority children in the United States, however, the numbers were lower (Kasper et al. 1993). This group screened 2523 children (mean age of 7.2 years) at 15 day care centers and 10 schools for musculoskeletal complaints. Of the 168 children who had a musculoskeletal problem, 8% had knee pain that was not associated with knee laxity, knock knee, or Osgood-Schlatter's disease.

Children with knee pain often describe a gradual onset and complain of dull aching over the peripatellar area (Goldberg 1991). They also tend to report that pain is worse after activity, climbing stairs, squatting, and sitting for long periods (Passo 1982; Goldberg 1991). Many children experience this pain bilaterally. In a recent study of 110 patients aged 10–29 years, Al-Rawi and Nessan (1997) found that 57% had bilateral chondromalacia patellae. However, Fairbank and his colleagues (1984b) found an increased frequency of pain in the right knee in their study of 446 schoolchildren. Johnson (1997) has recently proposed that the features of a child's patellar pain reflect the cause. He suggests that children with pain due to a tight knee extensor mechanism experience little pain during activity, but persistent pain for days after activity, while children with pain due to subluxation experience brief pain during malengagement, followed by short-term tenderness.

In fact, many conditions may result in patellofemoral pain. Faulty mechanics, such as joint laxity, patellar instability, congenital synovial plica, hamstring tightness, and structural abnormalities of the foot have been suggested. While many factors may cause patellar pain, it is only when they result in changes to the cartilage that the term chondromalacia patellae is appropriate (Thabit and Micheli 1992).

To examine the role of joint laxity, Al-Rawi and Nessan (1997) used the method described by Carter and Wilkinson (1964) to determine the hypermobility of 115 patients aged 10–29 and 110 controls matched for age, sex, height, and body weight. They found 93 hypermobile knee joints among the group with chondromalacia, compared to 28 hypermobile joints among the controls. They concluded that hypermobility of the knee joint contributes to chondromalacia patellae.

In contrast, Fairbank and his group (1984b) have proposed that chronic overloading is the root cause of patellar pain. In their study, the children who reported knee pain in the previous year did not differ from those without pain in the range of medial femoral rotation, the quadriceps angle, valgus angle, or patella alta ratio (patellar height/patellar tendon length). Knee pain was more common in those who were active in sports, which prompted the authors' speculation that repeated medial overloading was the dominant contributor to knee pain.

Although the cause of patellar pain may vary, the impact on children and adolescents seems to be similar. Sandow and Goodfellow (1985) found that almost all of 54 female adolescents presenting with some type patellofemoral knee pain still experienced some pain when followed 2–8 years after initial presentation. However, they also found that 46% had reduced severity and only 13% reported worsening of symptoms. Fritz et al. (1981) also found that the 28 adolescents aged 12–16 who attended an orthopedic clinic had similar difficulties, whether their patellar pain was associated with orthopedic problems, poor patellar tracking, mild chondro-malacia patellae, or no observable organic condition. Most reported that their pain had lasted more than 6 months, and half had missed school be-cause of it. One factor that did differ between the groups, however, was the percentage who had previously received unsuccessful treatment. All adoles-cents with no organic cause for their pain reported that they had undergone unsuccessful treatments, while 50% of the 17 with poor tracking or chon-dromalacia and 41% of those with orthopedic conditions reported previous unsuccessful treatments.

Although the proposed causes of patellar pain are numerous, the sug-gested treatments are rather homogeneous. Sandow and Goodfellow (1985) reported that 90% of their patients did not require surgery, which is gener-ally considered a treatment of last resort. According to Goldberg (1991), the goal of conservative treatment strategies is to control the associated pain and discomfort and to improve patellar tracking. NSAIDs and cryotherapy are the first choice for pain management, and knee taping, neoprene sleeves, and other measures of stabilizing or, in some cases, immobilizing the knee may be necessary (Goldberg 1991; Johnson 1997).

In summary, like back pain, knee pain occurs frequently and is not always the result of observable pathology. As in the case of back pain, the research most lacking is that addressing treatment.

GROWING PAINS

"Growing pains" have been known since earliest recorded medical his-tory, but relatively few literature references can be found for this relatively common problem. The most commonly used criteria are those proposed by Naish and Apley (1951). They described growing pains as pain occurring late in the day or at night for at least 3 months that is severe enough to wake a child or disrupt activities. The pain must not be in the joints, and there must be pain-free periods lasting from days to months. Finally, their criteria included negative laboratory and examination results. Growing pains are usually bilateral and are not accompanied by tenderness, redness, or swell-ing. In one study of 480 schoolchildren, nearly 75% reported pain in the leg, 30% pain in the knee, and 30% pain in more than one location (Keinanen-Kiukaanniemi et al. 1985).

Growing pains may be accompanied by restlessness, and some children with restless leg syndrome are misdiagnosed with growing pains (Walters et al. 1996). However, Ekbom (1975) concluded that the two conditions are distinct after studying a family in which three boys, all with severe growing pains, had a mother with restless leg syndrome and a history of growing pains in childhood. Growing pains are not accompanied by an abnormality of gait, nor do they develop into pathologic conditions. There is some evidence for a familial aggregation of growing pains (Oster 1972a; Ekbom 1975; Keinanen-Kiukaanniemi et al. 1985), but no well-designed studies have been conducted.

The reported incidence of growing pains varies greatly. Naish and Apley (1951), using strict criteria, found that about 4% of the children they studied had experienced growing pains, while Hawksley (1939), using undefined criteria, estimated that growing pains occurred in nearly 34% of the hospitalized children in his study (Table VI). Growing pains are not usually seen in pediatric rheumatology clinics (Bowyer and Roettcher 1996; Malleson et al. 1996). Some studies have found higher rates of growing pains in girls (Brenning 1960; Oster and Nielsen 1972), while others have reported no gender differences (Naish and Apley 1951; Keinanen-Kiukaanniemi et al. 1985; Abu-Arafeh and Russell 1996; Bowyer et al. 1996). Some authors have reported that growing pains most often occur between ages 8 and 12 (Naish and Apley 1951; Keinanen-Kiukaanniemi et al. 1985; Peterson 1986; Oberklaid et al. 1997). However, Oster and Nielsen (1972) found that while the rate of occurrence remained steady for boys aged 6–13, it peaked at 11 years for girls, and Bowyer and Roettcher (1996) found the average age of onset to be 3.4 years. For many children, growing pains appear to subside with time (Naish and Apley 1951).

The cause of growing pains is unknown. With advancing knowledge of rheumatic fever and rheumatoid arthritis, rheumatic causes have now been discredited. Similarly, growth per se has been discounted as a cause. Children with growing pains do not grow differently from those who do not have

Table VI
Prevalence of growing pains in children

Reference	Age Range	Sample	Prevalence
Hawksley 1939	4–14	505 hospitalized children	33.6%
Naish and Apley 1951	4–15	721 schoolchildren	4.2%
Brenning 1960	6–7	257 children	13.6%
	10–11	419 children	19.8%
Oster and Neilsen 1972	6–19	2178 schoolchildren	15.5%
Keinanen-Kiukaanniemi et al. 1985	10–12	480 schoolchildren	13.3%
Abu-Arafeh and Russell 1996	5–15	2165 schoolchildren	

growing pains, and these pains do not occur during periods of maximum growth (Oster 1972a; Leung and Robson 1991; Haasbeek and Wright 1993; Walco 1997). Three theories are current—that growing pains are caused by orthopedic abnormalities, psychosocial problems, or fatigue. Orthopedic abnormalities have been discounted because repeated assessments of these children have produced no findings (Leung and Robson 1991). Many early studies (Naish and Apley 1951; Oster and Nielsen 1972) endorsed a psychogenic model, and a recent study (Oberklaid et al. 1997) reached similar conclusions. But the latter has been sharply criticized (Walco 1997) because of the overinclusive way it defined growing pains. In addition, no studies using standardized measurement and appropriate design have investigated the psychogenic model (Walco 1997), and clear criteria for psychogenic pain are usually not met in children with growing pain.

Finally, fatigue was proposed as a cause by Bennie in 1894 and reiterated by Naish and Apley (1951), because pain was often worse after exertion in the children they studied. This observation was also made by Abu-Arafeh and Russell (1996), who reported that 49% of the children in their study said that exertion was the most common precipitant to their pains. But again, no well-designed studies have confirmed that fatigue plays a role.

Growing pains are typically managed by reassurance that the child will outgrow them or by nonspecific interventions such as heat, massage, and aspirin or acetaminophen. When children were asked what seems to help (Keinanen-Kiukaanniemi et al. 1985), almost all children reported moderate success for massage, while analgesics were successful for about 23%. Only 12% of the children sought medical attention. In a recent study, 18 pediatric orthopedic surgeons, 9 pediatric rheumatologists, 72 pediatricians, and 76 family physicians responded to questions concerning their assessment and treatment of growing pains (Macarthur et al. 1996). Thirty-seven percent of the responders recommended reassurance, massage, and analgesics; 30% recommended reassurance and massage; 16% recommended reassurance and analgesics; and 15% recommended reassurance alone.

There have been two trials of treatment for growing pains. Baxter and Dulberg (1988) randomly assigned 36 children 5–14 years old with no orthopedic abnormalities to either a stretching exercise regimen or a control group. In the study group, the parent stretched the quadriceps, hamstrings, and gastrosoleus muscles twice a day for 10 minutes. The control group was reassured that the condition was benign, and friction rubs and aspirin were suggested for pain relief. Over a 3-month period, the frequency of painful episodes decreased from a baseline of 10 per month to 1.2 per month in the stretching group, and to 7 per month in the control group. However, two factors may confound the results. First, the stretching group received parental attention twice a day, while the control group did not. Second, neither the parents nor the investigators were blind to treatment condition.

The second study, conducted in Sweden, was a double-blind placebo-controlled trial of selenium (Brahme-Isgren et al. 1995). Selenium deficiency has been associated with leg muscle pain (Kelly et al. 1988) and has also been implicated in the pathology of rheumatoid arthritis (Tarp et al. 1985; Peretz et al. 1991). The Swedish study found low selenium levels in 25 children aged 3–12 years with growing pains who had negative physical and neurological results. They were given either selenium or a placebo, and both their selenium levels and pain were monitored for up to 4 months. Pain was measured by (1) parent and child retrospective report of frequency and intensity of growing pains, and (2) the use of a diary of pain frequency and intensity. The authors report that the treatment group displayed both higher selenium levels and lower pain than did the control group. Although preliminary, these results suggest that selenium may play a role in the etiology of growing pains and that further studies to replicate and confirm these results would be valuable.

The lack of studies might be attributed to the view that growing pains are benign and transient, or perhaps to the fact that they are not experienced by adults. Most research into children's pain is spurred by investigations of adult manifestations of the same condition, and this condition lacks an adult model. Although it may be easy to overlook the pain experienced by these children, their pain and their suffering are not inconsequential.

OVERUSE INJURIES

Overuse injuries are most often due to repeated microtrauma that occurs faster than the body can heal, or to excessive physical stress (Bernhardt and Landry 1995). Micheli has noted that these injuries were once considered an adult phenomenon, but are becoming more common in children due to their increased participation in organized sports and the increasing pressure for excellence (Micheli 1983; Micheli and Klein 1991). Overuse injuries often occur at the spine, shoulder, elbow, knee, and heel.

Pain at the spine is most often due to spondylolysis, hyperlordotic mechanics, or disk herniation (Micheli 1983). Little Leaguer's shoulder, in which pain is experienced in the proximal humerus during throwing, is a common shoulder overuse injury. It is believed to result from widening of the physis of the proximal humerus (Carson and Gasser 1998), and the onset of pain is usually gradual. Elbow pain due to overuse occurs in ballplayers (Bernhardt and Landry 1995) and gymnasts (Maffulli et al. 1992). Little

League elbow involves chronic pain over the medial aspect of the elbow caused by repetitive valgus strain during throwing. In gymnasts, fragmentation of the olecranon epiphysis is seen with olecranon overuse injuries. Pain at the knee can be the result of chronic overloading, in which there is no clear physiological etiology (see previous section on knee pain). This pain often includes a dull, chronic aching that is worsened by stair climbing and long periods of sitting (Bernhardt and Landry 1995). Knee pain may also reflect Osgood-Schlatter's disease, which is characterized by pain over the tibial tubercle. The knee used for takeoff in the sport played may be more affected, and the syndrome is believed to result from microavulsion fractures produced by repetitive forces on the quadriceps or patellar tendon (Berhardt and Landry 1995). Finally, pain at the heel is often the result of a tight Achilles tendon, especially during periods of rapid growth, or of improper training or footwear (Micheli 1983). This condition has been called Sever's disease, and those affected experience a chronic ache in the heel that appears gradually.

Overuse injuries are not limited to one sport. A 12-month study at a high school found that 86% of 266 athletes aged 14 years suffered an injury (Weir and Watson 1996) and that overuse injuries were more frequent in contact sports, but also frequent in swimming, badminton, and athletics. Nielsen and Yde (1989) reported that 37% of the injuries in youth soccer clubs were due to overuse, and that 18% of the injuries of 221 adolescent handball players were classed as overuse (Yde and Nielsen 1990). In a more recent study, 2800 Little League players aged 7–18 were followed for one season (Pasternack et al. 1996); 19% of the 81 reported injuries were classed as overuse.

The most comprehensive clinical study of overuse musculoskeletal injuries in child athletes was conducted at an outpatient sports clinic in Finland (Kannus et al. 1988) and involved a 30-month follow-up of all competitive athletes under age 16 who visited the clinic. The most common sites of overuse injuries for the 74 boys aged 10–15 were the knee (28%), heel (11%), ankle (10%), and lower leg (8%). The most common sites for the 83 girls aged 8–15 were the knee (29%), lower back (12%), ankle (11%), and lower leg (10%). Diagnoses were given for 76% of the boys and 69% of the girls. The most common diagnosis for boys was Osgood-Schlatter's disease (18%), while for the girls it was nonspecific knee synovitis (16%), followed closely by shin splint syndrome (15%) and Osgood-Schlatter's disease (13%). The authors also reported that boys' injuries were more likely to be classed as exercise-induced growth disorders or osteochondritic pains, while girls were more likely to experience lower back problems.

Young athletes with overuse injuries may not seek immediate medical attention. In fact, Kannus and his colleagues (1988) found that the average time from onset of symptoms to the first clinic visit was 4.2 months for boys and 4 months for girls. Over one-third waited more than 6 months from the onset of symptoms before seeking medical attention. The duration of overuse injury pain appears to be relatively long. Carson and Gasser (1998) reported on 23 cases of "Little Leaguer's shoulder." The boys in their study, aged 11–16, experienced symptoms for an average of 7.7 months. In another report on 10 elite gymnasts aged 11–15 years with overuse injuries of the olecranon, the patients were followed for 12 months to 9 years (Maffulli et al. 1992). Radiographs showed an appearance similar to that found in the tibial tuberosity with Osgood-Schlatter's disease. All but one of the injuries responded to conservative management.

The contributors to overuse injury vary as widely as the types of injuries. Micheli (1983) discusses the role of training errors, muscle-tendon imbalance, anatomic malalignment, footwear and playing surfaces, and pre-existing injuries or disease states. Joint hypermobility may also be a general contributor to injury in young athletes (Grana and Moretz 1978; Klemp et al. 1984; Kujala et al. 1992), although a large study of 150 male and 114 female athletes 12–19 years old contradicts this proposal (Decoster et al. 1997). This group used the method described by Carter and Wilkinson (1964) and found that significantly more female athletes (22%) than male athletes (6%) were hypermobile. However, the overall prevalence of nearly 13% hypermobility was similar to rates reported in schoolchildren (Gedalia et al. 1985, 1993; Gedalia and Press 1991).

Growth has also been implicated in as a factor in patellar pain (Micheli 1983), Osgood-Schlatter's disease (O'Neill and Micheli 1988), olecranon injuries (Maffulli et al. 1992), and low back pain in athletes (Kujala et al. 1995). Micheli (1983) suggests that growth cartilage in children is less resistant to repeated microtrauma than it is in adults. He also suggests that it is more susceptible to shear, especially at the elbow, ankle, and knee. In addition, loss of flexibility and muscle and tendon tightness around the joints are more common during periods of rapid growth such as adolescence, and may make these areas more susceptible to what have been called "overgrowth" overuse injuries.

Sward and colleagues (1990) investigated changes in the thoraco-lumbar spine of athletes with back pain. They asked 142 top athletes aged 14–25 to complete a back pain questionnaire. The athletes also received an X-ray examination of the lower thoracic and entire lumbar spine. Nearly 65% of the athletes reported moderate to severe back pain. Radiologic abnormalities, including reduced disk height, Schmorl's nodes, and change of configuration of vertebral bodies, were found in 36–55% and were correlated with pain.

As with the other musculoskeletal pains previously discussed, no prospective data have been collected to confirm that hypermobility, growth, or spine changes are causative. Although these problems are associated with back pain to some degree, further evidence is needed before we can draw any conclusions about causality.

The most common treatment for overuse injuries is rest from the pain-related activity (Kannus et al. 1988; Maffulli et al. 1992; Carson et al. 1998). Physiotherapy and cryotherapy are also commonly used. Kannus and his colleagues reported that local corticosteroid or glycosaminoglycan injections were used in only 10% of boys and 4% of girls, and that only 4% of boys and 5% of girls required surgery, most commonly for knee injuries.

Because overuse injuries are so varied, research into their correlates, treatment, and consequences has been rather disjointed, which makes it difficult to reach conclusions about common symptoms, contributors, or treatments. What is clear, however, is that these injuries are more likely to occur in children who are active in sports. Many researchers have concluded that the strenuousness and repetitiveness of the sport, combined with a growing body, are the determining factors in overuse pain. On the surface, overuse pain may appear less chronic than other musculoskeletal pains. However, the children who experience these injuries experience a great deal of pain and many functional limitations, and in some cases never resume their previous level of activity.

SUMMARY

Musculoskeletal pain in children, although common, has been the subject of relatively little research. This scarcity is especially notable when it comes to research into treatments for these conditions.

It is often the case that children with pain of unknown origin are the most neglected because research is spurred by the "search for a cause." This trend is clearly seen in the musculoskeletal pains discussed. Although finding a cause is important, future studies should focus on relieving the suffering experienced by these children, given the documented negative effects of chronic pain on children's physiological and psychological functioning.

Moreover, because many pains are of unknown origin, debate and uncertainty frequently surround diagnosis. Pain of unknown origin is often characterized as psychogenic without any evidence for a psychological cause, such as pain associated with events or emotions. The occurrence of elevated levels of psychological distress in children with nonpathologic pain does not provide convincing evidence of psychogenicity because there is ample evidence that pain with clear physiological causes produces similar levels of distress (Raymer et al. 1984; Cunningham et al. 1987; Walker and Green 1989). A successful psychological treatment of pain does not provide evidence of psychological causation any more than successful treatment with morphine implies that morphine deficiency is the cause. All pain is inherently both psychological and physiological. Separating the psychological and physical aspects is artificial, although at times, focusing on one aspect or another may be useful. Researchers and clinicians should be constantly aware of the interplay and overlap between psychological and physiological factors and keep in mind that this matrix cannot readily be disentangled.

REFERENCES

Abu-Arafeh I, Russell G. Recurrent limb pain in schoolchildren. *Arch Dis Childhood* 1996; 74:336–339.

Afshani E, Kuhn JP. Common causes of low back pain in children. *Radiographics* 1991; 11:269–291.

Al-Rawi Z, Nessan AH. Joint hypermobility in patients with chondromalacia patellae. *Br J Rheumatol* 1997; 36:1324–1327.

Balagué F, Dutoit G, Walburger M. Low back pain in schoolchildren. *Scan J Rehab Med* 1988; 20:175–179.

Balagué F, Skrovon ML, Dutoit G, Walburger M. Low back pain in schoolchildren: a study of familial and psychological factors. *Spine* 1995; 20(11):1265–1270.

Baxter MP, Dulberg CS. "Growing pains" in childhood—a proposal for treatment. *J Pediatr Orthop* 1988; 8:402–406.

Beales JG, Keen JH, Holt PJ. The child's perception of the disease and the experience of pain in juvenile chronic arthritis. *J Rheumatol* 1983; 10:61–65.

Benestad B, Vinje O, Veierrd MB, Vandvik IH. Quantitative and qualitative assessments of pain in children with Juvenile Chronic Arthritis based on the Norwegian Version of the Pediatric Pain Questionnaire. *Scand J Rheumatol* 1996; 25:293–299.

Bennie PB. Growing pains. *Arch Pediatr* 1894; 1:337–47.

Bernhardt DT, Landry GL. Sports injuries in young athletes. *Adv Pediatr* 1995; 42:465–500.

Boisset-Pioro MH, Esdaile JM, Fitzcharles MA. Sexual and physical abuse in women with fibromyalgia syndrome. *Arthritis Rheum* 1995; 38:235–241.

Bowyer S, Roettcher P. Pediatric rheumatology clinic populations in the United States: results of a 3 year study. *J Rheum* 1996; 23(11):1968–1974.

Brahme-Isgren M, Brandt C, Waldenström J, Stenhammar L. Peroral selenium therapy in growth pain in children. *Lakartidningen* 1995; 92(40):3706–3708.

Breau L, McGrath PJ, Ju L. Fibromyalgia and Chronic Fatigue Syndrome in children and adolescents. *J Develop Behav Pediatrics* (in press).

Brenning R. Growing pains. *Acta Soc Med Uppsala* 1960; 65:185–201.

Burton AK. Low back pain in children and adolescents: to treat or not? *Bull Hosp Jt Dis* 1996; 55(3):127–129.

Burton AK, Clarke RD, McClune TD, Tillitson KM. The natural history of low back pain in adolescents. *Spine* 1996; 21(20):2323–2328.

Buskila D, Press J, Gedalia A, et al. Assessment of nonarticular tenderness and prevalence of fibromyalgia in children. *J Rheumatol* 1993; 20:368–370.

Buskila D, Neumann L, Carmi R. Analysis of genetic aspects in fibromyalgia families. *J Musculoskeletal Pain* [Abstract] 1995a; 3:(1)50.

Buskila D, Neumann L, Hershman E, et al. Fibromyalgia syndrome in children: an outcome study. *J Rheumatol* 1995b; 22(3):525–528.

Buskila D, Neumann L, Hazanov I, Carmi R. Familial aggregation in the Fibromyalgia Syndrome. *Semin Arthritis Rheum* 1996; 26(3):605–611.

Carson WG, Gasser SI. Little Leaguer's Shoulder: a report of 23 cases. *Am J Sports Med* 1998; 26(4):575–580.

Carter C, Wilkinson J. Persistent joint laxity and congenital dislocation of the hip. *J Bone Joint Surg* 1964; 46:40–45.

Coombs JA, Caskey PM. Back pain in children and adolescents: a retrospective review of 648 patients. *South Med J* 1997; 90(8):789–792.

Cunningham SJ, McGrath PJ, Ferguson HB, et al. Personality and behavioural characteristics in pediatric migraine. *Headache* 1987; 27:16–20.

Decoster LC, Vailas JC, Lindsay RH, Williams R. Prevalence and features of joint hypermobility among adolescent athletes. *Arch Pediatr Adolesc Med* 1997; 151:989–992.

Ekbom KA. Growing pains and restless legs. *Acta Pediatr Scand* 1975; 64:264–266.

Erball PS. The epidemiology of male adolescent low back pain in a north suburban population of Melbourne, Australia. *J Manipulative Physiol Ther* 1994a; 17(7):447–453.

Erball PS. Some anthropometric dimensions of male adolescents with idiopathic low back pain. *J Manipulative Physiol Ther* 1994b; 17(5):296–301.

Fairbank JC, Pynsent PB, Van Poortvliet JA, Phillips H. Influence of anthropometric factors and joint laxity in the incidence of adolescent back pain. *Spine* 1984a; 9:461–464.

Fairbank JC, Pynsent PB, Van Poortvliet JA, Phillips H. Mechanical factors in the incidence of knee pain in adolescents and young adults. *J Bone Joint Surg* 1984b; 66:685–693.

Fritz GK, Bleck EE, Dahl IS. Functional versus organic knee pain in adolescents: a pilot study. *Am J Sports Med* 1981; 9(4):247–249.

Gedalia A, Press J. Articular symptoms in hypermobile schoolchildren: a prospective study. *J Pediatr* 1991; 119:944–946.

Gedalia A, Person D, Brewer E, Gianini E. Hypermobility of the joints in juvenile episodic arthritis/arthralgia. *J Pediatr* 1985; 107:873–876.

Gedalia A, Press J, Klein M, Buskila D. Joint hypermobility and fibromyalgia in school children. *Ann Rheum Dis* 1993; 52:494–496.

Goldberg B. Chronic anterior knee pain in the adolescent. *Pediatr Annals* 1991; 20(4):186–193.

Gragg RA, Rapoff MA, Danovsky MB, et al. Assessing chronic musculoskeletal pain associated with rheumatic disease: further validation of the Pediatric Pain Questionnaire. *J Pediatr Psychol* 1996; 21:237–250.

Grana WA, Moretz J. Ligamentous laxity in secondary school athletes. *JAMA* 1978; 18:167–169.

Haasbeek JF, Wright JG. Getting to the bottom of growing pains. *Can J Diagn Ups* 1993; April:155–165.

Hawksley JC. The nature of growing pains and their relation to rheumatism in children and adolescents. *BMJ* 1939; Jan 28:155–157.

Hogeweg JA, Kuis W, Huygen ACJ, et al. The pain threshold in juvenile chronic arthritis. *Br J Rheumatol* 1995a; 34:61–67.

Hogeweg JA, Kuis W, Oostendorp RAB, Helders PJM. General and segmental reduced pain thresholds in juvenile chronic arthritis. *Pain* 1995b; 62:11–7.

Ilowite NT, Walco GA, Pochaczevsky R. Assessment of pain in patients with juvenile rheumatoid arthritis: relation between pain intensity and degree of joint inflammation. *Ann Rheum Dis* 1992; 51:343–346.

Insall J. "Chondromalacia Patellae": patellar malalignment syndrome. *Orthop Clin North Am* 1979; 10:117–127.

Insall J. Current concepts review: patellar pain. *J Bone Joint Surg* 1982; 64:147–152.

Jaworski TM. Juvenile rheumatoid arthritis: pain-related and psychosocial aspects and their relevance for assessment and treatment. *Arthritis Care Res* 1993; 6(4):187–196.

Johnson RP. Anterior knee pain in adolescents and young adults. *Curr Opin Rheumatol* 1997; 9:159–164.

Kannus P, Niittymaki S, Jarvinen M. Athletic overuse injuries in children. *Clin Pediatr* 1988; 27(7):333–337.

Kasper MJ, Robbins L, Root L, Peterson MGE, Allegante JP. A musculoskeletal outreach screening, treatment, and education program for urban minority children. *Arthritis Care Res* 1993; 6(3):126–133.

Keinanen-Kiukaanniemi S, Hakkinen J, Korhonen J, Kouvalainen K. Growing pains in school children. *Acta Pediatr Scand* 1985; (S322):27.

Kelly DA, Coe AW, Shenkin A, Lake BD, Walker-Smith JA. Symptomatic selenium deficiency in a child on home parenteral nutrition. *J Pediatr Gastroenterol Nutr* 1988; 7(5):783–786.

King HA. Evaluating the child with back pain. *Pediatr Clin North Am* 1986; 33:1489–1493.

Klemp P, Stevens JE, Isaacs S. A hypermobility study in ballet dancers. *J Rheumatol* 1984; 11:692–696.

Kristjánsdóttir G. Prevalence of self-reported back pain in school children: a study of sociodemographic differences. *Eur J Pediatr* 1996; 155:984–986.

Kujala UM, Salminen JJ, Taimela S, Oksanen A, Jaakkola L. Subject characteristics and low back pain in young athletes and nonathletes. *Med Sci Sports Exerc* 1992; 24:627–632.

Kujala UM, Taimela S, Erkintalo M, Salminen JJ, Kaprio J. Low back pain in adolescent athletes. *Med Sci Sports Exerc* 1995; 28(2):165–170.

Larsson BS. Somatic complaints and their relationship to depressive symptoms in Swedish adolescents. *J Child Psychol Psychiatry* 1991; 32:821–832.

Lavigne JV, Ross CK, Berry SL, Hayford JR. Evaluation of a psychological treatment package for treating pain in juvenile rheumatoid arthritis. *Arthritis Care Res* 1992; 5:101–110.

Leboef-Yde C, Kyvik KO. At what age does low back pain become a common problem? A study of 29,424 individuals aged 12–41 years. *Spine* 1998; 23(2):228–234.

Leung AKC, Robson WLM. Growing pains. *Can Fam Physician* 1991; 37:1463–1467.

Lovell DJ, Walco GA. Pain associated with juvenile rheumatoid arthritis. *Pediatr Clin North Am* 1989; 36:1015–1027.

Macarthur C, Wright JG, Srivastava R, Rosser W, Feldman W. Variability in physicians' reported ordering and perceived reassurance value of diagnostic tests in children with "growing pains." *Arch Pediatr Adolesc Med* 1996; 150:1072–1076.

Maffulli N, Chan D, Aldridge MJ. Overuse injuries of the olecranon in young gymnasts. *J Bone Joint Surg* 1992; 74(B):305–308.

Malleson PN, al Matar M, Petty RE. Idiopathic musculoskeletal pain syndromes in children. *J Rheumatol* 1992; 19:1786–1789.

Malleson PN, Fung MY, Rosenberg AM. The incidence of pediatric rheumatic diseases: results from the Canadian Pediatric Rheumatology Association disease registry. *J Rheumatol* 1996; 23(11):1981–1987.

Micheli LJ. Overuse injuries in children's sports: the growth factor. *Orthop Clin North Am* 1983; 14(2):337–360.

Micheli LJ, Klein JD. Sports injuries in children and adolescents. *Br J Sports Med* 1991; 25(1):6–9.

Mierau D, Cassidy JD, Yong-Hing K. Low-back pain and straight leg raising in children and adolescents. *Spine* 1989; 14(5):526–528.

Mikkelsson M, Salminen JJ, Kautiainen H. Non-specific musculoskeletal pain in preadolescents. Prevalence and 1-year persistence. *Pain* 1997a; 73:29–35.

Mikkelsson M, Sourander A, Piha J, Salminen JJ. Psychiatric symptoms in preadolescents with musculoskeletal pain and fibromyalgia. *Pediatrics* 1997b; 100(2 Pt 1):220–227.

Milling LS, Shaw WJ, Durniat K. Behavioral management of chronic back pain in children and adolescents. In: Roberts MC, Walker E (Eds). *Casebook of Child and Pediatric Psychology*. New York: Guilford Press, 1989, pp 380–403.

Moe N, Rygg M. Epidemiology of juvenile chronic arthritis in northern Norway: a ten-year retrospective study. *Clin Exp Rheumatol* 1998; 16:99–101.

Naish JM, Apley J. 'Growing pains': a clinical study of non-arthritic limb pains in children. *Arch Dis Child* 1950; 134–140.

Newcomer K, Sinaki M. Low back pain and its relationship to back strength and physical activity in children. *Acta Pediatr* 1996; 85:1433–1439.

Nielsen AB, Yde J. Epidemiology and traumatology of injuries in sports. *Am J Sports Med* 1989; 17(6):803–807.

Nissinen M, Helivaara M, Seitsamo J, Alaranta H, Poussa M. Anthropometric measurements and the incidence of low back pain in a cohort of pubertal children. *Spine* 1994:19(12):1367–1370.

Oberklaid F, Amos D, Liu C, Jarman F. "Growing pains": clinical and behavioral correlates in a community sample. *J Dev Behav Pediatr* 1997; 18(2):102–106.

O'Neill DB, Micheli LJ. Overuse injuries in the young athlete. *Clin Sports Med* 1988; 7:591–610.

Oster J. Growing pain: a symptom and its significance (a review). *Dan Med Bull* 1972a; 19:72–79.

Oster J. Recurrent abdominal pain, headache and recurrent limb pains in children and adolescents. *Pediatrics* 1972b; 50(3):429–436.

Oster J, Nielsen A. Growing pains: a clinical investigation of a school population. *Acta Paediatr Scand* 1972; 61:329–334.

Passo MH. Aches and limb pain. *Pediatr Clin N Am* 1982; 29:209–219.

Pasternack JS, Veenema KR, Callahan CM. Baseball injuries: a little league survey. *Pediatrics* 1996; 98(3):445–448.

Peretz AM, Neve JD, Famaey JP. Selenium in rheumatic diseases. *Semin Arthritis Rheum* 1991; 20(5):305–316.

Peterson H. Growing pains. *Ped Clin N Am* 1986; 33(6):1365–1372.

Rabinovich CE, Schanberg LE, Stein LD, et al. A follow up study of pediatric fibromyalgia patients [Abstract]. *Arthritis Rheum* 1990; 33(Suppl 9):S146.

Raymer D, Weininger O, Hamilton JR. Psychological problems in children with abdominal pain. *Lancet* 1984; 1:439–440.

Reid GJ, Lang BA, McGrath PJ. Primary juvenile fibromyalgia: psychological adjustment, family functioning, coping and functional disability. *Arthritis Rheum* 1996; 40(4):752–760.

Roizenblatt S, Tufik S, Goldenberg J, et al. Juvenile fibromyalgia: clinical and polysomnographic aspects. *J Rheumatol* 1997; 24(3):579–585.

Romano TJ. Fibromyalgia in children: diagnosis and treatment. *W V Med J* 1991; 87:112–114.

Ross CK, LaVigne J, Hayford JR, Dyer AR, Pachman LM. Validity of reported pain as a measure of clinical state in juvenile rheumatoid arthritis. *Ann Rheum Dis* 1989; 48:817–819.

Ross CK, Lavigne JV, Hayford JR, et al. Psychological factors affecting reported pain in juvenile rheumatoid arthritis. *J Pediatr Psychol* 1993; 18:561–573.

Salminen JJ, Maki P, Oksanen A, Pentti J. Spinal mobility and trunk muscle strength in 15-year-old schoolchildren with and without low-back pain. *Spine* 1992; 17(4):405–411.

Salminen JJ, Erkintalo M, Laine M, Pentti J. Low back pain in the young: a prospective three-year follow-up study of subjects with and without low-back pain. *Spine* 1995; 20(19):2101–2108.

Sandow MJ, Goodfellow JW. The natural history of anterior knee pain in adolescents. *J Bone Joint Surg* 1985; 67:36–38.

Schaller JG. Chronic childhood arthritis and spondylarthropathies. In: Calin A (Ed). *Spondylarthropathies*. New York: Grune and Stratton, 1984, pp 187–208.

Schanberg LE, Lefebvre JC, Keefe FJ, Kredich DW, Gil KM. Pain coping and the pain experience in children with juvenile chronic arthritis. *Pain* 1997; 73(2):181–189.

Sherry DD, Bohnsack J, Salmonson K, Wallace CA, Mellins E. Painless juvenile rheumatoid arthritis. *J Pediatr* 1990; 116:921–923.

Siegel DM, Janeway D, Baum J. Fibromyalgia syndrome in children and adolescents: clinical features at presentation and status at follow-up. *Pediatrics* 1998; 101(3):377–382.

Smedbråten BK, Natvig B, Rutle O, Bruusgaard D. Self-reported bodily pain in schoolchildren. *Scand J Rheumatol* 1998; 27:273–276.

Still GF. *The History of Paediatrics*. Oxford: Oxford University Press, 1931.

Sward LM, Hellstrom B, Jacobsson B, Nyman R. Acute injury of the vertebral ring apophysis and intervertebral disc in adolescent gymnasts. *Spine* 1990; 15:144–148.

Symmons DPM, Jones M, Osborne J, et al. Pediatric rheumatology in the United Kingdom: data from the British Pediatric Rheumatology Group national diagnostic register. *J Rheumatol* 1996; 23:1975–1980.

Taimela S, Kujala UM, Salminen JJ, Viljanen T. The prevalence of low back pain among children and adolescents. *Spine* 1997; 22(10):1132–1136.

Tarp U, Hansen JC, Overvad K, Thorling EB. Low selenium level in rheumatoid arthritis. *Scand J Rheumatol* 1985; 14(2):97–101.

Taylor ML, Trotter DR, Csuka ME. The prevalence of sexual abuse in women with fibromyalgia. *Arthritis Rheum* 1995; 38:229–234.

Thabit G, Micheli LJ. Patellofemoral pain in the pediatric patient. *Orthop Clin North Am* 1992; 23(4):567–585.

Thompson KL, Varni JW, Hanson V. Comprehensive assessment of pain in juvenile rheumatoid arthritis: an empirical model. *J Pediatr Psychol* 1987; 12:241–255.

Truckenbrodt H. Pain in juvenile chronic arthritis: consequences for the musculo-skeletal system. *Clin Exp Rheumatol* 1993; 11(Suppl 9):S59–S63.

Turner PG, Green JH, Galasko CSB. Back pain in childhood. *Spine* 1989; 14(9):812–814.

Vandvik IH, Eckblad G. The relationship between pain, disease severity and psychosocial function in patients with juvenile chronic arthritis (JCA). *Scad J Rheumatol* 1990; 19:295–302.

Vandvik IH, Forseth KO. A bio-psychosocial evaluation of ten adolescents with fibromyalgia. *Acta Paediatr* 1994; 83:766–771.

Varni JW, Thompson KL, Hanson V. The Varni/Thompson Pediatric Pain Questionnaire: I. Chronic musculoskeletal pain in juvenile rheumatoid arthritis. *Pain* 1987; 28:27–38.

Walco GA. Growing pains. *J Dev Behav Pediatr* 1997; 18(2):107–108.

Walco GA, Ilowite NT. Cognitive-behavioral intervention for juvenile primary fibromyalgia syndrome. *J Rheumatol* 1992; 19:1617–1619.

Walco GA, Varni JW, Ilowite NT. Cognitive-behavioral pain management in children with juvenile rheumatoid arthritis. *Pediatrics* 1992; 89:1075–1079.

Walker LS, Greene JW. Children with recurrent abdominal pain and their parents: more somatic complaints, anxiety, and depression than other patient families? *J Pediatr Psychol* 1989; 14:231–243.

Walters AS, Hickey K, Matzman J, et al. A questionnaire study of 138 patients with restless legs syndrome: the "night-walkers" survey. *Neurology* 1996; 4692–4695.

Weir MA, Watson AWS. A twelve month study of sports injuries in one Irish school. *Ir J Med Sci* 1996; 165(3):165–169.

Wolfe F, Smythe HA, Yunus MB, et al. The American College of Rheumatology 1990 criteria for the classification of fibromyalgia. *Arthritis Rheum* 1990; 33:160–172.

Wolfe F, Ross K, Anderson J, et al. The prevalence and characteristics of fibromyalgia in the general population. *Arthritis Rheum* 1995; 38:19–28.

Yde J, Nielsen AB. Sports injuries in adolescents' ball games: soccer, handball and basketball. *Br J Sports Med* 1990; 24:51–54.

Yunus MB, Masi AT. Juvenile primary fibromyalgia syndrome. A clinical study of thirty-three patients and matched normal controls. *Arthritis Rheum* 1985; 28:138–145.

Correspondence to: Patrick J. McGrath, PhD, Department of Psychology, Dalhousie University, Halifax, Nova Scotia, Canada B3H 4J1. Fax: 902-494-6585; email: Patrick.McGrath@dal.ca.

Chronic and Recurrent Pain in Children and Adolescents, Progress in Pain Research and Management, Vol. 13, edited by Patrick J. McGrath and G. Allen Finley, IASP Press, Seattle, © 1999.

10

Gender Variation in Children's Pain Experiences

Anita M. Unruh[a] and Mary Ann Campbell[b]

[a]School of Occupational Therapy, and [b]Psychology Department, Dalhousie University, Halifax, Nova Scotia, Canada

Interest in gender variation in pain experience has grown considerably in the last 5–10 years (Berkley 1992, 1993, 1997; Vallerand 1995; Unruh 1996; Derbyshire 1997; Riley et al. 1998). Much of the literature concerns gender variation in pain experience in adulthood. Researchers argue that important physiological differences place women at greater risk for pain (Berkley 1997) and that women are likely to report lower pain thresholds, lower pain tolerance, and higher pain ratings than men in an experimental context (Fillingim and Maixner 1995; Riley et al. 1998). Evidence indicates that women report more health care utilization and more short-term disability when they experience pain (Unruh 1996) and that they use more coping strategies (Unruh 1996), seek more social support (Unruh 1996; Unruh et al. 1999), and have a greater tendency to catastrophize pain events (Sullivan et al. 1999).

Gender differences are shaped by biological, psychological, social, and environmental dimensions (Unruh 1996). Biological mechanisms that affect gender differences in pain experience may begin to exert their influence in utero and continue with the maturation of the central and peripheral nervous systems and the onset of pubertal hormonal and structural changes. Berkley (1997) has argued that the animal literature provides considerable physiological evidence for sex differences in pain. These differences can be demonstrated in both young and mature rats (see Chapter 3 for a full discussion). Nevertheless, in the human clinical literature, gender differences may not be found or may be smaller than might have been expected on the basis of animal and experimental literature (Berkley 1997). Clearly, the biological, psychological, social, and environmental aspects of pain experience are interactive.

In this chapter, we will review the evidence for gender variation in pediatric pain, considering the prevalence of common recurrent pains and the risks for depression and disability. We will provide an overview of medication use, coping strategies, and health care utilization for pain, and discuss factors that might influence gender variation. The limitations that must be considered in a review of children, gender, and pain experience include the publication bias to report differences rather than similarities, as well as the failure of many researchers to perform gender-related data analysis (Unruh 1996).

PREVALENCE OF COMMON RECURRENT PAINS BY GENDER IN CHILDHOOD AND ADOLESCENCE

Children are not strangers to pain. Observational studies of incidents of everyday pain among preschoolers and young school-aged children yield mean rates between 0.34 and 0.41 incidents per hour per child (Fearon et al. 1996; von Baeyer et al. 1998). Neither Fearon nor von Baeyer found any gender difference for the rate of incidence or severity of pain.

We conducted searches of MEDLINE, Cinahl, and Psychlit to obtain epidemiological surveys of common recurrent pains in childhood or adolescence that provided gender-comparative outcomes. We excluded studies using primarily adult samples, unless the researcher(s) provided information about outcomes specifically concerned with gender variation for the pediatric portion of the sample.

HEADACHE AND MIGRAINE

Epidemiological studies of pediatric headache and migraine that report gender outcomes are summarized in Table I. Other summary tables of prevalence for pediatric and adult headache and migraine with gender-related information for the years 1937–1987 are given in Chen (1993). Prevalence of migraine and headache is similar for girls and boys in the school-age years (age 5–12) but is slightly higher in boys, with an increase in rates for girls during adolescence (Bille 1962, 1981; Dalsgaard-Nielsen et al. 1970; Oster 1972; Deubner 1977; Sillanpää 1983a,b; Passchier and Orlebeke 1985; Aro et al. 1987, 1989; Beiter et al. 1991; Larsson 1991; Mortimer et al. 1992; Kristjánsdóttir and Wahlberg 1993; Carlsson 1996). In adulthood, nausea, vomiting, and unilateral numbness or tingling are more common in women, while men are more likely to experience migraine with aura (Unruh 1996). Bille (1997) reported that visual disturbances were reported by 70% of the children with migraines in his original 1955 sample and were reported significantly more often by girls.

There is clearly some relationship between migraine and hormones, as the prevalence of migraine increases with puberty for girls and adult women and may be affected not only by menstruation and ovulation, but also by pregnancy and menopause (Somerville 1975; Ratinahirana et al. 1990; Bousser and Massiou 1993; Silberstein and Merriam 1993).

Stress is often argued to be an important causal factor in the higher prevalence of migraines for adolescent girls on the basis that girls seem to be more sensitive to interpersonal conflicts that might occur within the family, at school, or among peers (Aro 1987). Recently, Metsähonkala et al. (1998) found that stress and bullying at school and poor relationships with peers were reported more often by children who had migraines or headaches. For girls, stress was highly associated with migraine, whereas boys with migraine were more likely to report poor relationships with their peers ($P < 0.01$). Nevertheless, when headache-free subjects were matched with headache sufferers, significant associations were found between self-reports of stress and psychological symptoms for both groups (Carlsson et al. 1996). Unfortunately, very little information exists on gender variations in the pathophysiology of migraine (Burstein 1998).

FACIAL PAIN

The most common type of facial pain is temporomandibular joint dysfunction (TMD). Studies of pediatric orofacial pain that report gender outcomes are summarized in Table II. Increased rates of TMD pain and pain in the jaw muscles in women may emerge during adolescence (Wänman and Agerberg 1986a,b; Pilley et al. 1992). Widmalm et al. (1995) found that even among 4–6-year-old children, girls are significantly more likely than boys to have one or more oral parafunctions, which are thought to be risk factors for later occurrence of TMD. However, Riolo et al. (1987) found no gender difference in a sample aged 6–17 years.

MUSCULOSKELETAL AND BACK PAIN

Epidemiological studies of musculoskeletal pain that report gender distributions are given in Table III. In a comprehensive population study of musculoskeletal pain in schoolchildren over a 1-year period, Mikkelsson et al. (1997) found that 32% of children have musculoskeletal pain in at least one part of the body at least once a week. Further, about half of the children who had pain at least once a week continued to have pain at the 1-year follow-up. Reports of pain were most common in the lower extremities and the neck, but the only significant prevalence difference was a more frequent report of chest pain by girls ($P = 0.005$).

Table I
Gender variation in prevalence of headache and migraine among
children and adolescents

Reference		Outcome	
(Sample)	Variable(s)	Female	Male
Aro et al. 1987, 1989 (n = 999f, 1002m, mean age 15 y, Finland)	Prevalence of headache quite often, often, or continuously, during 1 y	14.9% ($P < 0.001$)	7.2%
Barea et al. 1996 (n = 266f, 272m, age 10–18 y, Brazil)	Prevalence of headache: lifetime	94.4%	92.3%
	in the last year	87.9% ($P < 0.002$)	77.9%
	in the last week	2:1 ($P < 0.001$)	
	in the last 24 h	2:1 ($P < 0.001$)	
	Prevalence of migraine: in the last year	10.3%	9.6%
	in the last week	5.6%	5.8%
	in the last 24 h	1.8%	0.7%
Beiter et al. 1991 (n = 652f, 691m, mean age 13.7 y, USA)	Headache frequency (at least weekly)	30% ($P < 0.0001$)	18%
Bille 1962, 1981 (n = 4553f, 4440m, age 7–15 y, Sweden)	Prevalence of migraine	4.5%	3.4%
		Prevalence similar in boys and girls aged 7–9 y at 2.5% but increased for girls after age 11 y. Duration of >12 h rare; occurred almost exclusively in girls.	
Carlsson 1996 (n = 556f, 628m, age 7–16 y, Sweden)	Prevalence of headache at least once a month:		
	grades 1–3	19.6% (n.s.)	18.1%
	grades 4–6	24.5% (n.s.)	26.3%
	grades 7–9	44.3% ($P < 0.001$)	25.5%
	Headache several times a week or daily:		
	grades 1–3	7.5% (n.s.)	4.9%
	grades 4–6	7.2% (n.s.)	3.8%
	grades 7–9	12.8% ($P < 0.001$)	0.7%

Table I
Continued

Reference (Sample)	Variable(s)	Outcome	
		Female	Male
Celentano et al. 1990 (n = 3851f, 2496m, age 12–29 y, one or more head-aches in past 4 wk, USA)	Four or more headaches in previous 4 wk	18.4% ($P < 0.001$)	10.6%
	Headache duration	Women reported headaches of significantly longer duration (P value not given).	
Dalsgaard-Nielsen et al. 1970 (n = 952f, 1075m, age 7–18 y, Denmark)	Prevalence of migraine	7.5%	6.9%
Deubner 1977 (n = 303f, 297m, age 10–20 y, USA)	Prevalence of migraine	22.1%	15.5%
	Prevalence of headache	82%	74%
Eminson et al. 1996 (n = 410f, 395m, age 11–16 y, UK)	Lifetime prevalence of headaches	35.3%	27.6%
Kristjánsdóttir and Wahlberg 1993 (n = 1045f, 1084m, ages 11–12 y and 15–16 y, Iceland)	Prevalence and frequency of headache	No gender difference in headache prevalence in 11–12-year-olds, but in older group girls had higher prevalence than boys ($P < 0.001$). Girls in both age groups reported more frequent headaches ($P < 0.001$).	
Larsson 1991 (n = 269f, 270m, age 13–18 y, Sweden)	Prevalence, frequency, and intensity of headache	Girls reported more headaches than boys ($P < 0.001$); frequency and severity were higher in girls than boys.	

(continued)

Table I
Continued

Reference		Outcome	
(Sample)	Variable(s)	Female	Male
Linet et al. 1989 (*n* = 5055f, 4394m, age 12–29 y, USA)	Headache in last 4 wk	76.5%	57.1%
	Four or more headaches in past month	14.0%	6.1%
	Average duration of most recent headache	8.2 h	5.9 h
	Duration of ≥6 h for most recent headache	27.6%	19.3%
	Mean pain intensity ≥6	5.4%	3.2%
Metsähonkala et al. 1998 (*n* = 486f, 491m, age 8–9 y, Finland)	Prevalence of migraine	43.2% with migraine and 49.7% with nonmigrainous headache were girls.	
Mortimer et al. 1992, 1993 (*n* = 6917f, 6397m, age 3–11 y, England)	Lifetime prevalence: headache	55%	56%
	migraine	5.1%	4.7%
		At 3–5 y of age, boys reported more headaches than girls ($P < 0.05$).	
Orji and Iloeje 1997 (*n* = 2184f, 2214m, age 6–13 y, Nigeria)	Lifetime prevalence of migraine	7.2%	6.3%
		(1.13:1 ratio)	
		Prevalence increased with age for girls and boys until age 12 and then increased for girls and decreased for boys. Change with puberty significant for both ($P < 0.02$).	
Oster 1972 (*n* = 8947f, 9215m, age 6–19 y, Denmark)	Prevalence of headache	22.7%	18.6%
Passchier and Orlebeke 1985 (*n* = 2300 schoolchildren age 10–17 y, The Netherlands)	Prevalence of headache during past year	Girls reported more headaches in elementary and secondary schools ($P < 0.001$), more frequent headaches ($P < 0.001$), headaches of greater intensity ($P < 0.01$). Girls in secondary school reported longer headaches ($P < 0.05$).	

Table I
Continued

Reference (Sample)	Variable(s)	Outcome	
		Female	Male
Sillanpää 1983a (n = 1873f, 1911m, age 13 y, Finland)	Frequency of headache: no headache	16%	20%
	once in previous year	14%	18%
	2–3 times a month	11%	8%
	once a week	6%	2%
	2–6 times a week	4%	2%
	Prevalence of migraine	14.5%	8.1%
Sillanpää 1983b (n = 1448f, 1473m, surveyed at age 7 and 14)	Prevalence of migraine: at age 7	2.5%	2.9%
	at age 14	8.6%	4.7%
Sparks 1978 (n = 3242f, 12,543m, age 10–18 y, England)	Prevalence of migraine: overall prevalence	2.5%	3.3%
	at least weekly	5%	9%
	several times a month	25%	18%
	severe	46%	37%
	lasting >6 h	39%	24%
Stang et al. 1992 (n = 6400 medical records for one county, ages 0–60+ y, USA)	Age-adjusted incidence of migraine per 100,000 person-years	294	137
		Highest incidence at age 20–24 y in females and 10–14 y in males	
Stewart et al. 1991 (n = 1018f, 392m, ages 12–29 y, USA)	Peak age-specific migraine incidence per 1000 person-years: with visual aura	14.1, age 14–17	6.6, age 5
	without visual aura	18.9, age 14–17	10.1, age 10–11

Table II
Gender variation in prevalence of facial and oral pain among children and adolescents

Reference (Sample)	Variable(s)	Outcome	
		Female	Male
Larsson 1991 (*n* = 269f, 270m, age 13–18 y, Sweden)	Prevalence of mouth-opening/chewing pain	No gender difference	
Motegi et al. 1992 (*n* = 4118f, 3219m, age 6–18 y, Japan)	Prevalence in temporomandibular disorders.	13% (n.s.)	11.1%
Pilley et al. 1992 (*n* = 398f, 393m, age 15 y, Sweden)	Pain around the TMJ Pain in jaw muscles	11% 4% More positive signs of craniomandibular disorders in girls	6% 4%
Riolo et al. 1987 (*n* = 614f, 631m, age 6–17 y, USA)	TMJ tenderness Muscle tenderness	No gender difference No gender difference	
Wänman and Agerberg 1986a,b (*n* = 139f, 146m, age 17 y, Sweden)	Tenderness on palpation	Girls more tender on palpation (*P* < 0.05); signs of clinical dysfunction more common in girls (*P* < 0.01)	
Widmalm et al. 1995 (*n* = 243f, 282m, mean age 5.1 y, U.S. Caucasian and African American children)	Prevalence of oral parafunctions (thumb sucking, nail biting, bruxism)	Caucasian 82% (*P* < 0.005); African American 71%	

Growing pains are a common musculoskeletal pain occurring in about 10–15% of children and are characterized by deep aching sensations in the muscles of the lower limbs late in the day or at night (Naish and Apley 1950; Goodenough 1998). Oster and Nielsen (1972) found growing pains to be more common among girls, but a recent review found no evidence for gender-based variations (Goodenough 1998).

The prevalence of back pain has been examined primarily in adolescent samples, and ranges from 25% to 38%. Although some studies have reported significantly higher prevalence rates for girls (Balagué et al. 1988; Salminen et al. 1992), others report more back pain for boys (e.g., Burton et al. 1996). Most epidemiological studies do not identify gender differences in prevalence rates of back pain (see Table IV) and do not distinguish between upper and lower back pain. However, anatomical differences between girls and boys may present different risks for pain in different locations of the back. Mikkelsson et al. (1997) reported significantly higher rates of upper back pain for girls but no gender difference for frequency of low back pain.

Several studies identify increased prevalence rates of back pain with

Table III
Gender variation in prevalence of musculoskeletal pain among
children and adolescents

Reference (Sample)	Variable(s)	Outcome	
		Female	Male
Buskila et al. 1993 (*n* = 159f, 179m, age 9–15 y, Israel)	Frequency of fibromyalgia	8.8%	3.8%
Eminson et al. 1996 (*n* = 410f, 395m, age 11–16 y, UK)	Lifetime prevalence of: joint pains pains in arms/legs	 39.6% 29.5%	 29.1% 33.6%
Fairbank et al. 1984b (*n* = 219f, 227m, age 13–17 y, England)	Prevalence of knee pain: in previous year at time of study	 31.5% 16%	 29.5% 26%
Larsson 1991 (*n* = 269f, 270m, age 13–18 y, Sweden)	Prevalence of limb pain	No gender difference	
Lee et al. 1985 (*n* = 11,606f, 11,417m, adults and children, all ages, Canada Health Survey)	Prevalence by age of musculoskeletal pains: 65+ y 15–64 y <15 y	 55.7% 19.4% 1.4%	 39.2% 14.6% 1.3%
Naish and Apley 1950 (*n* = 721 schoolchildren, age range not given, England)	Limb pain	4.7%	4.0%
Oberklaid et al. 1997 (*n* = 160, 51% female, mean age 8.5 y, Australia)	Prevalence of growing pains	No gender difference	
Oster and Nielsen 1972 (*n* = 1116f, 1062m, age 6–9 y, Denmark)	Growing pains	18.4%	12.5%
Vähäsarja 1995 (*n* = 451f, 405m, age 9–10 or 14–15 y, Finland)	Prevalence of chronic knee pain by age: 9–10 y 14–15 y	 3.1% 19.8%	 4.8% 16.8%

age, with rates of 1–6% in the school-age years (Taimela et al. 1997), but reaching 50% and higher by late adolescence (e.g., Balagué et al. 1988; Newcomer and Sinaki 1996; Taimela et al. 1997; Leboeuf-Yde and Kyvik 1998). Taimela et al. (1997) reported that girls were significantly more likely than boys to report recurrent or chronic low back pain.

Several researchers have found increased risk for back pain to be linked with sports and other physical activities, particularly those associated with musculotendinous or ligamentous strains caused by excessive loading (Burton et al. 1996; Kujala et al. 1996, 1997; Newcomer and Sinaki 1996; Leboeuf-Yde and Kyvik 1998). Some back pain may also be associated with menstrual

Table IV
Gender variation in prevalence of back pain among children and adolescents

Reference (Sample)	Variable(s)	Outcome	
		Female	Male
Balagué et al. 1988 (*n* = 875f, 840m, age 7–17 y, Switzerland)	Prevalence of back pain	38% (*P* < 0.005); increase from 19% to 70% with age	32%; increases from 14% to 57% with age
Burton et al. 1996 (*n* = 216, ~50%f, mean age 11.7 y, UK)	Lifetime prevalence of back pain prospectively over 5 y	11.6% at 11+ y, 50.4% at 15+ y. More common in boys, especially by age 15. Positive link between sports and back pain, only for boys.	
Eminson et al. 1996 (*n* = 410f, 395m, age 11–16 y, UK)	Lifetime prevalence of back pain	9.8%	6.9%
Fairbank et al. 1984a (*n* = 219f, 227m, age 13–17 y, England)	Prevalence of back pain	26.9%	24.6%
Hertzberg 1985 (*n* = 149f, 147m, age 16 y, Norway)	Muscular tension and tenderness on palpation in any part of spinal muscles or in cervical muscles	23.7% spinal; 21.7% cervical	10% spinal; 8% cervical
Leboeuf-Yde and Kyvik 1998 (*n* = 4884, age 12–17 y, Denmark)	Prevalence of low back pain	7% at 12 y, increasing to 50% by 18 y (f) or 20 y (m)	
Nissinen et al. 1994 (*n* = 408f, 451m, in fourth-grade children, age 11.8–13.8 y, Finland, 1986–1989)	Incidence of low back pain over 1 y	18.4%	16.9%
Olesen et al. 1992 (*n* = 601f, 641m, age 11–17 y, USA)	Prevalence of back pain in past 12 mo	30%	31%
Salminen et al. 1992 (*n* = 725f, 778m, age 14 y, Finland)	Prevalence of back pain in past 12 mo	33.9% (*P* = 0.002)	27%
Taimela et al. 1997 (*n* = 594f, 577m, age 7–10, 14, or 16 y, Finland)	Prevalence of (a) low back pain that interfered with school or leisure activities in the previous year; (b) recurrent or chronic low back pain	(a) 9.4%; (b) 33% (*P* = 0.009)	(a) 10.1%; (b) 26%

pain for older girls. Campbell and McGrath (under review) found that 72% of a sample of 289 adolescent girls reported back pain in association with menstrual pain in at least three cycles. Salminen et al. (1992) found that abdominal pain (which may have included menstrual pain) occurred significantly more often with low back pain for girls ($P = 0.03$).

ABDOMINAL PAIN

Faull and Nicol (1986) examined the prevalence of abdominal pain in school-aged children, but found no gender difference in reports of abdominal pain. In samples of adolescents, girls report higher rates of abdominal pain (Apley and Naish 1957; Oster 1972; Larsson 1991), but the higher prevalence in this age group may be due to menstrual pain. Aro et al. (1987, 1989) reported no gender difference for prevalence of abdominal pain when menstrual pain was excluded. Gender-comparative epidemiological studies of abdominal pain are given in Table V.

Table V
Gender variation in prevalence of abdominal pain among children and adolescents

Reference (Sample)	Variable(s)	Outcome	
		Female	Male
Apley and Naish 1957 ($n = 472$f, 528m, age 5–15 y, England)	Prevalence of recurrent abdominal pain with at least three attacks sufficient to interfere with activities	12.3%	9.5%
Aro et al. 1987, 1989 ($n = 999$f, 1002m, mean age 15 y, Finland)	Prevalence of abdominal pain, quite often, often, or continuously, during 1 y (excluding pain due to menstruation)	2.5%	2.5%
Eminson et al. 1996 ($n = 410$f, 395m, age 11–16 y, UK)	Lifetime prevalence of abdominal pain	38.7%	19.4%
Faull and Nicol 1986 ($n = 439$, gender distribution not given, age 6 y, England)	Prevalence of abdominal pain	No gender difference	
Larsson 1991 ($n = 269$f, 270m, age 13–18 y, Sweden)	Prevalence, frequency, and intensity of abdominal pain	Girls reported more abdominal pain than boys ($P < 0.001$) and reported more severe and frequent pain	
Oster 1972 ($n = 8947$f, 9215m, age 6–19 y, Denmark)	Prevalence of abdominal pain	16.7%	12.1%

MULTIPLE PAINS OF PRIMARILY PSYCHOLOGICAL ORIGIN

Several epidemiological studies have examined prevalence rates for multiple pains in conjunction with other physical symptoms thought to be of psychological origin. This clustering of symptoms is typically referred to as psychosomatic illness, somatization, or somatization disorder. The distinction between these terms is often unclear. Psychosomatic illness is not a diagnostic term, but can be defined as a physical condition caused or maintained by psychological or emotional factors (Brown 1993). Somatization disorder is a psychiatric diagnosis associated with multiple pains and somatic symptoms that cannot be fully explained by an underlying physical condition (American Psychiatric Association 1980, 1994). In these cases, psychological factors are considered to have primary causal and contributory roles. In clinical samples, somatization disorder may be associated with depression (Smith 1992).

Epidemiological studies of multiple pains and somatic symptoms have found similar prevalence rates for girls and boys in childhood (Ernst et al. 1984; Garber et al. 1991), but higher rates for girls in adolescence (Aro et al. 1987, 1989; Offord et al. 1987; Garber et al. 1991; Larsson 1991; Eminson et al. 1996). Eminson et al. (1996) found that the number of symptoms did not vary with age for boys but increased with age for girls. The higher prevalence of somatization disorder for females continues into adulthood (Morrison 1990).

The difficulty with this classification of pain is that the diagnosis relies on the exclusion of organic pathology rather than on positive evidence from studying psychological precursors and consequences (McGrath and Unruh 1987). Psychological difficulties may be the result rather than the cause of multiple pains and somatic symptoms (Merskey 1988).

CHRONIC PAIN PROBLEMS AND PAIN DUE TO DISEASE

Fortunately, children are less likely than adults to develop many serious acute or chronic health problems that are commonly associated with pain. The most common childhood disease that is accompanied by pain is juvenile chronic arthritis (JCA). In a survey of 400,600 children attending pediatric rheumatology clinics, Gäre et al. (1987) reported that girls predominated over boys in a ratio of 3:2 among children with JCA, with a ratio of 61:36 for the 0–4 age group, and 89:57 for children with mono- and pauciarticular JCA. Systemic disease occurred primarily in boys, and juvenile ankylosing spondylitis only occurred in boys. Approximately 25% of children with JCA have moderate to severe pain (Schanberg et al. 1997). However, it is not known whether gender influences the experience of pain in JCA. Hagglund et al. (1995) did not find any significant gender difference in pain intensity due to juvenile rheumatoid arthritis.

Chronic pain problems such as complex regional pain syndrome, type I (CRPS-I, also known as reflex sympathetic dystrophy) and fibromyalgia occur in childhood and adolescence, and as in the adult population, these problems are more prevalent among girls. Berde (1998) has reported that CRPS-I is five times more common in girls than in boys. It is rare among children less than 8 years of age, but increases markedly just before puberty. Many of these children are dancers, gymnasts, or competitive athletes (Berde 1998); however, such children may also be more likely to seek treatment. Buskila et al. (1993) reported that 6.2% of a sample of healthy schoolchildren, aged 9–15 years, had fibromyalgia. The difference between girls (8.8%) and boys (3.9%) was borderline significant. Although some researchers (e.g., Rollman 1998) argue that psychological factors such as hypervigilance play a role in the occurrence of fibromyalgia, there is ample evidence of biological mechanisms, at least in adulthood (Boissevain and McCain 1991; Russell et al. 1994; Bradley et al. 1996).

Some children experience pain associated with sickle cell disease (see Chapter 6). Shapiro et al. (1995), in a prospective diary study of 7 girls and 11 boys aged 8–17 years, found that pain was reported on 30% of days. Girls reported more pain than boys. Increasing age was also associated with the length of pain episodes. More severe pain was associated with school absences.

GENDER-SPECIFIC PAIN

Anatomical and hormonal differences leave girls vulnerable to the recurrent pain of menstruation. Epidemiological surveys of menstrual pain in adolescence are summarized in Table VI. Female adolescents typically begin menstruation around 10–15 years of age (Linkie 1982). Menstruation may be associated with cramp-like pain in the pelvic region and other discomforting symptoms (e.g., backache, nausea, headache, irritability; Fuchs 1982). Pain due to ovulation and breast tenderness may precede menstrual pain. In an epidemiological study of physical symptoms in adolescents, Eminson et al. (1996) reported that girls who had started to menstruate reported significantly more lifetime prevalence of physical symptoms than girls who had not yet experienced menarche.

Menstrual cramps typically occur over a 12–48-hour period with the onset of menstruation (Hoffman 1988). Primary dysmenorrhea is characterized

Table VI

Menstrual pain: prevalence, health care utilization, medication use, and disability among adolescent women

Reference (Sample)	Prevalence	Health Care Utilization	Medication Use	Disability
Andersch and Milsom 1982 (n = 596f, age 19 y, Sweden)	72.4% experienced painful menstruation; 223 women reported moderate to severe pain on a 10-point VAS.	22% had consulted a physician for dysmenorrhea and a further 23.9% wanted medical attention for dysmenorrhea.	38.2% regularly used analgesics or antispas-modics; 15.4% had reported poor effect from analgesics.	43.9% absent from school or work half day to full day; 7.5% absent for 2 d. Inability to work correlated with severity of menstrual pain.
Campbell and McGrath 1997 (n = 289f, age 14–21 y, Canada)	42% reported moderate pain over past three cycles; 5% had severe pain. Severity of pain increased with gynecological age.	—	70% used OTC medication; 57% used medication less frequently than recom-mended.	59% mildly, 36% moderately, 5% severely disabled by menstrual pain. Symptom severity associated with disability ($P < 0.001$).
Golub et al. 1958 (n = 16,183f, high school students, USA)	Prevalence of frequent dysmenorrhea ranged from 13.5% to 55.9%.	—	—	—
Klein and Litt 1981 (n = 1611f, age 12–17 y, Center of Health Statistics, USA)	59.7% reported menstrual pain; of this group 14% had severe, 37% moderate, and 49% mild pain. Prevalence increased with age.	14.5% with dysmenorrhea had ever sought out health care, including only 29% with severe dysmenorrhea. 30% of parents were unaware of their daughter's dysmenorrhea.	—	17% missed school because of mild cramps; 50% missed school because of severe cramps.

Study	Prevalence	Medication use	Absenteeism	Impact on daily activities
Pazy et al. 1989 (n = 75f, age 17 y, Israel)	60% reported moderate or severe menstrual cramps. 27% reported moderately to severely painful breasts in the premenstrual phase.		—	<25% of the sample (exact figures not specified) reported avoidance of social activities and lower school or work performances due to menstrual pain.
Shye and Jaffe 1991 (n = 545f, age 16–21 y, Israel)	70% had experienced menstrual pain some time in the past, but 41% had no pain in previous three cycles.		—	25% reported strong/very strong pain sufficient to discontinue work or school activities and require rest.
Teperi and Rimpela 1989 (n = 3370f, age 12–18 y, Finland)	48% of 12-year-olds and 79% of 18-year-olds reported menstrual pain	Correlated with pain severity and increasing chronological age. 18–21% of 16- and 18-year-olds used medication.	—	Absenteeism increased with age. 4–5% of 16-and 18-year-olds had often missed school due to menstrual pain in the previous 6 mo.
Widholm 1979 (Sample 1: n = 5458f, age 10–20 y)	38.5% occasionally had menstrual pain; 13% invariably had pain.		—	—
(Sample 2: n = 331f, age 13–20 y, Finland)	Prevalence range: 36–56.5%.	Ranged from 3.25% to 27%, associated with increasing age.	5–20.6%, associated with increasing age	2.7% frequently absent from school; 20.7% sometimes absent. Absenteeism increased with age.

Abbreviations: OTC = over-the-counter drugs; VAS = visual analogue scale.

as moderate to severe pain without organic pathology. Secondary dysmenorrhea is pelvic pain associated with an organic abnormality. Primary dysmenorrhea is more prevalent and tends to develop early in the post-menarche period, whereas secondary dysmenorrhea may occur after many years of pain-free menstruation (Fuchs 1982; Vargyas 1988). In addition to cramping pain, many women and adolescents experience other secondary physical and psychological symptoms such as headaches, irritability, backaches, and depressed mood (Scambler and Scambler 1985; Dicke 1988; Abidoye and Agbabiaka 1994), as well as nausea, vomiting, and diarrhea (Campbell and McGrath, under review). Decreased uterine blood flow, myometrial hyperactivity, and fluctuating levels of estrogen, progesterone, arginine vasopressin, and especially prostaglandins are implicated in primary dysmenorrhea (Dicke 1988), although the mechanisms are not well understood.

Menstrual pain or discomfort is fairly common among adolescents. The prevalence of menstrual pain or discomfort can range from 36% to 93% of post-menarche adolescent girls, depending on the age of the sample and the diagnostic criteria used (Widholm 1979; Klein and Litt 1981; Andersch and Milsom 1982; Teperi and Rimpela 1989; Shye and Jaffe 1991; Campbell and McGrath 1997). Older adolescents have a higher prevalence of menstrual discomfort than do younger teenage girls (Widholm 1979; Klein and Litt 1981; Teperi and Rimpela 1989). About half the adolescents who report menstrual pain or discomfort indicate that it is mild in severity (Klein and Litt 1981; Campbell and McGrath 1997), while 5–16% report severe pain (Klein and Litt 1981; Teperi and Rimpela 1989; Campbell and McGrath 1997). Further, the severity of dysmenorrhea increases with time since menarche (Andersch and Milsom 1982).

When pain and other symptoms associated with menstruation are mild and do not interfere with an adolescent's daily activities, they are typically viewed as a normal part of the menstrual process (Hoffman 1988). However, when these symptoms are moderate to severe and begin to limit daily activities, they should no longer be viewed as a normal element of the menstrual cycle.

PAIN DUE TO ABUSE

Girls and boys may also experience recurrent pain due to physical or sexual abuse. The consequences of abuse in childhood on subsequent pain experience are not well understood. Sexual abuse of girls has been associated with the development of chronic pelvic pain in adulthood (Walker et al. 1988; Toomey et al. 1993), but boys may also be at risk for future pain problems.

RELATIONSHIP OF STRESS AND DEPRESSION WITH PAIN

Stress and depression may be more closely associated with pain in girls than in boys. Headache and abdominal pain have been associated with depression in adolescent girls, whereas only headache was related to depression in boys (Larsson 1991). As the number of symptoms increases, the gender difference may disappear. For example, Garber et al. (1991) reported that four or more somatic symptoms were significantly associated with depression in both girls and boys in a sample of adolescents. Such studies typically do not inquire about menstrual pain, which may be associated with headache, abdominal pain, back pain, and depression. Campbell and McGrath (under review) found that 69% of adolescent girls in a community sample who experienced mild to moderately severe menstrual pain reported feeling depressed as one of their menstrual symptoms.

DISABILITY DUE TO PAIN

In health research, disability in childhood most often refers to limitations in activities or school absences. Gender variations in disability due to pain are summarized in Table VII. Higher rates of school absence due to pain for girls were reported by Bille (1962, 1981), Fairbank et al. (1984a), and Sparks (1978), but not by Lee et al. (1985). Salminen et al. (1992) found that girls reported significantly more limitations in their activities of daily living because of back pain. Mikkelsson et al. (1997) did not report any gender difference in disability or in school absence due to musculoskeletal pain.

Disability rates cannot be adequately understood without consideration of pain severity, duration, or frequency of occurrence. In several adult epidemiological studies, higher disability rates have been associated with greater pain severity and increased pain frequency (Philips 1977; Von Korff et al. 1990; Hasvold and Johnsen 1993). Mikkelsson et al. (1997) found that disability and school absence were most common among children who reported widespread pain and who experienced more frequent pain. The combined effect of possible headache, back pain, and musculoskeletal pain in association with menstrual pain for girls may also contribute to higher disability rates when samples include girls with a history of more severe menstrual pain.

DISABILITY DUE TO MENSTRUAL PAIN

Primary dysmenorrhea interferes significantly with the normal routine and activities of about 15–25% of adolescent girls (Holmlund 1990; Shye and Jaffe 1991) (see Table VI). According to Abidoye and Agbabiaka (1994),

Table VII
Gender variation in disability due to pain among children and adolescents

Reference (Sample)	Disability Measure	Outcome	
		Female	Male
1) Headache			
Attansio and Andrasik 1987 (*n* = 420f, 359m, mean age 18.6 y)	Restriction of daily activities	46.7%	35.9%
	Restriction of daily activities by at least half a day	14%	8%
Bille 1962, 1981 (*n* = 470f, 295m, age 7–15 y)	Mean no. school absences of ≤1 d:		
	with migraine	3.95	3.56
	with headache	3.15	3.35
	with no or infrequent headache	2.60	2.78
	Mean no. school absences of >1 d:		
	with migraine	1.88	1.25
	with headache	1.79	0.95
	with no or infrequent headache	1.03	1.13
	Total school absence due to migrainous vs. nonmigrainous headache	Girls had more absences due to migraine (*P* <0.01); no significant difference for boys	
Sparks 1978 (*n* = 3242f, 12,543m, age 7–18 y)	Absences from school per year:		
	none	32	51
	1–2	26	26
	3–5	23	13
	>5	19	10
	Number of days absent per attack:		
	none	33	53
	1	56	42
	≥2	11	5
2) Back Pain			
Fairbank et al. 1984a (*n* = 219f, 227m, age 13–17 y)	Time off school	15%	9%
Olsen et al. 1992 (*n* = 601f, 641m, age 11–17 y)	School absence; restriction from playing sports	No gender difference	
Salminen et al. 1992 (*n* = 725f, 778m, age 14 y)	Limitation in sitting, standing, participation in sports, rising from bed, sleep, making bed, putting on socks, during past year	Girls had more limitations in activities (*P* < 0.001).	

Table VII
Continued

		Outcome	
Reference (Sample)	Disability Measure	Female	Male
3) Musculoskeletal Pain			
Fairbank et al. 1984b (n = 219f, 227m, age 13–17 y)	Stopped playing games	16%	21%
Mikkelsson et al. 1997 (Sample 1: n = 444f, 423m, mean age 9.8 y)	Subjective Disability Index	No gender difference	
(Sample 2: 450f, 439m, mean age 11.8 y)	Criteria of Mikkelsson et al. (1996), score 0–5; school absence due to pain	No gender difference	

almost 40% of their 16–35-year-old sample of 180 female Nigerian students reported menstrual discomfort that limited their abilities because of interference with learning and thinking abilities. Notably, more than half (51–54%) of the adolescent girls who experience menstrual pain or discomfort are absent from school or work as a result (Alvin and Litt 1982; Andersch and Milsom 1982; Teperi and Rimpela 1989; Campbell and McGrath 1997). More severe menstrual pain is associated with increased disability (Campbell and McGrath 1997).

GENDER VARIATIONS IN MEDICATION USE

Understanding gender variations in medication use for pain in childhood is complicated by parental responsibility for their children's health care. Parents may not provide adequate medication for their children's pain, even for postsurgical pain, and even when the parent believes the child is in pain and has been given specific instructions about pain management (Finley et al. 1996; Chambers et al. 1997). It is not known whether provision of pain medication by a parent is influenced by the child's gender. Moreover, the mothers were the caregivers in these studies of parental behavior; it is unknown whether fathers would make similar decisions.

Researchers examining pain due to dental procedures have reported that girls used significantly more medication for pain; in both studies girls also reported more pain (Acs and Drazner 1992; Scheuer et al. 1996). Jones and

Chan (1992) found that girls did not use more medication to relieve pain following a tooth extraction, but there was no difference in reported pain severity.

In adolescence, girls and boys assume more responsibility for their use of medication. Bédard et al. (1997) found that medication use for pain in young adolescents (grades seven to nine) was related to catastrophizing in response to pain. High catastrophizers took more medication for pain than low catastrophizers for all types of pain. Girls were more likely than boys to catastrophize in response to pain.

Although many adolescent girls experience substantial menstrual pain, they do not appear to use medication in a way that will provide sufficient pain relief (see Table VI). NSAIDs such as ibuprofen and naproxen sodium relieve 60–100% of dysmenorrhea, and they are significantly more effective than a placebo (Chan et al. 1979; Henzel et al. 1980; Morrison et al. 1980; Jay et al. 1986). They are also associated with improvements in participation in daily activities (Henzel et al. 1980; Morrison et al. 1980). In a recent survey of over-the-counter (OTC) medication use, approximately 70% of a nonclinical sample of adolescents reported using OTC medications to manage their menstrual discomfort; OTC users tended to report greater symptom severity and disability (Campbell and McGrath 1997). However, the authors also found that although 75% of these teens had taken the recommended single dose of OTCs as indicated on the package label (i.e., 1–2 pills), 57% were taking tablets less often than the package label indicated. Only 17% of these teens had used a prescription medication to manage menstrual discomfort.

HEALTH CARE UTILIZATION

Health care utilization has been examined in various epidemiological studies addressing pain prevalence (summarized in Table VIII). As with medication use, use of health services by children and adolescents is influenced by the attitudes and expectations of parents and other caregivers. Some gender differences in health care use for pain may begin in childhood. Fifty percent of visits to school health services are made by only 8–12% of schoolchildren (Lewis and Lewis 1982). These children are often girls, first-born children, and children from a lower socioeconomic class. In a prospective record of camp infirmary visits by children and adolescents aged 8–18 years, significantly more visits were made by girls, usually for injury resulting from musculoskeletal or superficial skin trauma (Rudolf et al. 1992). Examination of infirmary records did not reveal any gender biases in the

Table VIII
Gender variation in health care utilization for pain among children and adolescents

Reference (Sample)	Variable(s)	Outcome	
		Female	Male
1) Headache and Migraine			
Celentano et al. 1990 (n = 3851f, 2496m, age 12–29 y)	Health care utilization in previous 12 mo for headache/migraine	15% ($P < 0.001$) Difference persisted after adjustment for other factors	6.5%
Linet et al. 1989 (n = 5055f, 4394m, age 12–29 y)	Health care utilization in previous 12 mo for headache/migraine	15%	6.5%
Balagué et al. 1988 (n = 875f, 840m, age 7–17 y)	Health care utilization for headache/migraine	No gender difference; frequency of pain and disability associated with health care utilization ($P < 0.0001$)	
2) Back Pain			
Cypress 1983 (n = 98,335 patient records, all ages, National Ambulatory Medical Care Surveys)	Annual rate of back pain per 1000 population	75 visits Rate higher for women at <15 y and 65+ y	77 visits
Fairbank et al. 1984a (n = 219f, 227m, age 13–17 y)	Health care utilization for back pain	31%	13%
Hertzberg 1985 (n = 152f, 150m, age 16 y)	One or more consultations in 9–12-y follow-up period for back pain	41%	16%
	One or more consultations in 9–12-y follow-up period.	28%	33%
Olsen et al. 1992 (n = 601f, 641m, age 11–17 y)	Lifetime health care utilization for back pain.	8% (95% CI = 7.4–8.7)	6.7%
3) Musculoskeletal Pain			
Fairbank et al. 1984b (n = 219f, 227m, age 13–17 y)	Health care utilization (physician)	22%	37%
Eminson et al. 1996 (n = 410f, 395m, age 11–16 y)	Health care utilization (doctor visit) for pain over past 6 or 12 mo	No gender difference on any variable	
Rudolf et al. 1992 (n = 211f, 187m, age 8–18 y, campers)	Hospital visits	Girls made more visits than boys ($P < 0.005$); musculoskeletal or skin trauma most common problem	

provision of symptomatic treatment, encouragement to return to the infirmary, or admission to the infirmary. However, in an epidemiological study of 11–16-year-olds, Eminson et al. (1996) found no gender differences in self-reported health care use in the previous 6 or 12 months.

Health care utilization practices for some pain problems may be influenced, in part, by embarrassment about certain aspects of the pain. Klein and Litt (1981) found that only 14.5% of adolescent girls seek medical assistance for menstrual pain, including only 29% of girls with severe dysmenorrhea. Teperi and Rimpela (1989) found that 31% of girls with severe pain did not even use any medication for pain relief. Klein and Litt (1981) reported that only 30% of these girls even told their mothers about their menstrual pain.

In a community study of pain over a 2-week period, Unruh et al. (1999) found that the single most important influence on seeking health care was the suggestion by someone else that one should. It may be that the higher rates of health care utilization of health services by women in adulthood is shaped in part by early life experiences that may make it more acceptable for girls and later for women to seek help for pain.

COPING WITH PAIN

Several studies have found that girls tend to show more emotional distress in response to pain as one of their coping strategies. In an observational study of everyday pain incidents on a playground among preschoolers, Fearon et al. (1996) found no gender differences in the severity or frequency of pain. However, girls were more likely to respond to pain with crying, screaming, or anger. In a replication of this study, von Baeyer et al. (1998) reported no significant differences in these behaviors, with the exception that boys displayed significantly more anger. Some unreliability in their measure of anger may have affected this outcome. In both studies, girls displayed more facial expressions of distress in response to pain, but the difference was significant only in Fearon et al. (1996).

Among school-aged children, girls are more likely to report that they cry, moan, or seek comfort when they have pain, while boys report more behavioral and cognitive distraction and more problem-solving than girls (Reid et al. 1998). In contrast, Brown et al. (1986) found no gender differences in school-aged children's reported coping strategies or in tendencies to focus on or exaggerate pain. However, the tendency for girls to exhibit more anxiety and more behavioral distress (particularly crying) is also reflected in several studies of pain during health procedures (LeBaron and Zeltzer 1984; Fowler-Kerry and Lander 1991; Bournaki 1997; Tesler et al. 1998) (see Table VII). In the adult literature, women report more emotion-focused coping than men (Reid et al. 1998), suggesting that over time girls are socialized to have more self-control over emotional expressions of pain such as crying.

There is also evidence in adult pain research that women use more catastrophizing than men (Sullivan et al. 1999), although this gender difference does not always occur (Unruh et al. 1999). Catastrophizing reflects emotive thinking that is concerned with ruminating, magnifying or exaggerating pain, and feeling helpless about pain (Sullivan et al. 1995). Catastrophizing is generally argued to be predictive of pain disability and poor coping (Turner and Clancy 1986; Bennett-Branson and Craig 1993). Nevertheless, Sullivan et al. (1999) maintain that catastrophizing may be adaptive for women and may be important in obtaining timely assistance and support for the management of pain. Catastrophizing may be related to how women and men learn to appraise pain, learning that may have origins in early life experiences (Unruh and Ritchie 1998).

Catastrophizing has had limited attention in pediatric pain research. Reid et al. (1998) found no gender difference in catastrophizing when children or adolescents were asked about the way they coped with pain in the previous 6 months. However, Bédard et al. (1997) found that girls had higher catastrophizing scores and that catastrophizing increased with age (grade seven to nine). These authors suggested that catastrophizing may have been higher for girls because they were experiencing more pain. High catastrophizers reported more severe and frequent headaches and more severe abdominal, ear and throat, muscle, joint, back, and menstrual pain than did low catastrophizers. Girls may develop more catastrophizing responses as the frequency and severity of pain increase with the onset of puberty.

The most consistent gender difference related to coping in adulthood is the more frequent use of social support and the greater number of coping strategies for any pain event (Unruh 1997). As girls enter puberty, they become increasingly more likely to experience pain, and may begin to develop a broader repertoire of coping strategies to manage pain promptly and minimize disability. Much is still to be understood about possible gender variations in coping with pain particularly in the transition from childhood to adolescence. It may be helpful to determine how coping with menstrual pain may differ from coping with other pain experiences in girls.

WHAT FACTORS MAY HAVE A BEARING ON GIRLS' AND BOYS' EXPERIENCE OF RECURRENT OR CHRONIC PAIN?

BIOLOGY

Until very recently, there was little research on gender variation in the biological mechanisms that may influence pain experience. However, gender differences in brain chemistry, metabolism, physical structures, and hormones influence the biological mechanisms of pain transmission, pain sensitivity, and pain perception (Unruh 1996). Ovarian steroids have numerous effects on the brain, beginning in utero and continuing through the aging process (McEwen 1998). These steroids not only affect reproductive function but also have a pervasive effect throughout the brain on catecholaminergic neurons, serotonergic pathways, and the basal forebrain cholinergic system (McEwen 1998). In various areas of the brain, neurons involved in pain modulation overlap with sex steroid receptors (Polleri 1992). Peripheral and central mechanisms of nociception may have some gender variation affecting the transmission of cutaneous, deep, and visceral pain as well as neuropathic pain.

Biological factors are clearly implicated in the greater risk for headache and migraine in girls and women, and may also have a bearing on their greater risk to develop CRPS-I and fibromyalgia.

In animals, biological effects on gender variation in pain behavior can be demonstrated early in life (Anand 1998), but there are no apparent consistent differences in humans (Breedlove 1998). The effect of biological factors on infants and children may be masked by other factors, or may have subtle effects that only become significant with the onset of puberty.

TEMPERAMENT

Temperament of children may also have some bearing on pain sensitivity and pain response. There is preliminary evidence that the child's temperament is related to pain behavior, and also may mediate the relationship between parental behavior and the child's pain behavior (Sweet 1998; Sweet et al. 1999). However, Sweet et al. (1999) found that while the child's temperament (difficult) and maternal behavior predicted the child's pain behavior during immunization at 6 months, by the age of 18 months maternal sensitivity was a more important predictor than the child's temperament. In other words, the child's socialization experience in response to the sensitivity of the mother may have influenced his or her ability to regulate emotional response to the pain (Sweet et al. 1999).

Unfortunately, research concerned with temperament and pain has given very little attention to gender as a possible mediating influence. Temperament and socialization, particularly for males, may have an important influence on pain response. For example, Séguin et al. (1996) found that boys who were assessed at ages 6, 10, 11, and 12 years and showed stable aggressiveness (as measured via the Social Behaviour Questionnaire, Tremblay et al. 1991), were also the least pain sensitive when compared to boys who were nonaggressive or exhibited unstable aggressiveness. There are several possible explanations for this outcome. The pairing of an aggressive temperament with decreased pain sensitivity in boys may have biological underpinnings. In addition, boys with aggressive temperaments may also have a vested interest in appearing tough and may receive social reinforcement for decreased pain sensitivity.

DIFFERENCES IN PAIN THRESHOLD, PAIN TOLERANCE, AND PAIN RATINGS

Pain threshold and pain tolerance are typically examined in experimental research. In most adult experimental pain research in which significant gender differences are reported, women are found to have lower pain threshold and tolerance, and higher pain ratings (Fillingim and Maixner 1995; Riley et al. 1998).

Ethical issues limit the use of experimental pain in pediatric pain research. The existing studies providing gender-related information are summarized in Table IX. There are two reported studies of electric shock, in both cases showing higher pain thresholds for male newborns (significant difference in only one study; Lipsitt and Levy 1959). Pain threshold declined over the first 4 days of life for female and male infants, suggesting increasing pain sensitivity either with maturity or with repeated exposure.

Miller et al. (1994) and Zeltzer et al. (1989) used cold water as the pain stimulus in samples of school-aged children. Miller et al. (1994) reported more pain response from girls, but the girls were significantly younger than the boys in this sample. Hence the gender difference may reflect developmental rather than gender difference. Zeltzer et al. (1989) found that girls gave significantly higher pain ratings and withdrew their arm sooner from the cold water than boys, but these differences disappeared when the water temperature was reduced from 15°C to 12°C.

Pressure has also been used in a few studies. Buskila et al. (1993) and Buchanan and Midgely (1987) reported significant gender differences in pain threshold (girls had lower thresholds). Walco and Dampier (1990) did not find a gender difference, but the comparison groups of healthy children and

Table IX

Gender-comparative experimental pediatric pain research

Reference (Sample)	Main Variables and Measures	Outcome	Methodological Notes
1) Electric Shock Pain Stimulus			
Lipsitt and Levy 1959: Study 1 ($n = 18$f, 18m neonates) Study 2 ($n = 20$f, 20m neonates)	Pain threshold, measured by extension of big toe or all toes and possible withdrawal of entire leg.	Boys had a higher pain threshold ($P < 0.05$); threshold for boys and girls decreased over the four days ($P < 0.01$). Pain threshold was higher for boys on first three days (n.s.) Pain threshold declined over the four days for boys and girls.	Test on four consecutive days beginning with first day of life on back calf of left leg. First shock administered at 5 V and increased at 5-V increments until point of reaction.
2) Cold Pain Stimulus			
Zeltzer et al. 1989. Study 1 ($n = 29$ children, age 6–12 y); Study 2 ($n = 37$ children, age 6–12 y) (29 of these children participated in session 2)	Pain rating on 11-point scale (1 = no bother, 10 = bother enough to withdraw arm). Premature arm withdrawal rate before 40 s. Effect of water temperature: two sessions separated by 3 mo at 15°C and 12°C. Effect of hypnosis on pain rating; subjects randomly assigned to hypnosis or control in both sessions.	Girls had higher pain ratings at 15°C ($P < 0.002$), but difference disappeared at 12°C. Difference in premature withdrawal rate for girls at 15°C but not 12°C for all conditions ($P < 0.05$). Males increased premature withdrawal with decrease in temperature ($P < 0.05$). Hypnosis group had lower ratings of discomfort only at 12°C. No gender effect.	Water maintained at 15°C or 12°C for max. 40 s. Experimenter gender not given. "Bother" may differ from pain, but may have been suitable for pediatric sample. Two baseline trials and two trials using hypnosis. Younger children withdrew arm significantly earlier than did older children.
Miller et al. 1994 ($n = 21$f, 23m, age 8–11 y, from a private school)	Threshold: raised hand when hurt first experienced. Tolerance: when subject cannot tolerate holding arm in water. Intensity of feeling during immersion. VAS rating of strength of feeling in the hand.	Female gender appeared to be related to responses on the cold pressor test, but girls were younger than boys in this sample ($P = 0.04$). No other information related to gender.	Forearm warmed at 37°C. Cold water bath maintained at 10°C.

3) Pressure or Ischemia Pain Stimulus

Study	Methods	Results	Comments
Bell and Costello 1964 (n = 34f, 40m, age 74 and 87 h)	Pain threshold: sum of movement of eyes, mouth, face, head, and hands.	Thresholds at both time intervals were correlated for all infants ($P <$ 0.01). No gender difference.	Middle of heel stimulated using 20 nylon monofilaments varying in diameter. Interobserver agreement = 0.92.
Buchanan and Midgely 1987 (high school students, age 17–19 y)			No significant difference in intra-observer error over 10 points in 18 subjects. Significant interobserver error only at one site ($P < 0.05$). Experimenter gender not given.
Study 1 (n = 26m, 26f)	Pain threshold (methods not described).	Females had lower pain threshold than did males ($P < 0.05$ at all five sites tested).	Multiple comparisons without control of alpha value.
Study 2 (n = 20m, 20f)	Pain threshold (methods not described).	No significant differences within gender for body site.	
Study 3 (n = 20m, 20f)	Effects of stress using two procedures: (1) Prior to test, subject told that second stimulus would be very painful; a confederate acted as if in extreme pain. (2) Subjects were blindfolded for the trial.	Decrease in pain threshold for males ($P < 0.05$) and females ($P < 0.05$) in response to stress.	
Walco et al. 1990 (n = 72m, 68f, age 5–15 y; n = 35 with sickle cell disease, 35 with asthma, 35 healthy; black, Asian, Caucasian, and Hispanic)	Pain threshold: child instructed to state when he or she felt hurt, pain, or uncomfortable. Clinical pain: VAS for present, worst, and average pain experience (rated only by adolescents). Effect of ethnicity.	No gender difference for pain threshold, but significant difference in pain threshold between children with clinical pain and healthy children. Pain thresholds were related to ethnicity of child, but no gender comparisons within ethnic group.	Experimenter gender not given. "Hurt," "pain," and "uncomfortable" may not be equivalent terms.
Buskila et al. 1993 (n = 179m, 159f, age 9–15 y)	Pain threshold: subjects asked to say when sensation is definitely not pressure but pain.	Pain threshold lower in girls than boys at tender points ($P < 0.001$) and control sites ($P < 0.001$).	Experimenter gender not given.

children with sickle cell disease or asthma may have obscured gender effects.

The existing experimental pediatric pain research is limited. Gender differences may not be common, but when they occur they may be similar to observed differences in the adult experimental pain research; that is, girls report lower pain thresholds and higher pain ratings than do boys. The study by Zeltzer et al. (1989) suggests that if the pain severity of the experimental stimulus increases, then gender differences in pain response among children may disappear.

It is difficult to study pain threshold or tolerance outside the experimental context. However, pain intensity can be examined for common health procedures such as heel lances, venipunctures, immunizations, and dental procedures. Grunau and Craig (1987) found that boys cried sooner and had more cry cycles than did girls in response to heel lances, but Owens and Todt (1984) found no gender difference for the same procedure. Although there is some evidence that girls anticipate having more pain from venipunctures (e.g., Fowler-Kerry and Lander 1991), no consistent gender differences have emerged in ratings of pain intensity for venipunctures, immunizations, or bone marrow aspirations (LeBaron and Zeltzer 1984; Lander et al. 1989; Fowler-Kerry and Lander 1991; Bournaki 1997). For the most part, there are also no gender differences in ratings of pain intensity for dental procedures (Jones 1984; Jones and Chan 1992), with the exception of invasive restorative procedures (Acs and Drazner 1992), or orthodontic treatment and placement of fixed dental appliances (Scheuer et al. 1996). Thus far, research about pain intensity in a nonexperimental context does not consistently demonstrate gender differences in ratings of pain intensity for children (except possibly for major dental procedures).

EARLY EXPERIENCES OF PAIN

Very little attention has been given to the possibility that childhood experiences of pain may affect gender variation in sensitivity and response to experiences of recurrent or chronic pain later in life. Such experiences may affect the development of physiological pain mechanisms and may shape learning about pain that influences later pain anxiety and coping behavior.

A common early pain experience for many boys in North America and some other societies is circumcision, usually in infancy, but in some societies in later childhood. It is typically performed without anesthesia or analgesia (Schoen and Fischell 1991). There is no firm evidence that neonatal circumcision influences gender differences in neonatal behavior (e.g., sleep, aggressiveness, crying, response to stimuli) (Brackbill and Schroder 1980). However, there is some emerging evidence from a post hoc analysis of a

randomized controlled trial and a prospective study that this early experience of pain may affect subsequent pain experiences of male infants during
routine vaccination given at 4–6 months (Taddio et al. 1995, 1997) (see
Chapter 4). Circumcised infants had significantly more pain as rated by a
blinded observer and pediatrician; they also had higher behavioral pain
scores and cried longer. Early experiences of unrelieved pain during circumcision may have long-lasting effects on pain perception and pain response for boys.

It is estimated that 4–5 million female infants and girls are annually
subjected to the cultural or religious practice of female genital mutilation,
also known as female circumcision (American Academy of Pediatrics 1998).
The procedure is performed primarily without anesthesia by a lay person or
midwife in African countries and in some parts of the Middle East and Asia,
but may also be requested from physicians by immigrants for their daugh-
ters (Dorkenoo 1996; American Academy of Pediatrics 1998; Ortiz 1998).
Female genital mutilation is associated with a variety of acute and chronic
complications that may involve considerable acute, recurrent, and chronic
pain (American Academy of Pediatrics 1998). Various organizations including the World Health Organization, the International Federation of Gyne-
cologists and Obstetrics, the American Academy of Pediatrics, and the College of Physicians and Surgeons of Ontario, Canada, caution their members
against performing any form of female genital mutilation (American Academy of Pediatrics 1998). Criminal laws prohibiting this practice have been
passed in Sweden, Norway, Australia, the United Kingdom, and the United
States (Key 1997; American Academy of Pediatrics 1998).

COGNITIVE DEVELOPMENT

Children's cognitive development influences their understanding of their
own and others' pain, the correlates of pain, and the way in which pain is
best managed and expressed. We have limited understanding of the way in
which gender might affect cognitive development and influence the child's
pain experience.

When preschoolers are exposed to displays of sadness, anger, or pain
by a familiar female experimenter, no gender differences are observed in
their responsive prosocial behaviors toward the experimenter (Denham et al.
1995). Children provide more prosocial responses when the experimenter
labels the emotion. Children are also more positively responsive to displays
of anger by an adult experimenter and least prosocial to pain. The children's
responses to displays of pain tend to be egocentric, reflecting their concern
that they themselves might also have pain. Their reaction demonstrates an

inability to know how to respond to the pain of someone else, at least an adult (e.g., by comforting or helping).

As children enter the school-age years, their cognitive understanding of pain continues to demonstrate few gender differences (Gaffney 1993). However, girls begin to use more affect-laden words to describe their pain and what they do when they have pain (Savedra et al. 1982), to show more emotional expression of pain, and to report more unpleasantness associated with pain such as needle pain (Goodenough et al. 1999). This tendency is a recurrent theme in research about the influence of family and peers on pain behavior. Girls demonstrate more behavioral distress toward pain from venipunctures, immunizations, and bone marrow aspirations (Jay et al. 1983; Fowler-Kerry and Lander 1991; Schechter et al. 1991; Fowler-Kerry and Day 1993), and more anxiety about dental procedures (Wright et al. 1980; Liddell and Murray 1989), although as discussed above, actual pain intensity ratings show no consistent differences.

THE FAMILY

Families may influence children's experiences of pain through family members' own experiences of pain and use of pain coping strategies, as well as caregiving behaviors that differentially support or repress pain responses. Much of this socialization process may be influenced by the gender of the parent and of the child.

Craig (1978) proposed that children learn about pain, in part, by observing the behavior of significant role models when they are in pain. Considerable research has sought to determine whether a family history of pain is more common among patients with chronic pain, with the underlying assumption that such patients may have a learned response to pain acquired in childhood and adolescence (e.g., Hasvold and Johnsen 1993). Further, since women are more likely to seek health care for pain (Unruh 1996; Unruh et al. 1999), and since girls are more responsive to social influences, family pain experiences may also contribute to gender differences in childhood and adult pain experiences. Studies have found increased family reports of pain among patients with chronic pain (Violin and Giurgea 1984; Ehde et al. 1991), and more pain models in the families of women who report pain (Edwards et al. 1985; Hasvold and Johnsen 1993; Lester et al. 1994). Nevertheless, it is not at all clear that girls have more pain models than do boys, particularly when models of menstrual pain are excluded (Koutanji et al. 1998). Other research suggests that fathers' rather than mothers' somatic symptoms are more consistently associated with children's symptoms (Walker et al. 1994).

Parents and other family members may also influence children more directly by the way in which a child is socialized to think about pain and behave when in pain. Some of this socialization process will be influenced by the mother's or father's own convictions about how a male or female should respond to and deal with pain. Although there is little research about gender-loaded personal attitudes about pain and their impact on the socialization of children, evidence suggests that expectations about pain are more central to our stereotypical ideas about how males ought to behave, than how we expect women to act. In particular, there is experimental, epidemiological, qualitative, and anecdotal evidence that men and boys believe they should be tough in the face of pain, particularly in the presence of other men (Otto and Dougher 1985; Levine and De Simone 1991; Schechter et al. 1991; Grunau et al. 1994; Zeman and Garber 1996; Unruh et al. 1999).

In a study of pain sensitivity and temperament in toddlers, Grunau et al. (1994) found that parents of toddlers rated their boys as less sensitive than girls to the pain of bumps, cuts, or common hurts. Schechter et al. (1991) reported that fathers were more likely than mothers to believe that comforting a child in pain encouraged the child to cry and that boys handled pain better than girls.

Several studies of school-aged children have been concerned with emotional expressions of pain. Zeman and Garber (1996) presented school-aged children with 12 stories based on four scenarios and inquired about emotional expression of anger, sadness, and physical pain in these vignettes. Children reported that they would control their emotional expression significantly more in the presence of peers than with either their mother or father, or when alone. Girls were more likely than boys to express pain, whereas boys were more likely to regulate expressions of pain. Similar results were reported by Fuchs and Thelen (1988). Zeman and Garber (1996) found that boys and girls also reported that they would be more likely to express pain to their mother than to their father. By the fifth grade, boys and girls were significantly less likely to express pain to their fathers than were younger children. Unfortunately, the authors did not specify whether boys would be less likely than girls to express pain to their fathers. The children indicated that they would express pain when the intensity of the pain was too great to control expression. They would also express pain if it would result in help and positive interpersonal benefit. Girls used more affective responses to all situations, and expected more positive interpersonal displays from others. Girls were more like to self-disclose, to directly seek help, and to alter emotional expressions sooner than boys and at a younger age. Girls' greater willingness to disclose pain suggests that, although like boys they take into account the reaction of the other person, girls appear to feel freer about expressing pain. The authors suggested that boys receive more negative consequences for expression of sadness or pain (Zeman and Shipman 1996). This research is consistent with Walker and Zeman's (1992) finding that girls perceive that they receive more sympathy and relief from responsibilities than boys when they are ill or have pain. These studies suggest that girls and boys may be socialized somewhat differently about expression of anger, sadness, and pain, may experience different consequences when they do so, and may learn to discriminate to whom expressions of pain are acceptable and under what conditions.

Gender variation in parents' expectations about pain and the resulting difference in caregiving can be difficult to assess. Mothers and other female caregivers may be more conscious of wanting to avoid socializing children in traditional gender-stereotyped roles. In particular, they may be much more tolerant of expressions of sadness and pain in boys than are fathers. The absence of an influence of child gender on women's caregiving for pain is demonstrated in the studies discussed previously about pain incidents on playgrounds. Fearon et al. (1996) found that preschool girls were given significantly more physical comfort than boys for pain, but when the children were matched by age and level of distress, there was no difference. Similarly, von Baeyer et al. (1998) did not report a gender difference. However, it must be noted that factors such as education, socioeconomic class, and culture may also influence women's expectations about pain and how they care for children.

Unfortunately, pain researchers have paid little attention to fathers. However, beliefs about male sensitivity and responsiveness to pain most likely influence men in their parenting, particularly of sons. Some experimental studies suggest that men, more than women, adjust their pain sensitivity in response to social cues such as the gender of the experimenter. Levine and De Simone (1991) found that when experimenters are attractive males or females, men give significantly lower pain intensity ratings to the female experimenter than the male, while experimenter gender had no significant effect on pain ratings given by the women. Otto and Dougher (1985) reported that men who rated themselves high on a measure of masculinity also had significantly higher pain thresholds. Ratings of femininity had no relationship to women's pain thresholds.

In a community survey of pain over a 2-week period, Unruh et al. (1999) found that women reported more crying, moaning, and seeking of comfort for pain than did men, but the report of these behaviors was significantly influenced by the gender of the questioner. Men did not report these behaviors to a male interviewer. This study found no gender difference in report of emotional upset due to pain. Men may be as emotionally upset about pain as women, but like boys, they are less likely to report crying or similar expressions of pain.

These studies suggest that pain expression and pain behavior for adult men may have some relationship to their perceptions of male roles. Some religious and cultural practices, particularly those concerning male circumcision, further reinforce possibly deeply entrenched views that endurance of pain may be one aspect of the gender role expected for males.

Thus far research that has examined the role of fathers has been concerned primarily with illness and misbehavior. In a vignette study, fathers expressed significantly more anger toward boys and more sympathy for pain for adolescent girls (Walker et al. 1995). Fathers' expectations of pain sensitivity and the pain response of men and the impact of these expectations on their parenting of sons should be further examined.

RESEARCH AND CLINICAL ISSUES

The current interest in sex, gender, and pain is likely to add significantly to our understanding of this area in the coming years. In the meantime, health care professionals should be attentive to the possibility of sex-role stereotyping about pain sensitivity and pain behavior and about the impact these stereotypes may have on the care provided to children and adolescents in pain. Evidence from adult pain research shows that the gender of the patient can have a negative influence on the prescription and administration of medication for pain (Unruh 1996). In the pediatric literature, more attention has been given to whether children are medicated differently than adults for painful procedures, but Beyer et al. (1983) found that boys and men were prescribed significantly more codeine following open heart surgery than girls or women, who were prescribed more acetaminophen. Gillies et al. (1999), in a study of postoperative pain in adolescents, found that boys' and girls' reactions to pain were perceived differently by health professionals. This difference may explain why more girls than boys received milder analgesics, even though girls experienced more pain. In addition, more inappropriate psychological explanations are given for women's pain problems (Unruh 1996), and the same problem may also occur for girls, with insufficient attention given to psychological factors for boys.

Gender variation in biological mechanisms does not appear to have a substantial influence on the pain experience of infants or young children, but such variation may be masked by strong social influences that encourage girls but discourage boys from emotional expression of pain. Puberty clearly alters the biological background to pain experience, particularly for headache and migraine, but possibly also for other pain problems such as musculoskeletal pains.

More research is needed to determine the short- and long-term consequences of circumcision without adequate pain management on boys. More importantly, there is growing evidence that untreated neonatal pain can have persistent effects that do not occur if analgesics are provided (Taddio 1998; see Chapter 4).

Several researchers have raised concern about the high proportion of adolescents who experience back pain. There is some evidence that risk factors for back pain may be different for females and males (Nissinen et al. 1994; Kujula et al. 1997). The role of sports and strenuous physical activity during the growth spurt needs more attention as a risk factor for back pain.

Roughly 30% of adolescent girls do not use medications to manage their menstrual discomfort. Some adolescents may not feel comfortable discussing their menstrual-related difficulties with a physician or a pharmacist in order to obtain the necessary information about effective pain management and access to prescription medications. Other adolescents may not be able to afford medications as they do not have access to health insurance. As a result, this treatment option may be unknown or out of reach to many adolescents. As well, some adolescents may choose not to take medications due to their side effects, a reluctance to take drugs, or because they do not believe the medication will help. In addition, about 9–22% of adolescents do not respond to prostaglandin-synthetase inhibitors (Andersch and Milsom 1982; Dicke 1988). Although oral contraceptives have been found to reduce menstrual pain in about 90% of treated patients by suppressing ovulation (Smith 1988), not all adolescents can tolerate them, and many may not want to take oral contraceptives, especially if they are not sexually active.

There is increasing evidence of gender differences in the physiological response of adults to pharmacological pain management (Gear et al. 1996; Miaskowski et al. 1998). Although this research is too preliminary to provide clinical guidelines, this issue must be considered in the adolescent population with the onset of puberty.

Sex-role stereotypes about pain experience should receive more research attention. We know very little about why a stoical response toward pain in males might be reinforced by men and perhaps also by women, and whether it is unique to humans or also prevalent in other species. We know little about the possible physiological or psychological benefits of crying when in pain and whether these benefits differ for females and males. Crying is typically thought to be a means of seeking help or attention, but may occur in the absence of other individuals.

Differences between girls and boys or women and men are often not as great as the differences within each gender. To understand the effect of gender, it is important also to discern why some girls and boys are atypical from others in their gender group.

In conclusion, gender variation in pain experience has had very limited attention until this decade. Most of the research is concerned with sex or gender differences in adulthood. The existing pediatric research suggests that there are few observable differences in infancy and young childhood. As children enter the school-aged years, they begin to show more difference in willingness to express pain, particularly affective responses. Socialization practices may influence boys to inhibit expressions of pain, while giving girls more freedom to express or inhibit pain responsivity.

Although reproductive hormones affect development of the central and peripheral nervous system at the beginning of life, their effects on the pain experience of infants and children may be subtle until the onset of puberty. Puberty appears to act as a catalyst to other physiological mechanisms that may place girls at greater risk for pain, particularly migraines, musculoskeletal pains, and rheumatological disorders. However, research is preliminary; we need to know more about the impact of reproductive hormones on physiological pain mechanisms at this time of life.

Many infants, children, and adolescents may experience pain that could be successfully managed with medical, psychological, and rehabilitative assistance. More research is essential on the identification of gender differences in pain prevalence, severity, and correlated factors. Without such knowledge, our attempts to understand the mechanisms maintaining and minimizing risk for pain and pain response will be difficult and incomplete.

REFERENCES

Abidoye RO, Agbabiaka BA. Incidence and management of menstrual disorders and foods implicated among Nigerian adolescents. *Int J Adoles Youth* 1994; 4:271–283.

Acs G, Drazner E. The incidence of postoperative pain and analgesic usage in children. *J Dent Child* 1992; January–February:48–52.

Alvin PE, Litt IF. Current status of the etiology and management of dysmenorrhea in adolescence. *Pediatrics* 1982; 70:516–525.

American Academy of Pediatrics, Committee on Bioethics. Female genital mutilation. *Pediatrics* 1998; 102:153–156.

American Psychiatric Association. DSM-III. *Diagnostic and Statistical Manual of Mental Disorders*. Washington, DC: American Psychiatric Association, 1980.

American Psychiatric Association. DSM-III. *Diagnostic and Statistical Manual of Mental Disorders*. Washington, DC: American Psychiatric Association, 1994.

Andersch B, Milsom I. An epidemiological study of young women with dysmenorrhea. *Am J Obstet Gynecol* 1982; 144:655–660.

Apley J, Naish N. Children with recurrent abdominal pains: a field survey of 1000 school children. *Arch Dis Child* 1957; 33:165–170.

Aro H. Life stress and psychosomatic symptoms among 14-to-16-year-old Finnish adolescents. *Psychol Med* 1987; 17:191–201.

Aro H, Paronen O, Aro S. Psychosomatic symptoms among 14–16 year old Finnish adolescents. *Soc Psychiatr* 1987; 22:171–176.

Aro H, Hänninen V, Paronen, O. Social support, life events and psychosomatic symptoms among 14–16-year-old adolescents. *Soc Sci Med* 1989; 29:1051–1056.

Attansio V, Andrasik F. Further examination of headache in a college student population. *Headache* 1987; 27:216–223.

Balagué F, Dutoit, G, Waldburger M. Low back pain in schoolchildren: an epidemiological study. *Scand J Rehab Med* 1988; 20:175–179.

Barea LM, Tannenhauser M, Rotta NT. An epidemiological study of headache among children and adolescents of southern Brazil. *Cephalalgia* 1996; 16:545–549.

Bédard GBV, Reid GJ, McGrath PJ, Chambers CT. Coping and self-medication in a community sample of junior high school students. *Pain Res Manage* 1997; 2:151–156.

Beiter M, Ingersoll G, Ganser J, Orr DP. Relationships of somatic symptoms to behavioral and emotional risk in young adolescents. *J Pediatr* 1991; 118:473–478.

Bell RQ, Costello NS. Three tests for sex differences in tactile sensitivity in the newborn. *Biol Neonate* 1964; 7:335–347.

Bennett-Branson SM, Craig KD. Postoperative pain in children: developmental and family influences on spontaneous coping strategies. *Can J Behav Sci* 1993; 25:355–383.

Berde C. Gender difference in CRPSI/RSD in children and adolescents. Paper presented at the NIH Gender and Pain Conference, April 7–8, 1998, Bethesda, MD.

Berkley KJ. Vive la différence! *Trends Neurosci* 1992; 15:331–332.

Berkley KJ. Sex and chronobiology: opportunities for a focus on the positive. *IASP Newsletter,* January/February 1993, pp 2–5.

Berkley KJ. Sex differences in pain. *Behav Brain Sci* 1997; 20:371–380.

Beyer JE, DeGood DE, Ashley LC, Russell GA. Patterns of postoperative analgesic use with adults and children following cardiac surgery. *Pain* 1983; 17:71–81.

Bille B. Migraine in schoolchildren. *Acta Pediatr Suppl* 1962; 51:1–151.

Bille B. Migraine in childhood and its prognosis. *Cephalalgia* 1981; 1:71–75.

Bille B. A 40-year follow-up of school children with migraine. *Cephalalgia* 1997; 17:488–491.

Boissevain MD, McCain GA. Toward an integrated understanding of the fibromyalgia syndrome. I. Medical and pathophysiological aspects. *Pain* 1991; 45:227–238.

Bournaki M-C. Correlates of pain-related responses to venipunctures in school-aged children. *Nurs Res* 1997; 46:147–154.

Bousser M-G, Massiou H. Migraine in the reproductive cycle. In: Olesen J, Tfelt-Hansen P, Welch KMA (Eds). *The Headaches.* New York: Raven Press, 1993, pp 413–419.

Brackbill Y, Schroder K. Circumcision, gender difference, and neonatal behavior: an update. *Dev Psychobiol* 1980; 13:607–614.

Bradley RA, Alberts KR, Alarcon GC, et al. Abnormal brain regional blood flow (rCBF) and cerebrospinal fluid (CSF) levels of substance P (SP) inpatients and non-patients with fibromyalgia (FM). *Arthritis Rheum* 1996; 39:S212.

Breedlove SM. The role of androgens in behavioral sex differences. Paper presented at the NIH Gender and Pain Conference, April 7–8, 1998, Bethesda, MD.

Brown JM, O'Keeffe J, Sanders SH, Baker B. Developmental changes in children's cognition to stressful and painful conditions. *J Pediatr Psychol* 1986; 11:343–357.

Brown L. *The New Shorter Oxford English Dictionary on Historical Principles,* Vol. 2. Oxford: Clarendon Press, 1993.

Buchanan HM, Midgeley JA. Evaluation of pain threshold using a simple pressure algometer. *Clin Rheumatol* 1987; 6:510–517.

Burstein R. The pathophysiology of migraine in women and men. Paper presented at the NIH

Gender and Pain Conference, April 7–8, 1998, Bethesda, MD.

Burton AK, Clarke RD, McClune TD, Tillotson KM. The natural history of low back pain in adolescents. *Spine* 1996; 21:2323–2328.

Buskila D, Press J, Gedalia A, Klein M, et al. Assessment of nonarticular tenderness and prevalence of fibromyalgia in children. *J Rheumatol* 1993; 20:368–370.

Campbell MA, McGrath PJ. Use of medication by adolescents for the management of menstrual discomfort. *Arch Pediatr Adolesc Med* 1997; 151:905–913.

Campbell M, McGrath PJ. Non-pharmacological strategies used by adolescents for the management of menstrual discomfort. *Clin J Pain*, under review.

Carlsson J. Prevalence of headache in schoolchildren: relation to family and school factors. *Acta Paediatr* 1996; 85:696–696.

Carlsson J, Larsson, B, Mark A. Psychosocial functioning in schoolchildren with recurrent headaches. *Headache* 1996; 36:77–82.

Celentano DD, Linet MS, Stewart WF. Gender differences in the experience of headache. *Soc Sci Med* 1990; 30:1289–1295.

Chambers CT, Reid GJ, McGrath PJ, et al. A randomized trial of a pain education booklet: effects on parents' attitudes and postoperative pain management. *Children's Health Care* 1997; 26:1–13.

Chan WY, Dawood MY, Fuchs F. Relief of dysmenorrhea with prostaglandins synthetase inhibitor ibuprofen: effect on prostaglandin levels in menstrual fluid. *Am J Obstetrics* 1979; 135:102–108.

Chen ACN. Headache: contrast between childhood and adult pain. *Int J Adol Med Health* 1993; 6:75–93.

Craig KD. Social modelling influences on pain. In: Sternbach RA (Ed). *The Psychology of Pain*. New York: Raven Press, 1978, pp 73–109.

Cypress BK. Characteristics of physician visits for back symptoms: a national perspective. *Am J Public Health* 1983; 73:389–395.

Dalsgaard-Nielsen T, Engberg-Pedersen H, Holm HE. Clinical and statistical investigations of the epidemiology of migraine: an investigation of the onset and its relation to sex, adrenarche, menarche and the menstrual cycle in migraine patients, and of the menarche age, sex distribution and frequency of migraine. *Dan Med Bull* 1970; 17:168–172.

Denham SA, Mason T, Couchoud EA. Scaffolding young children's prosocial responsiveness: preschoolers' responses to adult sadness, anger, and pain. *Int J Behav Dev* 1995; 18:489–504.

Derbyshire SWG. Sources of variation in assessing male and female responses to pain. *New Ideas Psychol* 1997; 15:83–95.

Deubner DC. An epidemiological study of migraine and headache in 10–20 year olds. *Headache* 1997; 17:173–180.

Dicke JM. Endometriosis, dysmenorrhea and pelvic pain. In: Rayburn F, Zuspan FP (Eds). *Drug Therapy in Obstetrics and Gynecology,* 2nd ed. Norwalk, CT: Appelton Century Crofts, 1988, pp 434–446.

Dorkenoo E. Combating female genital mutilation: an agenda for the next decade. *World Health Stat Q* 1996; 49:142–147.

Edwards PW, Zeichner A, Kuczmierczyk AR, Boczkowski J. Familial pain models: the relationship between family history of pain and current pain experience. *Pain* 1985; 21:379–383.

Ehde DM, Holm JE, Metzger BS. The role of family structure, functioning, and pain modelling in headache. *Headache* 1991; 31:35–40.

Eminson M, Benjamin S, Shortall A, Woods T. Physical symptoms and illness attitudes in adolescents. An epidemiological study. *J Child Psychol Psychiatr* 1996; 37:519–528.

Ernst AR, Routh DK, Harper DC. Abdominal pain in children and symptoms of somatization disorder. *J Pediatr Psychol* 1984; 9:77–86.

Fairbank JCT, Pynsent PB, Van Poortvliet JA, Phillips H. Influence of anthropometric factors and joint laxity in the incidence of adolescent back pain. *Spine* 1984a; 9:461–464.

Fairbank JCT, Pynsent PB, Van Poortvliet JA, Phillips H. Mechanical factors in the incidence of knee pain in adolescents and young children. *J Bone Joint Surg* 1984b; 66-B:685–693.

Faull C, Nicol AR. Abdominal pain in six-year-olds: an epidemiological study in a new town. *J Child Psychol Psychiatr* 1986; 27:251–260.

Fearon I, McGrath PJ, Achat H. "Booboos": the study of everyday pain among young children. *Pain* 1996; 68:55–62.

Fillingim RB, Maixner W. Gender differences in the responses to noxious stimuli. *Pain Forum* 1995; 4:209–221.

Finley GA, McGrath PJ, Forward SP, et al. Parents' management of children's pain following 'minor' surgery. *Pain* 1996; 64:83–83.

Fowler-Kerry S, Day D. Age and gender differences in children's coping with venipuncture. *Abstracts: 7th World Congress on Pain.* Seattle: IASP Publications, 1993, p 512.

Fowler-Kerry S, Lander J. Assessment of sex differences in children's and adolescent's self-reported pain from venipuncture. *J Pediatr Psychol* 1991; 16:783–793.

Fuchs F. Dysmenorrhea and dyspareunia. In: Friedman RC (Ed). *Behavior and the Menstrual Cycle.* New York: Marcel Dekker, 1982, pp 199–216.

Fuchs D, Thelen MH. Children's expected interpersonal consequences of communicating their affective state and reported likelihood of expression. *Child Dev* 1988; 59:1314–1322.

Gaffney A. Cognitive developmental aspects of pain in school-age children. In: Schechter NL, Berde CB, Yaster M (Eds). *Pain in Infants, Children, and Adolescents.* Baltimore: Williams and Wilkins, 1993, pp 75–85.

Garber J, Walker LS, Zeman J. Somatization symptoms in a community sample of children and adolescents: further validation of the Children's Somatization Inventory. *J Consult Clin Psychol* 1991; 3:588–595.

Gäre BA, Fasth A, Andersson J, et al. Incidence and prevalence of juvenile chronic arthritis: a population survey. *Ann Rheum Dis* 1987; 46:277–281.

Gear RW, Miaskowski C, Gordon NC, et al. Significantly greater analgesia in females compared to males after kappa-opioids. *Nature Med* 1996; 2:1248–1250.

Gillies ML, Smith LN, Parry-Jones WLI. Postoperative pain assessment and management in adolescents. *Pain* 1999; 79:207–215.

Golub LJ, Lang WR, Menduke H. The incidence of dysmenorrhea in high school girls. *Postgrad Med* 1958; 23:15–28.

Goodenough B. Growing pains. *Pediatr Pain Letter* 1998; 2:38–41.

Goodenough B, Thomas W, Champion GD, et al. Unravelling age effects and sex differences in needle pain: ratings of sensory intensity and unpleasantness of venipuncture pain by children and their parents. *Pain* 1999; 80:179–190.

Grunau RVE, Craig KD. Pain expression in neonates: facial action and cry. *Pain* 1987; 28:395–410.

Grunau RVE, Whitfield MF, Petrie JH. Pain sensitivity and temperament in extremely low-birth-weight premature toddlers and preterm and full-term controls. *Pain* 1994; 58:341–346.

Hagglund KJ, Schopp LM, Alberts KR, et al. Predicting pain among children with juvenile rheumatoid arthritis. *Arthritis Care Res* 1995; 8:36–42.

Hasvold T, Johnsen R. Headache and neck or shoulder pain—frequent and disabling complaints in the general population. *Scand J Prim Health Care* 1993; 11:219–224.

Henzel MR, Massey S, Hanson FW, et al. Primary dysmenorrhea: a therapeutic challenge. *J Reprod Med* 1980; 25:226–235.

Hertzberg A. Prediction of cervical and low-back pain based on routine school health examinations. *Scand J Prim Health Care* 1985; 3:247–253.

Hoffman PG. Primary dysmenorrhea and the premenstrual syndrome. In: Glass RH (Ed). *Office Gynecology,* 3rd ed. Baltimore: Williams and Wilkins, 1988, pp 209–229.

Holmlund U. The experience of dysmenorrhea and its relationship to personality variables. *Acta Psychiatr Scand* 1990; 82:182–187.

Jay SM, Ozolins M, Elliot CH, Caldwell S. Assessment of children's distress during painful medical procedures. *Health Psychol* 1983; 2:133–147.

Jay MS, Durant RH, Shoffitt T, Linder CW. Differential response by adolescents to naproxen sodium therapy for spasmodic and congestive dysmenorrhea. *J Adolesc Care* 1986; 7:395–400.

Jones ML. An investigation into the initial discomfort caused by placement of an archwire. *Eur J Orthod* 1984; 6:48–54.

Jones M, Chan C. The pain and discomfort experienced during orthodontic treatment: a randomized controlled clinical trial of two initial aligning arch wires. *Am J Orthod Dentofac Orthop* 1992; 102:373–381.

Key FL. Female circumcision/female genital mutilation in the United States: legislation and its implications for health providers. *J Am Med Womens Assoc* 1997; 52:179–180,187.

Klein JR, Litt IF. Epidemiology of adolescent dysmenorrhea. *Pediatrics* 1981; 68:661–664.

Koutantji M, Pearce SA, Oakley DA. The relationship between gender and family history of pain with current pain experience and awareness of pain in others. *Pain* 1998; 77:25–31.

Kristjánsdóttir G. Prevalence of pain combinations and overall pain: a study of headache, stomach pain and back pain among school-children. *Scand J Soc Med* 1997; 25:58–63.

Kristjánsdóttir G, Wahlberg V. Sociodemographic differences in the prevalence of self-reported headache in Icelandic school-children. *Headache* 1993; 33:376–380.

Kujala UM, Taimela S, Erkintalo M, et al. Low-back pain in adolescent athletes. *Med Sci Sports Exerc* 1996; 28:165–170.

Kujala UM, Taimela S, Oksanen A, Salminen JJ. Lumbar mobility and low back pain during adolescence: a longitudinal three-year follow-up study in athletes and controls. *Am J Sports Med* 1997; 25:363–368.

Lander J, Fowler-Kerry S, Hargreaves A. Gender effects in pain perception. *Percept Mot Skills* 1989; 68:1088–1090.

Larsson BS. Somatic complaints and their relationship to depressive symptoms in Swedish adolescents, *J Child Psychol Psychiatry* 1991; 32:821–832.

LeBaron S, Zeltzer L. Assessment of acute pain and anxiety in children and adolescents by self-reports, observer reports, and a behavior checklist. *J Consult Clin Psychol* 1984; 52:729–738.

Leboeuf-Yde C, Kyvik KO. At what age does low back pain become a common problem? A study of 29,424 individuals aged 12–41 years. *Spine* 1998; 23:228–234.

Lee P, Helewa A, Smythe HA, et al. Epidemiology of musculoskeletal disorders (complaints) and related disability in Canada. *J Rheumatol* 1985; 12:1169–1173.

Lester N, Lefebvre JC, Keefe FJ. Pain in young adults: 1. Relationship to gender and family pain history. *Clin J Pain* 1994; 10:282–289.

Levine FM, DeSimone LL. The effects of experimenter gender on pain report in male and female subjects. *Pain* 1991; 44:69–72.

Lewis C, Lewis M. Determinants of children's health related beliefs and behaviors. *Fam Community Health* 1982; 2:85–97.

Liddell A, Murray P. Age and sex differences in children's reports of dental anxiety and self-efficacy relation to dental visits. *Can J Behav Sci* 1989; 21:270–279.

Linet MS, Stewart WF, Celentano DD, et al. An epidemiologic study of headache among adolescents and young adults. *JAMA* 1989; 261:2211–2216.

Lipsitt LP, Levy N. Electrotactual threshold in the neonate. *Child Dev* 1959; 30:547–554.

Linkie DM. The menstrual cycle. In: Friedman RC (Ed). *Behavior and the Menstrual Cycle*. New York: Marcell Dekker, 1982, pp 1–21.

McEwen BS. Multiple ovarian hormone effects on brain structure and function. Paper presented at the NIH Gender and Pain Conference, April 7–8, 1998, Bethesda, MD.

McGrath PJ, Unruh AM. *Pain in Children and Adolescents*. New York: Elsevier, 1987.

Merskey H. Regional pain is rarely hysterical. *Arch Neurol* 1988; 45:915–918.

Metsähonkala L, Sillanpää M, Tuominen J. Social environment and headache in 8-to-9-year-old children: a follow-up study. *Headache* 1998; 38:222–228.

Miaskowski C, Levine JD, Gear R, et al. Gender differences in response to analgesic medications. Paper presented at the NIH Gender and Pain Conference, April 7–8, 1998, Bethesda, MD.

Mikkelsson M, Salminen JJ, Kautianinen, H. Joint hypermobility is not a contributing factor to musculoskeletal pain in preadolescents. *J Rheumatol* 1996; 23:1963–1967.

Mikkelsson M, Salminen JJ, Kautianinen, H. Non-specific musculoskeletal pain in preadolescents. Prevalence and 1-year persistence. *Pain* 1997; 73:29–35.

Miller A, Barr RG, Young SN. The cold pressor test in children: methodological aspects and the analgesic effect of intraoral sucrose. *Pain* 1994; 56:175–183.

Morrison J. Managing somatization disorder. *Dis Mon* 1990; October:539–591.

Morrison JC, Ling FW, Forman EK, et al. Analgesic efficacy of ibuprofen for treatment of primary dysmenorrhea. *South Med J* 1980; 73:999–1002.

Mortimer MJ, Kay J, Jaron A. Epidemiology of headache and childhood migraine in an urban general practice using Ad Hoc, Vahlquist and IHS criteria. *Dev Med Child Neurol* 1992; 34:1095–1101.

Mortimer MJ, Kay J, Jaron A. Clinical epidemiology of childhood abdominal migraine in an urban general practice. *Dev Med Child Neurol* 1993; 35:243–248.

Motegi E, Miyazaki H, Ogura I, et al. An orthodontic study of temporomandibular joint disorders. Part 1: Epidemiological research in Japanese 6–18 year olds. *Angle Orthod* 1992; 62:249–255.

Naish JM, Apley J. Growing pains: a clinical study of non-arthritic limb pains in children. *Arch Dis Child* 1950; 26:134–140.

Newcomer K, Sinaki M. Low back pain and its relationship to back strength and physical activity in children. *Acta Paediatr* 1996; 85:1433–1439.

Nissinen M, Heliövaara M, Seitsamo J, et al. Anthropometric measurements and the incidence of low back pain in a cohort of pubertal children. *Spine* 1994; 19:1367–1370.

Oberklaid F, Amos D, Liu C, et al. "Growing pains": clinical and behavioral correlates in a community sample. *Dev Behav Pediatr* 1997; 18:102–106.

Offord DR, Boyle MH, Szatmari P, et al. Ontario Child Health Study. Six–month prevalence of disorder and rates of service utilization. *Arch Gen Psychiatry* 1987; 44:832–836.

Olsen TL, Anderson RL, Dearwater SR, et al. The epidemiology of low back pain in an adolescent population. *Am J Public Health* 1992; 82:606–608.

Orji GI, Iloeje SO. Childhood migraine in Nigeria. 1: A community-based study. *WAJM* 1997; 16:208–217.

Ortiz ET. Female genital mutilation and public health: lessons from the British experience. *Health Care Women Int* 1998; 19:119–129.

Oster J. Recurrent abdominal pain, headache and limb pains in children and adolescents. *Pediatrics* 1972; 50:429–436.

Oster J, Nielsen A. Growing pains: a clinical investigation of a school population. *Acta Pediatr Scand* 1972; 61:329–334.

Otto MW, Dougher MJ. Sex differences and personality factors in responsivity to pain. *Percept Motor Skills* 1985; 61:383–390.

Owens ME, Todt EH. Pain in infancy: neonatal reaction to a heel lance. *Pain* 1984; 20:77–86.

Passchier J, Orlebeke JS. Headache and stress in schoolchildren: an epidemiological study. *Cephalalgia* 1985; 5:167–176.

Pazy A, Yedlin N, Lomranz J. The measurement of perimenstrual distress. *J Psychol* 1989; 123:571–583.

Philips C. Headache in a general practice. *Headache* 1977; 16:322–329.

Pilley JR, Mohlin B, Shaw WC, Kingdon A. A survey of craniomandibular disorders in 800 15-year-olds; a follow-up study of children with malocclusion. *Eur J Orthod* 1992; 14:152–161.

Polleri A. Pain and sex steroids. In: Sicuteri F (Ed). *Advances in Pain Research and Therapy,* Vol. 20. New York: Raven Press, 1992, pp 253–259.

Ratinahirana H, Darbois Y, Bousser MG. Migraine and pregnancy: a prospective study in 702 women after delivery. *Neurology* 1990; 40(Suppl):437.

Reid GJ, Gilbert CA, McGrath PJ. The Pain Coping Questionnaire: preliminary validation. *Pain* 1998; 76:83–96.

Riley JL, Robinson ME, Wise EA, et al. Sex differences in the perception of noxious experimental pain: a meta-analysis. *Pain* 1998; 74:181–187.

Riolo ML, Brandt D, TenHave TR. Associations between occlusal characteristics and signs and symptoms of TMJ dysfunction in children and young adults. *Am J Orthod Dentofacial Orthop* 1987; 92:467–477.

Rollman GB. Hypervigilance: the interaction of psychobiology and cognition. Paper presented at NIH Gender and Pain Conference, April 7–8, 1998, Bethesda, MD.

Rudolf MCJ, Tomanovich O, Greenberg J, et al. Gender differences in infirmary use at a residential summer camp. *Dev Behav Pediatr* 1992; 13:261–265.

Russell IJ, Orr MD, Littman B, et al. Elevated cerebrospinal fluid levels of substance P in patients with fibromyalgia syndrome. *Arthritis Rheum* 1994; 37:1593–1601.

Salminen JJ, Pentti J, Terho P. Low back pain and disability in 14-year-old schoolchildren. *Acta Paediatr* 1992; 81:1035–1039.

Savedra MC, Gibbons PT, Tesler MD, et al. How do children describe pain? A tentative assessment. *Pain* 1982; 14:95–104.

Scambler A, Scambler G. Menstrual symptoms, attitudes and consulting behavior. *Soc Sci Med* 1985; 20:1065–1068.

Schanberg LE, Lefebvre JC, Keefe FJ, et al. Pain coping and the pain experience in children with juvenile chronic arthritis. *Pain* 1997; 73:181–189.

Schechter NL, Bernstein BA, Beck A, et al. Individual differences in children's responses to pain: role of temperament and parental characteristics. *Pediatrics* 1991; 87:171–177.

Scheuer PA, Firestone Ar, Bürgin WB. Perception of pain as a result of orthodontic treatment with fixed appliances. *Eur J Orthod* 1996; 18:349–357.

Schoen EJ, Fischell AA. Pain in neonatal circumcision. *Clin Pediatr* 1991; 30:429–432.

Séguin JR, Pihl RO, Boulerice B, et al. Pain sensitivity and stability of physical aggression in boys. *J Child Psychol* 1996; 37:823–834.

Shapiro BS, Dinges DF, Orne EC, et al. Home management of sickle cell-related pain in children and adolescents: natural history and impact on school attendance. *Pain* 1995; 61:139–144.

Shye D, Jaffe B. Prevalence and correlates of premenstrual symptoms: a study of Israeli teenage girls. *J Adolesc Health* 1991; 12:217–224.

Silberstein S, Merriam GR. Sex hormones and headache. *J Pain Symptom Manage* 1993; 8:98–114.

Sillanpää M. Prevalence of headache in prepuberty. *Headache* 1983a; 23:10–14.

Sillanpää M. Changes in the prevalence of migraine and other headaches during the first seven school years. *Headache* 1983b; 23:15–19.

Smith GR. The epidemiology and treatment of depression when it coexists with somatoform disorders, somatization, or pain. *Gen Hosp Psychiatry* 1992; 14:265–272.

Smith RP. Primary dysmenorrhea and the adolescent patients. *Adolescent Pediatr Gynecol* 1988; 1:23–30.

Somerville BW. Estrogen-withdrawal migraine. *Neurol* 1975; 25:239–244.

Sparks JP. The incidence of migraine in schoolchildren: a survey by the Medical Officers of Schools Association. *Practitioner* 1978; 221:407–411.

Stang PE, Yanagihara T, Swanson JW, et al. Incidence of migraine headache: a population-based study in Olmstead County, Minnesota. *Neurology* 1992; 42:1657–1662.

Stewart WF, Linet MS, Celentano, DD, et al. Age-and sex-specific incidence rates of migraine with and without visual aura. *Am J Epidemiol* 1991; 134:1111–1120.

Sullivan MJL, Bishop SR, Pivik J. The Pain Catastrophizing Scale: development and validation. *Psychol Assess* 1995; 7:524–532.

Sullivan MJL, Tripp DA, Santor D. Gender differences in pain and pain behavior: the role of catastrophizing. *Cog Ther Res*, 1999, in press.

Sweet SD. Child temperament and child pain behavior. *Pediatr Pain Letter* 1998; 2:2–5.

Sweet SD, McGrath PJ, Symons D. The roles of child reactivity and parenting context in infant pain response. *Pain* 1999: 80:655–661.

Taddio A. Clinical evidence for long-term effects of pain in neonates. *Pediatr Pain Letter* 1998; 2:5–8.

Taddio A, Goldbach M, Ipp M, et al. Effect of neonatal circumcision on pain responses during vaccination in boys. *Lancet* 1995; 345:291–292.

Taddio A, Katz J, Ilersich AL, Koren G. Effect of neonatal circumcision on pain response during subsequent routine vaccination. *Lancet* 1997; 349:599–603.

Taimela S, Kujala UM, Salminen JJ, Viljanen T. The prevalence of low back pain among children and adolescents: a nationwide, cohort-based questionnaire survey in Finland. *Spine* 1997; 22:1132–1136.

Teperi J, Rimpela M. Menstrual pain, health and behaviour in girls. *Soc Sci Med* 1989; 29:163–169.

Tesler MD, Holzemer WL, Savedra MC. Pain behaviors: postsurgical responses of children and adolescents. *J Pediatr Nurs* 1998; 13:41–47.

Toomey TC, Hernandez JT, Gittelman DF, Hulka JF. Relationship of sexual and physical abuse to pain and psychological assessment variables in chronic pelvic pain patients. *Pain* 1993; 53:105–109.

Tremblay RE, Loeber R, Gagnon C, et al. Disruptive boys with stable and unstable high fighting behavior patterns during junior elementary school. *J Abnormal Child Psychol* 1991; 19:285–300.

Turner JA, Clancy S. Strategies for coping with chronic low back pain. Relationship to pain and disability. *Pain* 1986; 24:355–362.

Unruh AM. Gender variations in clinical pain experience. *Pain* 1996; 65:123–167.

Unruh AM. Why can't a woman be more like a man? *Behav Brain Sci* 1997; 20:467–468.

Unruh AM, Ritchie JA. Development of the Pain Appraisal Inventory: psychometric properties. *Pain Res Manage* 1998; 3:105–110.

Unruh AM, Ritchie JA, Merskey H. Does gender affect appraisal of pain and pain coping strategies? *Clin J Pain* 1999; 15:31–40.

Vähäsarja V. Prevalence of chronic knee pain in children and adolescents in northern Finland. *Acta Paediatr* 1995; 84:803–805.

Vallerand AH. Gender differences in pain. *J Nurs Scholar* 1995; 27:235–237.

Vargyas JM. Dysmenorrhea. In: Mishell DN, Brenner PF (Eds). *Management of Common Problems in Obstetrics and Gynecology,* 2nd ed. Montvale, NJ: Medical Economics Books, 1988, pp 326–331.

Violon A, Giurgea D. Familial models for chronic pain. *Pain* 1984; 18:199–203.

von Baeyer CL, Baskerville S, McGrath PJ. Everyday pain in three- to five-year-old children in day care. *Pain Res Manage* 1998; 3:111–116.

Von Korff M, Dworkin SF, LeResche L. Graded chronic pain status: an epidemiological evaluation. *Pain* 1990; 40:279–291.

Walco GA, Dampier CD. Pain in children and adolescents with sickle cell disease. A descriptive study. *J Pediatr Psychol* 1990; 15:643–658.

Walker E, Katon W, Harrop-Griffiths J, et al. Relationship of chronic pelvic pain to psychiatric diagnoses and childhood sexual abuse. *Am J Psychiatry* 1988; 145:75–80.

Walker LS, Zeman JL. Parental response to child illness behavior. *J Pediatr Psychol* 1992; 17:49–71.

Walker LS, Garber J, Greene JW. Somatic complaints in pediatric patients: a prospective study of the role of negative life events, child social and academic competence, and parental somatic symptoms. *J Consult Clin Psychol* 1994; 62:1213–1221.

Walker LS, Garber J, Van Slyke DA. Do parents excuse the misbehavior of children with physical or emotional symptoms? An investigation of the pediatric sick role. *J Pediatr Psychol* 1995; 20:329–345.

Wänman A, Agerberg G. Mandibular dysfunction in adolescents. I. Prevalence of symptoms. *Acta Odontol Scand* 1986a; 44:47–54.
Wänman A, Agerberg G. Mandibular dysfunction in adolescents. II. Prevalence of signs. *Acta Odontol Scand* 1986b; 44:55–62.
Widholm O. Dysmenorrhea during adolescence. *Acta Obstet Gynecol Scand* 1979; 87:61–66.
Widmalm SE, Christiansen RL, Gunn SM. Oral parafunctions as temporomandibular disorder risk factors in children. *Pedodontics* 1995; 13:242–246.
Widmalm SE, Christiansen RL, Gunn SM, Hawley LM. Prevalence of signs and symptoms of craniomandibular disorders and orofacial parafunction in 4–6-year-old African-American and Caucasian children. *J Oral Rehabil* 1995; 22:87–93.
Wright FAC, Lucas JO, McMurray NE. Dental anxiety in five-to-nine-year-old children. *J Pedodontics* 1980; 4:99–115.
Zeltzer LK, Fanurik D, LeBaron S. The cold pressor pain paradigm in children: feasibility of an intervention model (part II). *Pain* 1989; 37:305–313.
Zeman J, Garber J. Display rules for anger, sadness, and pain: it depends on who is watching. *Child Dev* 1996; 67:957–973.
Zeman J, Shipman K. Children's expression of negative affect: reasons and methods. *Dev Psychol* 1996; 32:842–849.

Correspondence to: Anita M. Unruh, PhD, MSW, OT(C), Associate Professor, School of Occupational Therapy, Dalhousie University, Halifax, Nova Scotia, Canada B3H 3J5. Tel: 902-494-2601; Fax: 902-494-1229; email: aunruh@ is.dal.ca.

Chronic and Recurrent Pain in Children and Adolescents, Progress in Pain Research and Management, Vol. 13, edited by Patrick J. McGrath and G. Allen Finley, IASP Press, Seattle, © 1999.

11

Pharmacotherapy in Long-Term Pain: Current Experience and Future Direction

Navil F. Sethna

Department of Anesthesia and Pain Treatment Service, Children's Hospital, Boston, and Department of Anesthesia, Harvard Medical School, Boston, Massachusetts, USA

Treatment of chronic pain in adults is based on integrating the expertise of clinicians with the best available clinical evidence from randomized controlled trials. Decisions that affect the care of children with chronic pain syndromes are extrapolated from experience with adults, limited controlled trials, surveys, and physicians' preferences. This approach often results in ineffective or inappropriate management of pain in children. Even in adults, pharmacological approaches to chronic pain management have limited effectiveness and do not completely alleviate pain in some patients, but leave patients with chronic suffering and disability (Fields 1994).

To date, the many methodological, societal, ethical, and economical constraints on testing analgesics in children have limited treatment advances for this population (Berde 1991). In recent years, many of these constraints have been loosened by coordinated education efforts at all levels of the health professions, the community, and government to facilitate appropriate analgesic research in children. A change in direction at the federal level has placed a high priority on pain relief for children and has prompted the U.S. Food and Drug Administration to encourage pediatric analgesic trials, particularly in conditions that primarily occur in childhood. This change in federal policy and advances in pharmacological analytical techniques have spurred industry to support pediatric analgesic trials despite the relatively small market for these products.

Over the last decade, the use of opioids, NSAIDs, local anesthetics, tricyclic antidepressants, and anticonvulsants in children and adolescents has become increasingly common as more chronic pain syndromes are recognized and treated at younger ages. Pain specialists have reasonably applied findings from the adult literature, particularly in those painful disorders that are somewhat similar in children and adults, such as migraine headache. Nevertheless, in the absence of data to support efficacy and safety, valid concerns are often raised about the effects of long-term drug use on a child's physical and psychological development.

Despite increasing interest in pediatric chronic pain management, pharmacological interventions are based on limited empirical data. Some exceptions are opioids and NSAID trials in cancer, sickle cell disease, and rheumatoid arthritis (Shapiro 1989; Giannini and Cawkwell 1995; Collins and Berde 1997). For all other chronic and recurrent pain syndromes in childhood, the knowledge base is insufficient and in some instances nonexistent. Therefore, clinicians often respond to the needs of children in pain and their families by exercising clinical judgment and prescribing medications despite lack of efficacy data or approval for pediatric use.

Given the age-related complexities of disease processes, developmental status, and pharmacological variations, and the difficulties of conducting pediatric analgesic trials, considerable problems lie ahead, and others undoubtedly will arise.

This chapter addresses pharmacological therapies for chronic conditions in children for which there has been encouraging progress in clinical treatment.

ANTIDEPRESSANTS

Adult clinical studies suggest that antidepressants produce analgesia in various types of painful conditions independent of their antidepressant effects (Max 1994a). The analgesic effect has been demonstrated in several randomized placebo-controlled trials of painful diabetic neuropathy and postherpetic neuralgia, but is less evident with other painful conditions (Sindrup et al. 1992; Watson et al. 1992; Max 1994a,b; McQuay et al. 1996). In a recent evidence-based assessment of randomized controlled trials of the effectiveness of antidepressants in neuropathic pain, McQuay and Moore (1998) concluded that, relative to placebo, 30% of patients will obtain more than 50% pain relief, 30% will have minor adverse reactions, and 4% will have to discontinue treatment because of major adverse effects. The evidence of efficacy is less persuasive for the alleviation of pain in other chronic conditions of possible nociceptive or combined nociceptive and neuropathic pain, such as tension-type headache, migraine, facial pain, chronic back pain, and rheumatological pain (Magni 1991; Onghena and Van Houdenhove 1992).

INDICATIONS AND EFFICACY IN CHILDREN

Despite lack of placebo-controlled trials for chronic painful disorders in pediatric patients, tricyclic antidepressants (TCA) have been increasingly used in the past 15 years as adjuvant analgesics or as alternatives when pain is unresponsive to more conventional analgesics. TCA therapy is offered to many children with severe, distressing, and difficult to treat painful states, even if pain relief is mediocre, because TCA may ameliorate the insomnia and reactive depression that are often prominent sequelae of chronic pain syndromes.

The effectiveness of antidepressants in children is still to be determined, but it is reasonable to prescribe them for painful conditions where these drugs have demonstrated efficacy in adults. Such conditions include neuropathic pains, cancer-related and chemotherapy-induced neuropathies, diabetic neuropathy, causalgia, phantom pain, myofascial pain disorders, fibromyalgia, rheumatic disorders, migraines, chronic daily headache, abdominal pain, and complex regional pain syndrome, type I (CRPS-I).

CHOICE OF AN ANTIDEPRESSANT

The choice of a particular drug is primarily based on the relative risk and benefit and personal experience. There is no significant demonstrable difference in the analgesic effect of the tricyclic antidepressants (Max 1994a; Watson 1994; McQuay et al. 1996). The newer selective serotonin reuptake inhibitor (SSRI) antidepressants are better tolerated and have a better side-effect profile, so they appear to be a promising alternative. However, the limited controlled data on painful neuropathies suggest that SSRIs may be less effective than TCAs (Max et al. 1992). Clinical observation concerning their use in other painful conditions is also clearly preliminary but promising (Power-Smith and Turkington 1993; Saper et al. 1994; Goldenberg et al. 1996; Schreiber et al. 1996).

Nortriptyline and desipramine are preferred over amitriptyline and imipramine due to fewer anticholinergic and sedating effects; however, for patients with pain and sleep disturbance, a more sedating agent like amitriptyline, trazodone, or doxepin is prudent. Trazodone is not recommended in young males because of the rare occurrence of priapism. If sedation is a problem, the patient is advised to gradually increase the dose at 2- or 3-day intervals and to take the drug at bedtime to minimize the inconvenience of any drowsiness. Tolerance to sedation usually develops over time. Persistent sedation might warrant a lower dose. The persistence of other side effects would suggest a switch to an alternative with less anticholinergic effect (Table I).

Table I
Dosage of antidepressants for chronic pain management

Drug	Dose $(mg \cdot kg^{-1} \cdot d^{-1})$	Sedation Effect	Anticholinergic Effect
Amitriptyline†	0.25–2	High	High
Nortriptyline†	0.25–1	Moderate	Moderate
Imipramine†	0.25–2	Moderate	High
Desipramine	0.25–2	Low	Low
Doxepin†	0.25–2	High	High
Trazodone	0.25–2	High	Very low

*The higher doses are still within the lower range of anti-
depressant dose.
†Available in liquid form.

In children and adolescents with cardiac conduction disorders, a pediatric cardiologist should be consulted before initiating TCA therapy. TCA's
anticholinergic effects may produce tachycardia or aggravate preexisting
conduction abnormalities. No antidepressants should be prescribed during
the first trimester of pregnancy. Obstetricians and psychiatrists should be
consulted before prescribing any antidepressants to pregnant women.

DOSING REGIMEN

The effective analgesic dose is unknown, so a process of trial and error
is necessary. Individual dose tailoring is essential, given the wide variation
in responses to the same antidepressant. An antidepressant is started at a low
dose and gradually increased over several days until reasonable analgesia is
achieved or intolerable adverse effects occur. Analgesia is frequently achieved
within a few days to a week. Twice-daily doses may be necessary in prepubertal children and some adolescents because of wide variations in clearance compared to adult patients (Geller et al. 1984). A drug is considered
ineffective if antidepressant dose range is attained without pain relief. If
analgesia is inadequate but adverse effects occur, an alternative TCA should
be considered. Patient education regarding the side effects and periodic
contact with the patient or parents are necessary for optimal individualization of dosage regimen and safety.

No data are available about the correlation between plasma levels of
antidepressants and their analgesic effect in chronic painful conditions in
children. While some investigators have found significant correlation between dose and blood concentration, others observed weak or no correlation, so there is no clear reason for therapeutic monitoring (Max 1994b).

Clinical response is the best guide to dosing of antidepressants; periodic blood concentration monitoring is reserved for assessment of compliance, antidepressant therapeutic concentration, and altered metabolism due to slow clearance or drug interaction.

SIDE EFFECTS

TCAs produce transient anticholinergic effects including dry mouth, which occurs in most patients early in the treatment, tachycardia, dizziness, and postural hypotension. With the development of tolerance, these effects resolve without dosage adjustment. Constipation and urinary hesitancy are less common in children and occur later in the therapy, usually with high doses. Increased appetite and weight gain are of concern and a cause for discontinuation of therapy in female adolescents. Lack of energy and day-time sedation "hangover" are the most common dose-limiting side effects. Other anticholinergic side effects are blurred vision and worsening of nar-row-angle glaucoma.

Cardiac antidepressant effect is of greatest concern. The atrioventricu-lar conduction delay is clinically inconsequential in most patients, but may pose a risk in patients with preexisting conduction and rhythm defects (ven-tricular and supraventicular tachycardia, second-degree heart block, bundle branch blocks, and Wolff-Parkinson-White syndrome as well as other re-entry disturbances). Sudden deaths have been reported in a small number of children receiving desipramine, probably due to prolonged QT syndrome. Considerable uncertainty surrounds the causal relationship of TCA and sud-den death, but close monitoring of TCA cardiac effect is mandatory in all patients. A good medical history and baseline ECG are recommended to rule out pre-existing conduction defects, and vital signs should be measured at each visit. Serial ECG and monitoring of cardiac status, and serum drug concentration are recommended as the daily dose approaches the lower range of antidepressant dosage (Riddle et al. 1993; Wilens et al. 1996).

One study evaluated plasma concentration and ECG effects in a large number of children treated with nortriptyline. Nortriptyline produced a pre-dictable and linear increase of serum concentration with dose escalation. An average dose of 2 mg/kg yielded a mean serum level of 105.5 ± 7 ng/mL. This dose of nortriptyline also produced asymptomatic ECG-delayed car-diac conduction including increased heart rates and mild increases in PR and QRS intervals (Wilens et al. 1993). Other rare but serious complications include lowering of seizure threshold and hypersensitivity reactions such as bone-marrow depression and hepatic dysfunction.

Table II
Some substrates and inhibitors of cytochrome P (CYP) isoenzymes

CYP-2D6	CYP-3A3/4	CYP-1A2	CYP-2C9	CYP-2C19
Substrates				
Paroxetine	Imipramine	Imipramine	Warfarin	Imipramine
Sertraline		Caffeine	Phenytoin	Propranolol
Venlafaxine	Alprazolam	Theophylline	Tolbutamide	Diazepam
Desipramine	Triazolam	Clozapine	Diclofenac	Mephenytoin
Nortriptyline	Midazolam		Mefenamic acid	Omeprazole
				Hexobarbital
Clozapine	Clozapine		Piroxicam	
Risperidone			Naproxen	
Haloperidol	Terfenadine		Ibuprofen	
Thioridazine	Astemizole			
Perphenazine	Cisapride			
Propranolol				
Metoprolol	Diltiazem			
Timolol	Verapamil			
	Nifedipine			
Encainide				
Flecainide	Carbamazepine			
Propafenone	Erythromycin			
Codeine	Cyclosporin			
	Lidocaine			
	Acetaminophen			
	Quinidine			
Potent Inhibitors				
Quinidine	Ketoconazole		Sulfaphenazole	
Fluoxetine	Itraconazole			
Norfluoxetine	Grapefruit juice			
Paroxetine	Erythromycin			

Source: Riesenmann (1995); reprinted with permission.

DRUG INTERACTIONS

TCAs and the new SSRI antidepressants inhibit hepatic cytochrome P-450 isoenzymes. This effect is of relevance to a variety of drug interactions in clinical practice (Table II; Riesenman 1995).

WITHDRAWAL REACTIONS

Abrupt discontinuation of TCA is associated with a distinct withdrawal syndrome. As with opioids and other psychoactive drugs, the likelihood of a withdrawal reaction and its severity vary with the dose and duration of TCA therapy. Withdrawal reactions can be minimized by gradual decrease of the dose over days and weeks. Clinical manifestations include both central and peripheral anticholinergic rebound such as insomnia, dreams, headache, sweating, nausea, vomiting, abdominal cramps, and diarrhea (Geller et al. 1987).

ANTICONVULSANTS

Anticonvulsants are used effectively alone or in combination with TCAs to treat neuropathic pain. In placebo-controlled adult studies, carbamazepine substantially diminished pain from trigeminal neuralgia. Both carbamazepine and phenytoin significantly decreased pain associated with diabetic neuropathy. Carbamazepine and sodium valproate also are effective prophylactics for reducing the intensity and duration of migraine pain. Clonazepam has demonstrated significant reduction of pain in patients with mandibular joint dysfunction (McQuay et al. 1996; Young et al. 1997). However, controlled clinical trials are lacking as to the optimal drug, dose, and indications in various painful conditions. Major limitations to use of anticonvulsants are such common disturbing side effects as drowsiness, dizziness, and unsteady gait, and the infrequent but potentially serious side effects of bone marrow depression and hepatic dysfunction.

Although anticonvulsants are suggested for children with conditions similar to those in which these agents have been effective in adults, we lack data from controlled clinical trials in children. Most dosage regimens are empirical, as with anticonvulsive therapy. The dosing regimen should be individualized based on clinical response, untoward effects, drug interaction, and periodic monitoring of complete blood count and liver function (Lacouture et al. 1984; Virani et al. 1997).

Recent clinical experience offers a promising new anticonvulsant, gabapentin, in treatment of neuropathic pain of both paroxysmal and continuous types (Rosner et al. 1996; Mackin 1997). Gabapentin presents a worthwhile alternative to the conventional anticonvulsants because of its safer profile. Preclinical studies have identified several possible mechanisms for the effects of gabapentin on centrally facilitated pain states (Field et al. 1997; Gillin and Sorkin 1998).

Gabapentin may be a useful adjunct for treating neuropathic pain, particularly for post-traumatic painful peripheral neuropathies. The published reports cover a small number of patients and present retrospective reviews and limited data that do not allow adequate evaluation of efficacy. Recently, two controlled trials of gabapentin demonstrated efficacy similar to that of TCA in symptomatic treatment of chronic post-herpetic neuralgia and painful diabetic neuropathy (Backonja et al. 1998; Rowbotham et al. 1998).

Gabapentin has a high bioavailability, does not bind to plasma proteins, is not metabolized by the liver, and is eliminated unchanged by the kidneys (Andrews and Fischer 1994). To date no hypersensitivity or other systemic reactions have been observed. No studies have directly compared gabapentin to other anticonvulsants for treatment of neuropathic pain, and no data are available on its relative safety during long-term therapy. A preliminary open-label study in children aged 4 to 12 years showed that a gabapentin dose of less than 35 mg·kg^{-1}·d^{-1} was well tolerated during a 6-week treatment period (Leiderman et al. 1993; Trudeau et al. 1996).

The most frequent adverse effects reported in children are mild to moderate somnolence and dizziness. Children with complex behavioral and neurological history may be at risk for behavioral perturbations similar to those described with other conventional anti-epileptic drugs. The intensification of these behaviors apparently responds to dose adjustment or discontinuation of gabapentin (Wolf et al. 1995; Lee et al. 1996).

OPIOIDS

Although there is consensus among physicians on the appropriateness of opioid therapy in chronic painful conditions of nociceptive origin (i.e., associated with recognizable somatic or visceral tissue lesion), their use in neuropathic and nonmalignant chronic pain remains controversial (McQuay 1997). The use of opioids in children is limited to conditions where chronic pain is persistent and is evoked by a known nociceptive pathology (e.g., cancer, sickle cell disease, arthritis), and to a lesser extent as a short-term trial in conditions where pain is of uncertain pathophysiology.

All children with childhood malignancy will certainly experience some acute and intermittent pain during the course of their illness. Unlike in adults with cancer, treatment-related rather than cancer-related pain prevails in children (Elliott et al. 1991). In children, leukemias, cerebral tumors and sarcomas predominate, whereas carcinomas are common in adults. Chronic pain is experienced when the disease progresses unchecked by anticancer therapy and infiltrates somatic, visceral, and neural tissue to produce nociceptive and neuropathic pain states. Recurrence of malignancy usually causes rapid deterioration of the child's health and shortens the duration of palliative care, so the debilitating painful state may last for a relatively short time compared to adults with cancer.

Some long-term cancer survivors may develop chronic pain states from irreversible damage to somatic, visceral, and/or neural tissue from the cumulative effect of cancer therapy (chemotherapy and postsurgical and postradiation pain syndromes). Such conditions include causalgia of the lower extremity, stump pain, peripheral neuropathy, post-herpetic neuralgia, enteritis and proctitis, steroid-induced avascular osteonecrosis, osteoradion-ecrosis, and myofascial pain syndromes, to list a few (Collins and Berde 1997).

Despite the differences between adulthood and childhood malignancies and regardless of the nature of pain, most children's pains are controllable. Opioids constitute the primary analgesics for managing childhood malignancy pain irrespective of the underlying pathophysiology. The general principle of administrating analgesics follows the analgesic ladder of proceeding from oral weak non-opioid or opioid analgesics and gradually moving directly to strong opioids such as morphine for severe pain (Jadad and Browman 1995; Collins and Berde 1997).

As in adults, μ-agonist opioids are used initially in children with severe pain. All opioids are administered in incremental doses until adequate analgesia is achieved or intolerable adverse effects occur. Morphine is the preferred drug for management of chronic moderate to severe cancer pain in children because there is a wide clinical experience with its use, it has been investigated in children of all ages, and it is available in all formulations. A recent meta-analysis of pharmacokinetic parameters of morphine in neonates and children estimated a volume of distribution of 2.8 ± 2.6 L/kg, which was unrelated to age, while the elimination half-life and clearance were related to age (Table III).

Table III
Pharmacokinetic parameters of opioids in children and adults

Age	Steady-State Volume of Distribution (L/kg)	Clearance $(mL \cdot min^{-1} \cdot kg^{-1})$	Elimination Half-life (h)
*Morphine**			
Preterm neonates	2.8 ± 3†	2.2	9.0 ± 3
Full-term neonates	2.8 ± 3†	8.1 ± 3	6.5 ± 3
Infants and children	2.8 ± 3†	23.6 ± 9	2 ± 2
Adults	1–2	3.2	3–5
Fentanyl			
Full-term neonates (<1 wk)	3–7.9	9–28	3–7.9
Infants 2–12 mo	2.3–4.5	18–30.6	1–3.9
Children 1–6 y	1.4–3	11.5–12.8	2.4–4
Adults	4	12–15	3.6–4.4

Source: Olkkola et al. (1995); Kart et al. (1997).
*Pharmacokinetic parameters in infants and children are derived from meta-analysis.
†Values are obtained from meta-analysis.

An alternative opioid is considered if the child develops dose-limiting intolerable side effects or inadequate analgesia. Sequential trials of several opioids may be necessary to find the optimal drug and route of administration. Meperidine is not recommended for long-term management of cancer pain because of the risk of accumulation of normeperidine, an active metabolite that is associated with central nervous system (CNS) excitation and seizures as well as the potential for interaction with commonly used drugs (Kaiko et al. 1983; Kussman and Sethna 1998).

Methadone has a long half-life of elimination (mean of 19 hours in children over the age of 1 year) and requires careful dosage adjustment to avoid prolonged side effects. Its analgesic effectiveness in children is comparable to that of morphine after a single dose, but it is much more potent with repeated doses. It has incomplete cross-tolerance with other μ-opioid receptor agonists and so offers an important therapeutic option in the management of terminal-cancer-related pain refractory to other opioids (Crews et al. 1993).

Oxycodone is a semisynthetic μ-receptor agonist with physiochemical properties and analgesic potency comparable to morphine but with higher oral bioavailability (60%). The pharmacokinetic parameters in children aged 2–10 years resemble those observed in adults but with higher clearance and shorter mean elimination half-life of 1.8 hours (vs. 3.7 hours in adults) (Olkkola et al. 1994).

The goal of opioid therapy in children is to reach the optimal dose to maximize pain control and minimize the side effects. Untoward effects are inherent consequences of dose escalation and prolonged opioid therapy and thus should be preemptively treated. As with adults, effective opioid therapy strategies include administration routes via intravenous and subcutaneous infusion, transdermal fentanyl, and oral immediate-release and sustained-release formulations (Miser and Miser 1989; Goldman 1990; Collins and Berde 1997).

The use of sustained-release morphine in younger children is hampered by difficulty in swallowing large tablets. A lower strength tablet and controlled release suspension formulation, which are now available in the United Kingdom and other countries, may resolve this challenge. The widely published equianalgesic doses in adults are used as guidelines in pediatric practice but have not been substantiated in children. The opioid relative potency ratios are under reevaluation even in adults (Table IV) (Collins et al. 1996a).

Randomized clinical trials are clearly needed to evaluate the pharmacokinetics, dose equivalence, optimal route of administration, and clinical safety and efficacy of various opioids in children. Unfortunately, the number of children with cancer pain and stable analgesic requirements is usually not large enough to support well-controlled clinical trials at a single institution.

Table IV
Opioid analgesic doses

Drug	Dose (mg)* i.m.	p.o.	Potency Ratio (i.m.:p.o.)	Elimination Half-life (h)	Duration of Action (h)
Morphine	10	30	1:3	2–3.5	3–4
		60†	1:6†		
Codeine	130	200	1:1.5	2–3	2–4
Oxycodone	15	30	1:2	3–4	2–4
Hydromorphone	1.5	7.5	1:5	2–3	2–4
Methadone	10‡	20‡	1:2	15–120	4–8
Meperidine	75	300	1:4	2–3	2–4
Oxymorphone	1	10 (rectal)	1:10	2–3	3–4
Levorphanol	2	4	1:2	12–16	4–8
Tramadol	100	120	1:1.2	3–4	4–6
Fentanyl	0.1§	–	–	1–2†	1–3†

Source: Cherny (1996), reprinted with permission.
Abbreviations: i.m. = intramuscular; p.o. = per os.
*By convention, relative potency is expressed in comparison to 10 mg of i.m. morphine. These doses are approximate and are intended to serve as guidelines only.
†Derived from single-dose study.
‡Derived from single-dose study. At steady state, potency relative to morphine is probably 1–3:10.
§Empirically, transdermal fentanyl 100 μg/h approximately equals i.m. morphine 2–4 mg/h and is prescribed every 48–72 h.
Editor's note: Inclusion of i.m. equivalents is not a recommendation to use i.m. administration in children, and merely represents the data on parenteral dosing. Parenteral administration of analgesics in children should be by a nonpainful route.

Consequently, multicenter and perhaps multinational efforts are necessary to fully evaluate opioid pharmacokinetics, pharmacodynamics, and dosage guidelines in children with cancer.

Opioid withdrawal syndrome occurs after abrupt discontinuation of therapeutic doses of opioid in children and should not be equated to addiction (psychological dependence) (Miser et al. 1986). Withdrawal syndrome can be prevented by gradual tapering of an opioid or supplanting it with a tapering schedule of methadone. Addiction is a rare consequence of opioid use for medical reasons. However, inadequate opioid therapy in children may invoke drug-seeking behavior that can be misconstrued as addiction.

In general, clearance of most opioids from the body is slower during the first 1–3 months of life due to hepatic enzyme immaturity, and clearance is further prolonged in premature infants and by concurrent illness (Pokela et al. 1994; Lynn et al. 1998). Therefore, dose adjustment to offset the low clearance and careful observation are advised.

The general clinical impression has been that neonates and young infants are more susceptible to opioid-induced respiratory depression. An earlier study showed that the fentanyl response of infants aged 3 months and older appears similar to that of adults (Hertzka et al. 1989). A more recent study found no age-related differences in respiratory effect at similar serum morphine concentration during morphine infusion in children after cardiac surgery (Lynn et al. 1993). Nevertheless, close monitoring remains necessary in all patients receiving opioids, due to the wide variability of individual response.

CONTROL OF SEVERE PAIN IN CHILDREN WITH TERMINAL MALIGNANCY

Most children with cancer can obtain satisfactory analgesia with opioids, although a few children in the advanced stages of cancer experience inadequate analgesia despite dose escalation of opioids. In a recent study of children with terminal malignancy, 6% of children (12 of 199) required massive opioid dosing (defined as > 3 mg·kg^{-1}·h^{-1} of intravenous morphine equivalent) for control of pain associated with spread of malignancy to the peripheral and central nervous systems (Fig. 1) (Collins et al. 1995, 1996b). Some of these children further required sedation or neural axis infusion of opioids and local anesthetics when systemic opioids did not produce satisfactory analgesia with retention of alertness.

Possible causes for diminished response to opioid analgesia in advanced

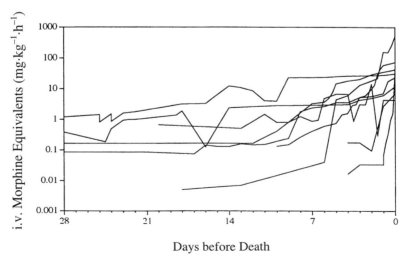

Fig. 1. Logarithmic escalation of opioid dose in patients requiring massive doses of opioid in terminal pediatric cancer (Collins et al. 1995; reprinted with permission).

cancer pain are attributable to alterations in patient-related pharmacokinetics, progression of the disease, opioid-resistant neuropathic pain, and development of tolerance. In children, adjuvant drugs are used for a variety of indications similar to those identified in adult cancer management. CNS stimulants such as oral dextroamphetamine and methylphenidate are used safely and effectively to enhance opioid analgesia and improve alertness in children with terminal cancer (Yee and Berde 1994). These agents inhibit the reuptake of dopamine (methylphenidate) and dopamine and norepinephrine (dextroamphetamine) in the cerebral cortex. A recommended initial dose in children aged 6–12 years is 2.5 mg before breakfast and lunch, increasing at weekly intervals to the desired effect. The dose-response of these adjuvant drugs and others has not been characterized, so it is prudent to start with low doses and gradually titrate to the desired effect or until unacceptable adverse effects occur. Both dextroamphetamine and methylphenidate are primarily excreted in the urine and to a lesser extent in the feces as metabolites and as the unchanged drug. Adverse effects include palpitation, increased blood pressure, anorexia, insomnia, lower seizure threshold and possible increased plasma concentration of TCA.

In some children, pain may not be controlled satisfactorily despite aggressive systemic pharmacological agents and invasive therapy, and continued escalation of pharmacological therapy eventually results in blunting of consciousness and deep sedation. In the few children for whom aggressive systemic opioid and adjuvant therapy along with other nonpharmacological and psychological modalities fail to control pain satisfactorily, neural axis blockade with local anesthetics and opioids, or neurolytic nerve blockade may be necessary (Tobias 1993; Cooper et al. 1994; Staats and Kost-Byerly 1995; Collins et al. 1996b).

HUMAN IMMUNODEFICIENCY VIRUS (HIV) INFECTION PAIN

Physicians are becoming more aware of the chronic pain associated with pediatric HIV infection, a condition characterized by inflammatory processes that involve virtually every body system due to dysregulation of the immune system. There are no systematic studies on the causes and prevalence of pain in children with HIV infection. A recent survey showed that pain is a significant issue in children with HIV infection and that more than half the children and their caregivers reported an alarming degree of pain-related psychological and functional morbidity. All the principles of analgesic pharmacology and strategies outlined in pediatric cancer pain are applicable to the management of painful states associated with pediatric HIV/AIDS (Hirschfeld et al. 1996; Weisman et al. 1998).

NONSTEROIDAL ANTI-INFLAMMATORY DRUGS (NSAIDS)

A few NSAIDs have been evaluated and shown to be valuable co-anal-
gesics in the treatment of severe cancer and sickle cell disease pain, but the
sequelae of long-term use of their combination with opioids need further
assessment. In juvenile chronic arthritis, NSAIDs are used as primary agents
to provide both analgesia and anti-inflammatory action (Leak et al. 1988;
Duffy et al. 1989; Hollingworth 1993). Although these drugs share certain
pharmacological and therapeutic actions, some are better tolerated than others. Newer NSAIDs generally have similar efficacy to aspirin but fewer side
effects. Few studies have compared the efficacy and side effects of different
NSAIDs in children (Brewer et al. 1982; Haapasaari et al. 1983; Kvien et al.
1984; Garcia-Morteo et al. 1987). Therefore, selection of the appropriate
NSAID often depends on toxicity, age of the patient, concurrent disease,
concomitant drug administration, convenient formulation (elixir or once- or
twice- daily administration), and clinician's preference. Individual differences in response to these drugs may require a trial-and-error approach to
find the most effective agent and appropriate dosage for a particular patient.

Open trials of ibuprofen and naproxen for 12 weeks to 6 months in
children with juvenile rheumatoid arthritis (JRA) documented satisfactory
pain control at the termination of the therapy (Laxer et al. 1988; Giannini et
al. 1990). A randomized controlled trial in a small number of children found
greater than 50% pain relief and overall clinical improvement and better
tolerance with piroxicam compared to naproxen (Garcia-Morteo et al. 1987).
A larger multicenter study of piroxicam versus naproxen, also in JRA, showed
no significant difference in efficacy or adverse effects (Williams et al. 1986).

The evidence for a good correlation between clinical effects and drug
plasma levels is scarce with NSAIDs. The best correlation of such a relationship and toxic manifestations has been observed with the salicylates in JRA.
Although salicylates have demonstrated efficacy for severe juvenile arthritis, they are now less extensively used because of the relatively higher incidence of adverse effects, including the potential for Reye's syndrome
(Everson and Krenzelok 1986).

Acetaminophen is a weak anti-inflammatory agent but is widely prescribed to children for its analgesic and antipyretic efficacy and low incidence of side effects. It is the preferred NSAID for children of all ages
because of a wide margin of safety. Primary biodegradation occurs via hepatic conjugation with sulphation and glucuronidation and renal excretion.
Bioavailability is more reliable after oral than rectal administration, which
leads to slow, erratic, and incomplete absorption and unpredictable peak

Table V
NSAIDs used in children

Drug	Age	Oral Dose $(mg \cdot kg^{-1} \cdot d^{-1})$	Frequency per Day	Elimination Half-life (h)	Drug Interaction and Comments
Aceta-minophen	Neonates	30	6	3.5	Phenobarbital, rifampin, phenytoin, or ethanol may enhance hepatic toxicity. May accumulate in children with fever and fasting.
	Infants and children	60	6	2	
	Infants and children	35–45 (rectal)	1		
Ibuprofen	3 mo–12 y	20–40	4	2.3 ± 0.5	Interaction with digoxin, metho-trexate, probenecid, salicylate. A higher dose (40 $mg \cdot kg^{-1} \cdot d^{-1}$) is used for rheumatic disorders in children.
Naproxen	>5 y	10–15	2	11–15	Aspirin, aluminum hydroxide, probenecid. Largely renal excretion.
Tolmetin	≥2 y	15–30	3	4.5–6	Aspirin
Choline magnesium trisalicylate	>1 y	30–60	3–4	~30	Other NSAIDs. Monitor salicylate blood level.
Diclofenac	>2 y	1–3	3	1.2–1.8	Aspirin, salicylates, lithium, digoxin, and other NSAIDs.

Source: Haapasaari et al. (1983); Walson and Mortensen (1989); Skeith and Jamali (1991); Brown et al. (1992); Autret et al. (1993); Montgomery et al. (1995).

plasma concentrations that are lower relative to oral administration. Acetaminophen plasma clearance is delayed in nconates because of limited glucuronidation capacity, so a lower dosage should be used (Table V) (Autret et al. 1993). Except for acute acetaminophen overdose, serious toxicity is relatively infrequent in children compared to its occurrence with aspirin and other NSAIDs.

ADVERSE EFFECTS

The high protein-binding capacity of NSAIDs (except for acetaminophen) primarily determines the age- and disease-related alterations in pharmacokinetics, efficacy, toxicity, and drug interactions (Walson and Mortensen 1989). The true incidence and risk of NSAID-related adverse effects in children are not known. As with adults, the most common adverse effect associated with NSAIDs is gastroenteropathy. Recent retrospective reviews have called attention to abdominal complaints (pain, heartburn, dyspepsia, and nausea) in children receiving long-term NSAIDs because of the risk of gastrointestinal injury. The estimated incidence of this complication was comparable to the rate reported in adults with arthritis, but the relative risk of life-threatening complications was small (Dowd et al. 1995; Li Voti et al. 1997).

Co-administration of misoprostol (a synthetic prostaglandin E_1 analogue) at an average dose of 10 µg/kg appeared to protect gastrointestinal mucosa and was effective in resolving symptoms and reducing occult blood loss from the gastrointestinal tract in 82% of children ages 7 years and older receiving long-term NSAIDs (Gazarian et al. 1995).

Other less frequent adverse effects related to cyclooxygenase enzyme inhibition include facial and skin scarring, elevation of liver enzymes, inhibition of platelet aggregation, acute renal failure, increased bleeding time, and anaphylaxis (Kordonouri et al. 1994; Wallace et al. 1994).

COX-2 INHIBITORS

Recent synthesis of more selective COX-2 (cyclooxygenase-2) inhibitors holds great promise for the advancement of therapy for inflammatory conditions such as rheumatic diseases (Van and Botting 1995). The inhibition of COX-1 enzyme by the traditionally used NSAIDs (e.g., aspirin, indomethacin) diminishes inflammation and impairs release of prostaglandins responsible for protective physiological functions in many body tissues, including gastrointestinal mucosa, kidney, and platelets, resulting in side effects. Unlike the COX-1 enzyme, the recently discovered COX-2 enzyme is induced only at the site of pathology by inflammatory mediators. Inhibition of prostaglandin biosynthesis by COX-2 inhibitors results in selective reduction of the inflammatory process with minimal perturbation of widely expressed COX-1 enzyme. Many of the currently available NSAIDs have greater inhibitory effects on COX-1 than COX-2, whereas the newer COX-2 inhibitors preferentially inhibit COX-2. It is suggested that the future COX-2 inhibitor NSAIDs will have an even greater selectivity to inhibit COX-2 relative to COX-1, and thus will offer a better benefit/risk ratio compared to the commercially available NSAIDs (Distel et al. 1996).

MISCELLANEOUS DRUGS

DRUGS FOR CHRONIC OR RECURRENT HEADACHE

Migraine is the most common cause of chronic or recurrent headache in prepubescents (see Chapter 7). Migraine pain is usually severe, lasting for several hours, and a recent epidemiological study suggests that its prevalence is increasing (Lipton 1997). Many drugs are used for symptomatic and prophylactic therapy, but very few well-controlled trials have been published to establish useful clinical guidelines.

Placebo-controlled double-blind randomized crossover trials of treatment of acute migraine episodes in a small number of children found variable efficacy of antimigraine drugs. Both acetaminophen (15 mg/kg) and ibuprofen (10 mg/kg) were effective for treating moderate and severe migraines, but a single dose of ibuprofen was twice as effective as acetaminophen in aborting migraine headache within 2 hours in more than half the children (Hämäläinen et al. 1997c). Two oral doses of dihydroergotamine (20 and 40 µg/kg) were clinically superior relative to placebo in a pilot study of a small number of children, but the difference did not achieve a statistical significance. Possible reasons for low efficacy are inadequate dosage, poor bioavailability, small sample size, and intrapatient variability (Hämäläinen et al. 1997b).

Unlike with adults, oral sumatriptan (5-hydroxytryptamine 1D agonist) in doses of 50 mg/0.75–1.5 m^2 failed to interrupt acute migraine attacks. This finding may reflect differences in pathogenesis or pharmacogenetics between child and adult migraine (Hämäläinen et al. 1997a).

An open-label prospective study demonstrated greater efficacy and a low recurrence rate after subcutaneous sumatriptan administration (60 µg/kg) in children older than 6 years with severe migraine. Overall headache reduction to mild or none was achieved in 78% of children. This improved efficacy via the subcutaneous route could be ascribed to greater bioavailability compared to the oral route (Linder 1996).

Most commonly used prophylactic agents (e.g., amitriptyline 0.25 mg·kg^{-1}·d^{-1} and cyproheptadine 2–4 mg·kg^{-1}·d^{-1}) lack proof of efficacy. Flunarizine (5 mg·kg^{-1}·d^{-1}), propranolol (2–4 mg·kg^{-1}·d^{-1}), and trazodone (0.25–2 mg·kg^{-1}·d^{-1}) are the only agents with positive results in controlled studies (Ludvigsson 1974; Sorge et al. 1982; Igarashi et al. 1992).

The prophylactic use of flunarizine (a calcium channel blocker) and propranolol (a nonselective adrenergic blocker) has produced significant reduction in the frequency of migraine episodes with both drugs in a double-blind study. The greater reduction in the severity of headache occurred with propranolol. The most frequent side effect was progressive fatigue, which

Table VI
Drugs used for migraine headache treatment in children

Trial	Efficacy	Comparison	Comments
Symptomatic Treatment			
RCT, DB, CO	Oral acetaminophen 15 mg/kg vs. ibuprofen 10 mg/kg	Ibuprofen twice as effective as acetaminophen	Abort headache within 2 h
RCT, DB, CO	Oral dihydroergotamine, 20 and 40 µg/kg	No different than placebo	Nausea and vomiting the only side effects
RCT, DB, CO	Oral sumatriptan	No difference from placebo	Response different from adults
Open label	Subcutaneous sumatriptan		84% good to excellent
Prophylactic Treatment			
RCT, DB, CO	Oral flunarizine	Flunarizine better than placebo	Daytime sedation
RCT, DB, CO	Oral trazodone vs. propranolol	Similar effect	Approx. 75% reduction in frequency and duration of episodes
Retrospective	Oral phenytoin	Effective	Effective in the presence of epileptiform EEG abnormality

Source: Compiled from multiple trials (Ludvigsson 1974; Camfield et al. 1978; Millichap 1978; Sorge et al. 1982; Lutschg and Vassella 1990; Battistella et al. 1993; Linder 1996; Hämäläinen et al. 1997a,b,c).
Abbreviations: CO = crossover trial; DB = double-blind trial; RCT = randomized controlled trial.

required interruption of therapy in the propranolol group (Lutschg and Vassella 1990).

An 8-month, double-blind, placebo-controlled crossover trial of trazodone in juvenile migraine prophylaxis showed significant reduction in both the frequency and the duration of episodes without side effects (Battistella et al. 1993). Anticonvulsants are also used for managing juvenile migraine headache. Phenytoin is particularly useful in migraines associated with epileptiform EEG abnormalities (Table VI) (Camfield et al. 1978; Millichap 1978).

More studies should be conducted using the International Headache Society's revised classification for pediatric headache. This would help to improve the sensitivity of clinical diagnosis and help researchers to evaluate the benefits of some of the traditional and newer antimigraine medications on subcategories of symptoms or patients (Winner et al. 1997).

DRUGS IN OTHER CHRONIC PAIN STATES

The role of the other heterogeneous group of drugs, including bretylium tosylate (for intravenous Bier block), local anesthetic (for systemic and regional administration), mexiletine (oral local anesthetic), phentolamine, prazosin, phenoxybenzamine, clonidine (for transdermal, parenteral, and epidural administration), calcitonin, baclofen, SSRI antidepressants, and topical NSAIDs and capsaicin, remains to be determined in the pediatric population, particularly in preadolescent patients. As with adults, the underlying pathophysiology in most chronic pain syndromes is unclear and may have multiple underlying mechanisms, so these therapies are prescribed empirically and are based on anecdotal clinical experience with no long-term treatment outcomes.

LONG-ACTING LOCAL ANESTHETICS

Development of a slow-release formulation of local anesthetics is a promising strategy to attain analgesia for days to weeks after surgery or for management of chronic painful states such as neuropathies. Preliminary animal studies based on incorporation of suspensions of bupivacaine into injectable polymer microspheres demonstrated a safe and effective means to provide prolonged peripheral nerve block for up to 2 weeks (Malinovsky et al. 1995; Curley et al. 1996; Drager et al. 1998).

CONCLUSION

In summary, as with adults, the current knowledge of chronic pain therapies in children clearly reveals gaps in our understanding of pain neurobiology. The assessment of various painful conditions should consider a broad view of multiple pathophysiological factors. Treatment approaches may necessitate the use of various drugs with the same or different mechanisms of action, sequentially or in combination. There is an urgent need for higher quality clinical trials to establish the efficacy of empirically used drugs and to discover safe and effective alternatives. Pediatric clinical trials are also needed to assess the utility of current and emerging therapies for chronic pain. Despite the limitations researchers face, chronic pain in children is a worthy challenge, and the implementation of various pharmacological modalities within the biopsychological model allows many patients to obtain sufficient relief and return to a more meaningful way of life.

REFERENCES

Andrews CO, Fischer JH. Gabapentin: a new agent for the management of epilepsy. *Ann Pharmacother* 1994; 28(10):1188–1211.

Autret E, Dutertre JP, Breteau M, et al. Pharmacokinetics of paracetamol in the neonate and infant after administration of propacetamol chlorhydrate. *Dev Pharmacol Ther* 1993; 20(3–4):129–134.

Backonja M, Beydoun A, Edwards KR, et al. Gabapentin for the symptomatic treatment of painful neuropathy in patients with diabetes mellitus: a randomized controlled trial. *JAMA* 1998; 280(21):1831–1836.

Battistella PA, Ruffilli R, Cernetti R, et al. A placebo-controlled crossover trial using trazodone in pediatric migraine. *Headache* 1993; 33(1):36–39.

Berde CB. Pediatric analgesic trials. In: Max MB, Portenoy RK (Eds). *Advances in Pain Reseach and Therapy.* New York: Raven Press, 1991, pp 445–455.

Brewer EJ, Giannini EH, Baum J, et al. Aspirin and fenoprofen (Nalfon) in the treatment of juvenile rheumatoid arthritis: results of the double-blind trial. A segment II study. *J Rheumatol* 1982; 9(1):123–128.

Brown RD, Wilson JT, Kearns GL, et al. Single-dose pharmacokinetics of ibuprofen and acetaminophen in febrile children. *J Clin Pharmacol* 1992; 32(3):231–241.

Camfield PR, Metrakos K, Andermann F. Basilar migraine, seizures, and severe epileptiform EEG abnormalities. *Neurology* 1978; 28(6):584–588.

Cherny NI. Opioid analgesics: comparative features and prescribing guidelines. *Drugs* 1996; 51(5):713–737.

Collins JJ, Berde CB. Management of cancer pain in children. In: Pizzo PA, Poplack DG (Eds). *Principles and Practice of Pediatric Oncology.* Philadelphia: Lippincott-Raven, 1997, pp 1183–1199.

Collins JJ, Grier HE, Kinney HC, Berde CB. Control of severe pain in children with terminal malignancy. *J Pediatr* 1995; 126(4):653–657.

Collins JJ, Geake J, Grier HE, et al. Patient-controlled analgesia for mucositis pain in children: a three-period crossover study comparing morphine and hydromorphone. *J Pediatr* 1996a; 129(5):722–728.

Collins JJ, Grier HE, Sethna NF, Wilder RT, Berde CB. Regional anesthesia for pain associated with terminal pediatric malignancy. *Pain* 1996b; 65(1):63–69.

Cooper MG, Keneally JP, Kinchington D. Continuous brachial plexus neural blockade in a child with intractable cancer pain. *J Pain Symptom Manage* 1994; 9(4):277–281.

Crews JC, Sweeney NJ, Denson DD. Clinical efficacy of methadone in patients refractory to other mu-opioid receptor agonist analgesics for management of terminal cancer pain. Case presentations and discussion of incomplete cross-tolerance among opioid agonist analgesics. *Cancer* 1993; 72(7):2266–2272.

Curley J, Castillo J, Hotz J, et al. Prolonged regional nerve blockade. Injectable biodegradable bupivacaine/polyester microspheres. *Anesthesiology* 1996; 84:1401–1410.

Distel M, Mueller C, Bluhmki E, Fries J. Safety of meloxicam: a global analysis of clinical trials. *Br J Rheumatol* 1996; 35(Suppl 1):68–77.

Dowd JE, Cimaz R, Fink CW. Nonsteroidal antiinflammatory drug-induced gastroduodenal injury in children. *Arthritis Rheum* 1995; 38(9):1225–1231.

Drager C, Benziger D, Gao F, Berde CB. Prolonged intercostal nerve blockade in sheep using controlled-release of bupivacaine and dexamethasone from polymer microspheres. *Anesthe-*

siology 1998; 89:969–979.

Duffy CM, Laxer RM, Silverman ED. Drug therapy for juvenile arthritis. *Compr Ther* 1989; 15(10):48–59.

Elliott SC, Miser AW, Dose AM, et al. Epidemiologic features of pain in pediatric cancer patients: a co-operative community-based study. *Clin J Pain* 1991; 7(4):263–268.

Everson GW, Krenzelok EP. Chronic salicylism in a patient with juvenile rheumatoid arthritis. *Clinical Pharmacy* 1986; 5(4):334–341.

Field MJ, Holloman EF, McCleary S, Hughes J, Singh L. Evaluation of gabapentin and S-(+)-3-isobutyl GABA in a rat model of postoperative pain. *J Pharmacol Exp Ther* 1997; 282(3):1242–1246.

Fields HL. Relief of unnecessary suffering. In: Fields HL, Liebeskind JC (Eds). *Pharmacological Approaches to the Treatment of Chronic Pain: New Concepts and Critical Issues.* Seattle: IASP Press, 1994, pp 1–10.

Garcia-Morteo O, Maldonado-Cocco JA, Cuttica R, Garay SM. Piroxicam in juvenile rheumatoid arthritis. *Eur J Rheumatol Inflamm* 1987; 8(1):49–53.

Gazarian M, Berkovitch M, Koren G, Silverman ED, Laxer RM. Experience with misoprostol therapy for NSAID gastropathy in children. *Ann Rheum Dis* 1995; 54(4):277–280.

Geller B, Cooper TB, Chestnut E, Abel AS, Anker JA. Nortriptyline pharmacokinetic parameters in depressed children and adolescents: preliminary data. *J Clin Psychopharmacol* 1984; 4(5):265–269.

Geller B, Cooper TB, Carr LG, Warham JE, Rodriguez A. Prospective study of scheduled withdrawal from nortriptyline in children and adolescents. *J Clin Psychopharmacol* 1987; 7(4):252–254.

Giannini EH, Cawkwell GD. Drug treatment in children with juvenile rheumatoid arthritis: past, present, and future. *Pediatr Clin North Am* 1995; 42(5):1099–1125.

Giannini EH, Brewer EJ, Miller ML, et al. Ibuprofen suspension in the treatment of juvenile rheumatoid arthritis. Pediatric Rheumatology Collaborative Study Group. *J Pediatr* 1990; 117(4):645–652.

Gillin S, Sorkin LS. Gabapentin reverses the allodynia produced by the administration of anti-GD2 ganglioside, an immunotherapeutic drug. *Anesth Analg* 1998; 86(1):111–116.

Goldenberg D, Mayskiy M, Mossey C, Ruthazer R, Schmid C. A randomized, double-blind crossover trial of fluoxetine and amitriptyline in the treatment of fibromyalgia. *Arthritis Rheum* 1996; 39(11):1852–1859.

Goldman A. The role of oral controlled-release morphine for pain relief in children with cancer. *Palliative Med* 1990; 4(4):279–286.

Haapasaari J, Wuolijoki E, Ylijoki H. Treatment of juvenile rheumatoid arthritis with diclofenac sodium. *Scand J Rheumatol* 1983; 12(4):325–330.

Hämäläinen ML, Hoppu K, Santavuori P. Sumatriptan for migraine attacks in children: a randomized placebo-controlled study. Do children with migraine respond to oral sumatriptan differently from adults? *Neurology* 1997a; 48(4):1100–1103.

Hämäläinen ML, Hoppu K, Santavuori PR. Oral dihydroergotamine for therapy-resistant migraine attacks in children. *Pediatr Neurol* 1997b; 16(2):114–117.

Hämäläinen ML, Hoppu K, Valkeila E, Santavuori P. Ibuprofen or acetaminophen for the acute treatment of migraine in children: a double-blind, randomized, placebo-controlled, crossover study. *Neurology* 1997c; 48(1):103–107.

Hertzka RE, Gauntlett IS, Fisher DM, Spellman MJ. Fentanyl-induced ventilatory depression: effects of age. *Anesthesiology* 1989; 70:213–218.

Hirschfeld S, Moss H, Dragisic K, Smith W, Pizzo PA. Pain in pediatric human immunodeficiency virus infection: incidence and characteristics in a single-institution pilot study. *Pediatrics* 1996; 98(3 Pt 1):449–452.

Hollingworth P. The use of non-steroidal anti-inflammatory drugs in paediatric rheumatic diseases. *Br J Rheumatol* 1993; 32(1):73–77.

Igarashi M, May WN, Golden GS. Pharmacologic treatment of childhood migraine. *J Pediatr*

1992; 120(4 Pt 1):653–657.

Jadad AR, Browman GP. The WHO analgesic ladder for cancer pain management. Stepping up the quality of its evaluation. *JAMA* 1995; 274(23):1870–1873.

Kaiko R, Foley K, Grabinski M, et al. Central nervous system excitatory effects of meperidine in cancer patients. *Ann Neurol* 1983; 13:180–185.

Kart T, Christrup LL, Rasmussen M. Recommended use of morphine in neonates, infants and children based on a literature review: Part 1: Pharmacokinetics. *Paediatr Anaesth* 1997; 7(1):5–11.

Kordonouri O, Dracou C, Papadellis F, et al. Glomerular microproteinuria in children treated with non-steroidal anti-inflammatory drugs for juvenile chronic arthritis. *Clin Exper Rheumatol* 1994; 12(5):567–571.

Kussman BD, Sethna NF. Pethidine-associated seizure in a healthy adolescent receiving pethidine for postoperative pain control. *Paediatr Anaesth* 1998; 8(4):349–352.

Kvien TK, Hoyeraal HM, Sandstad B. Naproxen and acetylsalicylic acid in the treatment of pauciarticular and polyarticular juvenile rheumatoid arthritis. Assessment of tolerance and efficacy in a single-centre 24-week double-blind parallel study. *Scan J Rheumatol* 1984; 13(4):342–350.

Lacouture PG, Gaudreault P, Lovejoy FH, Jr. Chronic pain of childhood: a pharmacologic approach. *Pediatr Clin North Am* 1984; 31(5):1133–1151.

Laxer RM, Silverman ED, St.-Cyr C, Tran MT, Lingam G. A six-month open safety assessment of a naproxen suspension formulation in the therapy of juvenile rheumatoid arthritis. *Clin Ther* 1988; 10(4):381–387.

Leak AM, Richter MR, Clemens LE, Hall MA, Ansell BM. A crossover study of naproxen, diclofenac and tolmetin in seronegative juvenile chronic arthritis. *Clin Exp Rheumatol* 1988; 6(2):157–160.

Lee DO, Steingard RJ, Cesena M, et al. Behavioral side effects of gabapentin in children. *Epilepsia* 1996; 37:87–90.

Leiderman D, Garofalo E, La Moreaux L. Gabapentin patients with absecne seizure: two double-blind, placebo controlled studies [Abstract]. *Epilepsia* 1993; 34(Suppl 6):45.

Li Voti G, Acierno C, Tulone V, Cataliotti F. Relationship between upper gastrointestinal bleeding and nonsteroidal anti-inflammatory drugs in children. *Pediatr Surg Int* 1997; 12(4):264–265.

Linder SL. Subcutaneous sumatriptan in the clinical setting: the first 50 consecutive patients with acute migraine in a pediatric neurology office practice. *Headache* 1996; 36(7):419–422.

Lipton RB. Diagnosis and epidemiology of pediatric migraine. *Curr Opin Neurol* 1997; 10(3):231–236.

Ludvigsson J. Propranolol use in prophylaxis of migraine in children. *Acta Neurol Scand* 1974; 50:109–115.

Lutschg J, Vassella F. The treatment of juvenile migraine using flunarizine or propranolol. *Schweiz Med Wochenschr* 1990; 120(46):1731–1736.

Lynn AM, Nespeca MK, Opheim KE, Slattery JT. Respiratory effects of intravenous morphine infusions in neonates, infants and children after cardiac surgery. *Anesth Analg* 1993; 77:695–701.

Lynn A, Nespeca MK, Bratton SL, Strauss SG, Shen DD. Clearance of morphine in postoperative infants during intravenous infusion: the influence of age and surgery. *Anesth Analg* 1998; 86(5):958–963.

Mackin GA. Medical and pharmacologic management of upper extremity neuropathic pain syndromes. *J Hand Ther* 1997; 10(2):96–109.

Magni G. The use of antidepressants in the treatment of chronic pain. A review of the current evidence. *Drugs* 1991; 42(5):730–748.

Malinovsky JM, Bernard JM, Le Corre P, et al. Motor and blood pressure effects of epidural sustained-release bupivacaine from polymer microspheres: a dose-response study in rabbits. *Anesth Analg* 1995; 81:519–524.

Max MB. Antidepressants as analgesics. In: Fields HL, Liebeskind JC (Eds). *Pharmacological Approaches to the Treatment of Chronic Pain: New Concepts and Critical Issues.* Seattle: IASP Press, 1994a, pp 229–246.

Max MB. Treatment of post-herpetic neuralgia: antidepressants. *Ann Neurol* 1994b; 35(3):S50–53.

Max MB, Lynch SA, Muir J, et al. Effects of desipramine, amitriptyline, and fluoxetine on pain in diabetic neuropathy. *N Engl J Med* 1992; 326(19):1250–1256.

McQuay HJ. Opioid use in chronic pain. *Acta Anaesthesiol Scand* 1997; 41(1 Pt 2):175–183.

McQuay H, Moore A. Antidepressants in neuropathic pain. In: McQuay H, Moore A (Eds). *An Evidence Based Resource for Pain Relief.* Oxford, New York, Tokyo: Oxford University Press, 1998, pp 231–241.

McQuay HJ, Tramer M, Nye BA, et al. A systematic review of antidepressants in neuropathic pain. *Pain* 1996; 68(2–3):217–227.

Millichap JG. Recurrent headaches in 100 children. Electroencephalographic abnormalities and response to phenytoin (Dilantin). *Child's Brain* 1978; 4(2):95–105.

Miser AW, Miser JS. The treatment of cancer pain in children. *Pediatr Clin North Am* 1989; 36(4):979–999.

Miser AW, Chayt KJ, Sandlund JT, et al. Narcotic withdrawal syndrome in young adults after the therapeutic use of opiates. *Am J Dis Child* 1986; 140(6):603–604.

Montgomery CJ, McCormack JP, Reichert CC, Marsland CP. Plasma concentrations after high-dose (45 mg·kg^{-1}) rectal acetaminophen in children. *Can J Anaesth* 1995; 42(11):982–986.

Olkkola KT, Hamunen K, SeppäläT, et al. Pharmacokinetics and ventilatory effects of intravenous oxycodone in postoperative children. *Br J Clin Pharmacol* 1994; 38:71–76.

Olkkola KT, Hamunen K, Maunuksela E-L. Clinical pharmacokinetics and pharmacodynamics of opioid analgesics in infants and children. *Clin Pharmacokinet* 1995; 28(5):385–404.

Onghena P, Van Houdenhove B. Antidepressant-induced analgesia in chronic non-malignant pain: a meta-analysis of 39 placebo-controlled studies. *Pain* 1992; 49(2):205–219.

Pokela M-L, Olkkola KT, SeppäläT, Koivisto M. Age-related morphine kinetics in infants. *Dev Pharmacol Ther* 1994; 20:26–34.

Power-Smith P, Turkington D. Fluoxetine in phantom limb pain. *Br J Psychiatry* 1993; 163:105–106.

Riddle MA, Geller B, Ryan N. Another sudden death in a child treated with desipramine. *J Am Acad Child Adolesc Psychiatry* 1993; 32(4):792–797.

Riesenman C. Antidepressant drug interactions and the cytochrome P450 system: a critical appraisal. *Pharmacotherapy* 1995; 15(6 Pt 2):84S–99S.

Rosner H, Rubin L, Kestenbaum A. Gabapentin adjunctive therapy in neuropathic pain states. *Clin J Pain* 1996; 12(1):56–58.

Rowbotham M, Harden N, Stacey B, Bernstein P, Magnus-Miller L. Gabapentin for the treatment of postherpetic neuralgia: a randomized controlled trial. *JAMA* 1998; 280(21):1837–1842.

Saper JR, Silberstein SD, Lake AR, Winters ME. Double-blind trial of fluoxetine: chronic daily headache and migraine. *Headache* 1994; 34(9):497–502.

Schreiber S, Backer MM, Yanai J, Pick CG. The antinociceptive effect of fluvoxamine. *Eur Neuropsychopharmacol* 1996; 6(4):281–284.

Shapiro BS. The management of pain in sickle cell disease. *Pediatr Clin North Am* 1989; 36(4):1029–1045.

Sindrup SH, Brøsen K, Gram LF. The mechanism of action of antidepressants in pain treatment: controlled cross-over studies in diabetic neuropathy. *Clin Neuropharmacol* 1992; 15(1):380A–381A.

Skeith KJ, Jamali F. Clinical pharmacokinetics of drugs used in juvenile arthritis. *Clin Pharmacokinet* 1991; 21(2):129–149.

Sorge F, Barone P, Steardo L, Romano MR. Amitriptyline as a prophylactic for migraine in children. *Acta Neurologica* 1982; 4(5):362–367.

Staats PS, Kost-Byerly S. Celiac plexus blockade in a 7-year-old child with neuroblastoma. *J*

Pain Symptom Manage 1995; 10(4):321–324.

Tobias JD. Indications and application of epidural anesthesia in a pediatric population outside the perioperative period. *Clin Pediatr* 1993; 32(2):81–85.

Trudeau V, Myers S, LaMoreaux L, et al. Gabapentin in naive childhood absence epilepsy: results from two double-blind, placebo-controlled, multicenter studies. *J Child Neurol* 1996; 11(6):470–475.

Van JR, Botting RM. New insights into the mode of action of anti-inflammatory drugs. *Inflamm Res* 1995; 44:1–10.

Virani A, Mailis A, Shapiro LE, Hear NH. Drug interactions in human neuropathic pain pharmacotherapy. *Pain* 1997; 73:3–13.

Wallace CA, Farrow D, Sherry DD. Increased risk of facial scars in children taking nonsteroidal antiinflammatory drugs. *J Pediatr* 1994; 125(5):819–822.

Walson PD, Mortensen ME. Pharmacokinetics of common analgesics, anti-inflammatories and antipyretics in children. *Clin Pharmacokinet* 1989; 1:116–137.

Watson CP. Antidepressant drugs as adjuvant analgesics. *J Pain Symptom Manage* 1994; 9(6):392–405.

Watson CP, Chipman M, Reed K, Evans RJ, Birkett N. Amitriptyline versus maprotiline in postherpetic neuralgia: a randomized, double-blind, crossover trial. *Pain* 1992; 48(1):29–36.

Weisman SJ, Bernstein B, Schechter NL. Consequences of inadequate analgesia during painful procedures in children. *Arch Pediatr Adolesc Med* 1998; 152(2):147–149.

Wilens TE, Biederman J, Spencer T, Geist DE. A retrospective study of serum levels and electrocardiographic effects of nortriptyline in children and adolescents. *J Am Academy Child Adolesc Psychiatry* 1993; 32(2):270–277.

Wilens TE, Biederman J, Baldessarini RJ, et al. Cardiovascular effects of therapeutic doses of tricyclic antidepressants in children and adolescents. *J Am Academy Child Adolesc Psychiatry* 1996; 35(11):1491–1501.

Williams PL, Ansell BM, Bell A, et al. Multicentre study of piroxicam versus naproxen in juvenile chronic arthritis, with special reference to problem areas in clinical trials of nonsteroidal anti-inflammatory drugs in childhood. *Br J Rheumatol* 1986; 25(1):67–71.

Winner P, Wasiewski W, Gladstein J, Linder S. Multicenter prospective evaluation of proposed pediatric migraine revisions to the IHS criteria. Pediatric Headache Committee of the American Association for the Study of Headache. *Headache* 1997; 37(9):545–548.

Wolf SM, Shinnar S, Kang H, Gil KB, Moshe SL. Gabapentin toxicity in children manifesting as behavioral changes. *Epilepsia* 1995; 36:1203–1205.

Yee JD, Berde CB. Dextroamphetamine or methylphenidate as adjuvants to opioid analgesia for adolescents with cancer. *J Pain Symptom Manage* 1994; 9(2):122–125.

Young WB, Silberstein SD, Dayno JM. Migraine treatment. *Sem Neurol* 1997; 17(4):325–333.

Correspondence to: Navil F. Sethna, MB, ChB, Pain Treatment Service, Department of Anesthesia, Children's Hospital, 300 Longwood Avenue, Boston, MA 02115, USA. Tel: 617-355-6995; Fax: 617-355-7887; email: Sethna@a1.tch.harvard.edu.

Index

Locators in *italic* refer to figures.
Locators followed by t refer to tables.

A

Abdominal pain, recurrent, 141–167
    assumptions concerning
        child-centered, 153–154
        developmental discontinuity, 155–156
        problem-based, 152–153
    case reports, 75–76
    characteristics, 142
    classification, 149–150
    clinical observations, 142–143
    course of, *152*
    defined, 141–142
    disability from, 148–149
    dysfunctional model, 145
    family environment, 144–145
    gastrointestinal disorders, 149–150
    gender in, 209, 209t
    history of research, 141–152
    individual differences, 146–147
    literature, changes in, 151t
    long-term outcomes, 165–166
    multivariate models, 145, 148–149
    psychological factors, 143–144
    psychosocial factors
        child characteristics, 153–154, 160–161
        community, 164
        context of, *154*
        culture, 164–165
        described, 156–157, 160
        family, 161–163
        health care system, 163–164
        model, *158–159*
        pain outcome, 149
        peers, 163
        research methods, 146
        school environment, 163
    research in, 151–152, 166–167
    severity of, 147–148
    sick role in, 157, 160–161
    and stressful life events, 144
    subgroups of, 149–150
    in tertiary care patients, 153
    treatment program design, 150–151
Abdominal Pain Index, 147
Abuse, physical, 179–180, 214. *See also* Sexual abuse
Acetaminophen
    adverse effects, 108
    therapeutic use, 256–257
        headache, 131
        migraine, 131, 259
        sickle cell pain, 107
Acute pain, neonatal, 49–50
Adenosine, 93–94
Adjuvant drugs, 110
Adrenocorticotropic hormone (ACTH), 44 45
A-fibers, 21, 23
African American Oucher scale, 104
African Americans, 99–100
Aggression, 223
Alfentanil, 88
Allodynia
    adenosine for, 93–94
    A-fiber pathways, 23
    diagnosis, 80–81
    ketamine for, 92
    in neuropathic pain, 78–79
Alpha-amino-3-hydroxy-5-methyl-4-isoxazolepropionic acid. *See* AMPA receptors
Amethocaine, 107
Amino acids, excitatory
    developmental aspects, 16–17
    and NMDA receptor complex, 15–16
    in pain transmission, 14–17
Amitriptyline, 92, 245, 259
AMPA receptors, 14, 16
Amputation, 84
Analgesia and analgesics
    antidepressants used for, 244
    for complex regional pain syndrome, type I, 91, 92t
    in infants, 70

267